CASE CONCEPTUALIZATION AND TREATMENT PLANNING

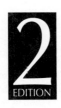

2
EDITION

CASE CONCEPTUALIZATION AND TREATMENT PLANNING

INTEGRATING THEORY WITH CLINICAL PRACTICE

PEARL S. BERMAN
Indiana University of Pennsylvania

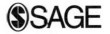

Los Angeles | London | New Delhi
Singapore | Washington DC

For information:

SAGE Publications, Inc.
2455 Teller Road
Thousand Oaks, California 91320
E-mail: order@sagepub.com

SAGE Publications India Pvt. Ltd.
B 1/I 1 Mohan Cooperative
    Industrial Area
Mathura Road, New Delhi 110 044
India

SAGE Publications Ltd.
1 Oliver's Yard
55 City Road
London EC1Y 1SP
United Kingdom

SAGE Publications Asia-Pacific
    Pte. Ltd.
33 Pekin Street #02-01
Far East Square
Singapore 048763

Printed in the United States of America

Library of Congress Cataloging-in-Publication Data

Berman, Pearl, 1955-
Case conceptualization and treatment planning : integrating theory with clinical practice / Pearl S. Berman. — 2nd ed.
        p. cm.
Includes bibliographical references.
ISBN 978-1-4129-6889-8 (cloth : alk. paper)
ISBN 978-1-4129-6890-4 (pbk. : alk. paper)
    1. Psychiatry—Case formulation. 2. Psychiatry—Differential therapeutics.
I. Title. [DNLM: 1. Psychology, Clinical—methods. 2. Diagnosis, Differential.
3. Patient Care Planning. 4. Psychotherapy—methods. WM 105 B516ca 2010]

RC473.C37B47 2010
616.89—dc22   2009037021

This book is printed on acid-free paper.

09   10   11   12   13   10   9   8   7   6   5   4   3   2   1

Acquisitions Editor:	Kassie Graves
Editorial Assistant:	Veronica Novak
Production Editor:	Karen Wiley
Copy Editor:	Melinda Masson
Typesetter:	C&M Digitals (P) Ltd.
Proofreader:	Jenifer Kooiman
Cover Designer:	Bryan Fishman
Marketing Manager:	Stephanie Adams

Contents

Preface

This book is designed to help clinicians develop effective case conceptualization and treatment planning skills. *Clinicians* is a general term used to refer to individuals who have obtained, or are in the process of obtaining, professional training in psychology, counseling, education, or social work departments at universities, medical centers, or training institutes.

The goals of case conceptualization are to provide a clear, theoretical explanation for *what the client is like* as well as theoretical hypotheses for *why the client is like this*. Based on this conceptualization, the clinician develops a treatment plan that will help the client change. The treatment plan also provides a mechanism for assessing client progress in the change process. When progress is not being made, the conceptualization is a resource for assessing barriers to progress. Case conceptualization and treatment planning skills have always been important in providing quality care to clients. These skills are even more vital in today's managed care market, as they can be used to document the need a client has for treatment and to support interventions for brief, intermediate, or long-term services.

The model this text presents addresses skill building in three areas of clinical practice: integrating psychological theory, integrating domains of human complexity, and organizing and writing effectively using your own personal style. Exercises will be provided to aid this skill building.

The psychological theories highlighted in the text include behavioral, cognitive, feminist, emotion-focused, family systems, dynamic, constructivist, and transtheoretical. The domains of human complexity introduced include age, gender, race and ethnicity, sexual orientation, socioeconomic status, and violence. The intent of practicing case conceptualization and treatment planning skills using diverse theoretical orientations and incorporating many domains of human complexity is to encourage clinicians to think about clients in an in-depth and flexible manner.

This is not a *know it all* book. There are many psychological theories and many domains of human complexity that might be relevant to a particular client beyond those presented in this text. In addition, clinicians will not become experts in any of the systems of psychotherapy or domains of human complexity that are introduced. The clinician who seeks to master the full richness of any of these knowledge bases will need further reading and extensive study. This is a *know how to* book. This book teaches a process that can be used in integrating any theory, any domain of complexity, and any new knowledge base into clinical work. It is implicit to this approach that clinicians need to keep up-to-date on new developments within the treatment literature and integrate this new knowledge into their work, to maintain ethical and effective treatment. This text will also help clinicians sharpen their professional writing skills.

Overview of Chapters

Chapter 1 will provide a discussion of the case conceptualization and treatment planning process used within the text. In addition, it includes a discussion of personal writing styles. Six styles of writing case conceptualizations and treatment plans are modeled within the text to help clinicians identify their own style. These styles have been labeled assumption-based, thematically based, historically based, symptom-based, interpersonally based, and diagnosis-based. In addition, three formats for presenting treatment goals are modeled. These formats have been labeled the basic format, the problem format, and the SOAP format.

The text instructions for case conceptualizations and treatment plans use a variety of key words to explain important concepts. The intent is for readers to use the key word that is most congruent with the way they think about and understand information. This variety of key words is maintained in the exercise instructions contained in Chapters 3 through 10. You can locate specific client examples or exercises quickly by theoretical perspective using the table of contents. To locate case conceptualization and treatment plan examples quickly by domain, conceptualization style, or treatment goal style, use Table 1.1.

Chapter 2 will provide clinicians with an introduction to the following domains of human complexity: age, gender, race and ethnicity, sexual orientation, socioeconomic status, and violence. This quick reference information, as well as the additional resources that are recommended, can be used by clinicians in the integration exercises that follow in Chapters 3 through 10. To locate domains of complexity quickly as they relate to presenting problems, referral sources, or treatment settings, see Table 2.1. To locate additional work that helps you compare different theories and different domains of complexity for particular clients, see Table 2.2.

Chapters 3 through 10 follow a parallel format. First, the case conceptualization and treatment planning process is modeled from a specific theoretical viewpoint integrating one domain of human complexity. Second, clinicians are given the opportunity to develop a theoretically driven case conceptualization and treatment plan that integrates a domain of human complexity. Exercises are provided to aid clinicians in this process. Finally, an exercise is provided to help clinicians critically think about theory, complexity, ethics, and personal growth using the specifics from a particular client case. Recommended resources for further skill building are provided including book references, Internet Web sites, and audiovisual materials.

The client interviews used within Chapters 3 through 10 have been simulated by the author of this text. Any similarities between the simulated clients and real individuals are coincidental. These interviews all take place after an earlier, brief appointment in which the limits of confidentiality, fees, and other treatment issues have been discussed. These clients, unlike many of those in real life, will always provide the clinician with enough information to formulate a conceptualization based on the first interview. Why the interview format? It is through interviews that clinicians gather information about clients in "real-world" settings. Although the text author shifts her perspective in different theoretical chapters, her own personal style is likely to still pervade all the interviews in the text. Do your best to put yourself into the role of the clinician even though your own style may differ significantly from hers.

Chapter 3 provides practice integrating behavioral theory into clinical practice. Interview 1 is with an assaultive, White man who is filled with rage. A sample behavioral case conceptualization and treatment plan is presented, using a historically based style and integrating the Domain of Violence. Interview 2 is with a White, teen male who hates himself and is phobic of mirrors. Exercises follow to help the clinician integrate the Domain of Age into a behavioral case conceptualization and treatment plan.

Chapter 4 provides practice integrating cognitive theory into clinical practice. Interview 1 is with a White widow struggling to grieve but inhibited in this process by her rigid gender beliefs. A sample cognitive case conceptualization and treatment plan using a diagnosis-based writing style and integrating the Domain of Gender is presented. Interview 2 is with a White, teen male struggling with his sexual identity. Exercises follow to help the clinician integrate the Domain of Sexual Orientation into a cognitive conceptualization and treatment plan.

Chapter 5 provides practice integrating feminist theory into clinical practice. Interview 1 is with a White man struggling to understand why his wife left him. A sample feminist case conceptualization and treatment plan using an assumption-based writing style and integrating the Domain of Race and Ethnicity is provided. Interview 2 is with a White mother of two who has recently remarried. Exercises follow to help the clinician integrate the Domain of Socioeconomic Status into a feminist case conceptualization and treatment plan.

Chapter 6 provides practice integrating emotion-focused theory into clinical practice. Interview 1 is with a White woman struggling to integrate her sexual identity into her interpersonal relationships. A sample emotion-focused case conceptualization and treatment plan using an interpersonally based writing style and integrating the Domain of Sexual Orientation is provided. Interview 2 is with an abused, White teen female who is struggling with fears of intimacy. Exercises follow to help the clinician integrate the Domain of Violence into an emotion-focused case conceptualization and treatment plan.

Chapter 7 provides practice integrating dynamic theory into clinical practice. Interview 1 is with a Mexican American teen male facing a drug conviction as he struggles to be a man. A sample dynamic case conceptualization and treatment plan using a symptom-based writing style and integrating the Domain of Race and Ethnicity is provided. Interview 2 is with a White man complaining of emotional detachment. Exercises follow to help the clinician integrate the Domain of Gender into a dynamic case conceptualization and treatment plan.

Chapter 8 provides practice integrating family systems theory into clinical practice. Interview 1 is with a White mother and daughter. The daughter is immature and caught in her parents' divorce war. A sample family systems case conceptualization and treatment plan is provided, using an assumption-based writing style and integrating the Domain of Age. Interview 2 is with a bereaved African American couple. Exercises follow to help the clinician integrate the Domain of Race and Ethnicity into a family systems case conceptualization and treatment plan.

Chapter 9 provides practice integrating constructivist theory into clinical practice. Interview 1 is with an African American college student who believes he was wrongly accused of violent behavior. A sample constructivist case conceptualization and treatment plan using a symptom-based style and integrating the Domain of Socioeconomic Status is provided. Interview 2 is with a Mexican American mother accused of child abuse. Exercises follow to help the clinician integrate the Domain of Violence into a constructivist case conceptualization and treatment plan.

Chapter 10 provides practice integrating transtheoretical theory into clinical practice. Interview 1 is with a White man who abused his son. A sample transtheoretical case conceptualization and treatment plan using a thematically based writing style and integrating the Domain of Violence is provided. Interview 2 is with a Sioux woman who complains of malaise. Exercises follow to help the clinician integrate the Domain of Race and Ethnicity into a transtheoretical case conceptualization and treatment plan.

Chapter 11 provides a discussion and extension of the model for developing case conceptualizations and treatment plans using, as an example, a Sioux woman who was a victim of physical and sexual abuse as a child. The following issues are discussed: increasing clinical effectiveness through attention to common factors, individualizing treatment to provide quality care, changing case conceptualizations and treatment plans over time, and red flag guidelines for developing case conceptualizations and treatment plans.

The final section of the text is a complete reference list of all scholarly work that has been cited in the theoretical discussions or recommended as further resources.

Acknowledgments

I would like to thank the doctoral students of Indiana University of Pennsylvania for inspiring me to write this book and for completing many questionnaires to help me improve the exercise instructions and the case examples. I would also like to thank specific graduate students and colleagues who provided me with in-depth feedback on certain chapters within the book: Dr. Beverly Goodwin, Dr. Kim Husenits, Ms. Catherine Swiderski, and Mr. Martin Pino. I would also like to thank specific graduate students who provided assistance for the instructor's manual of this text including Catherine Swiderski, Martin Pino, Rachel Andaloro, Janna Foster, Adrianne Fuller, Jennifer Hambaugh, Sarah Hasker, Megan Hoag, Susan Jefferson, Kelly Kovack, Shannon Lamoreaux, Alicia Puskar, Terra N. Sanderson, Erica Smith, Leslie Smith, Harmony Sullivan, Lauren Swenson, Shelly Thielges, Christopher Vrabel, and Jillian Zeitvogel.

I would also like to thank Ms. Lindsay Oliveria and Ms. Lindsey Grove for their unfailing patience in manuscript preparation.

Finally, no words could ever completely express my deep gratitude to my husband Michael and my daughters Irene and Rachel for their love, support, and belief in me.

One

Developing Case Conceptualizations and Treatment Plans

This book was designed to help you develop effective case conceptualization and treatment planning skills. In this chapter, a structure for developing these tools is introduced that includes four steps: (a) selecting the theoretical perspective that is most appropriate to the client; (b) utilizing a premise, supporting material, and a conclusion as key features of a case conceptualization; (c) utilizing a treatment plan overview, long-term goals, and short-term goals as key features in developing a treatment plan; and (d) developing an effective personal writing style that is comfortable for you and may be motivating to your client.

The text provides exercises for helping you through these steps while paying close attention to the extratherapeutic factors that the client brings into treatment including his or her strengths and resources. The exercises also stress writing treatment goals in a manner that helps the client see them as relevant and credible, creates a sense of hope and expectancy, and builds trust between you and the client. These factors are critical to developing a positive therapeutic alliance and in achieving a positive treatment outcome (Hubble, Duncan, & Miller, 1999).

Developing conceptualizations is time-consuming, so why not just go directly to the treatment plan? When there is no careful conceptualization,

1

there may be treatment chaos. For example, assume that Veona, a White female in her mid-30s, comes in to consult with you because her teenage son has just been arrested and she doesn't know what to do. She expresses a lot of fears for his safety in jail. Since she presents with this crisis, you go into crisis management mode and provide her with emotional support and advice about how to get legal representation. You intend to do a careful intake at the next session. Week 2 arrives, however, and before you can try to do this, she presents with a new crisis; her relationship with her significant other seems to be breaking up, and she's desperate for help in saving it. You try to initiate a conversation about her son, but she quickly diverts back to this relationship crisis. You go into crisis management mode and give her emotional support to calm her down and try to initiate a constructive conversation about her relationship issues. You're determined to conduct your intake in the next session. However, the client comes in drunk. You make several attempts to find out what happened with her teenage son and her significant other but quickly give up and send her home. Your plan is to be very firm when she comes in for her fourth session; thus, before she has a chance to tell you anything, you indicate the need to conduct a thorough intake. Veona interrupts you and indicates she is about to become homeless if she can't find the money to pay her rent by tomorrow. She used her rent money to pay the attorney you had recommended she get to represent her son. Frustrated, you go into crisis intervention mode and try to connect the client with community resources so that she won't become homeless.

Treatment is in a state of chaos because you don't know whether Veona's son is out of jail or not, you don't know if Veona is still with her significant other, and you don't know if she has a long-standing problem with alcohol or if her drunkenness was just a reaction to extreme stress. You may also be exhausted from all these crises.

Rewind and assume that while acknowledging the seriousness of her son's difficulties, when she brings them up, you still carry out an intake during the first session. Based on this intake, you come up with a behavioral conceptualization to capture what you consider to be her basic issues. The following is the premise or theory-driven introduction to this conceptualization:

Veona is a 35-year-old Caucasian woman who was raised by parents who modeled aggressive expressions of anger and aggressive or neglectful problem solving. Either Veona's parents ignored how she was behaving or what was happening to her or they overreacted to her mistakes and developmental struggles and used abusive punishment. Veona survived this history by developing a people-pleasing style where she carefully observed the people around her and tried to meet their needs so that they would accept her and not hurt her. Her passive approach to her own needs led to an early pregnancy outside of marriage. As she raised her son alone, she sought to be a "better parent" than she had had herself. She strove to attend to all of her son's needs and deny him nothing. As she had no role models for effective parenting, her wish to be loving led her to overindulge the desires of her son. Her desire to avoid abusive parenting practices has led her to avoid setting limits on her son's behavior. Veona's strengths lie in her sincere desire to be a good parent, her ability to observe and predict the moods of others, and her average level of intelligence that allows her to understand the consequences of her son's present behavior. At this time, Veona is very aware that she and her son are having serious difficulties, but she is not aware of how her permissive and people-pleasing style is related to these difficulties.

After completing the full conceptualization process, you decide that Veona would profit from a treatment plan that will teach her communication and problem-solving skills. Your long-term goals are as follows:

LONG-TERM GOAL 1: Veona will learn how to recognize and express her feelings assertively.

LONG-TERM GOAL 2: Veona will learn to express concerns in a relationship without blaming others.

LONG-TERM GOAL 3: Veona will learn how to negotiate solutions that respect the needs of self and others.

LONG-TERM GOAL 4: Veona will learn how to recognize her goals for a relationship.

LONG-TERM GOAL 5: Veona will learn how to break down goals into small steps that can be accomplished.

When Veona comes in for Session 2, if she wants to talk about her son's legal problems, you will (a) work on Veona communicating clearly to the police and her teen and (b) help Veona set goals around the arrest situation. If she wants to discuss imminent relationship failure, you will (a) work on Veona communicating clearly to her significant other and (b) help Veona set goals around the relationship. In both situations, you are not ignoring the crisis Veona wants to discuss. However, you are helping her build the skills she needs no matter what "issue" she wants to talk about. As she progresses through the treatment plan, her new skills may help her avert a life full of emergencies. Thus, while the process of developing a case conceptualization and treatment plan is time-consuming at first, over time it will increase the likelihood you will provide effective and time-efficient treatment. The four-step case conceptualization and treatment planning process will now be discussed in detail using the case of Pat.

Selecting a Theoretical Perspective

Pat is a 25-year-old European American male with a history of violent behavior toward men and verbal abuse of women. He was recently released from jail and given 2 years of probation. He served 3 years of a 2- to 5-year prison sentence for assault. He was sentenced after beating a man unconscious in a drunken brawl following a football game. This was Pat's first time in jail; however, he had been arrested 2 years earlier for participation in a bar fight. Pat was raised in a violent home where he witnessed domestic violence and was a victim of child abuse. He is presently involved in a new intimate relationship with Alice, a 19-year-old European American female; this relationship is in its second month.

Pat's past intimate relationships have never lasted beyond 6 months. He meets these women in his neighborhood and, after a brief dating period, invites them to move in. He says that he always finds the relationships satisfying but that the women always disappear one day when he is at work. He reports they move out of the neighborhood and he never sees them again. Pat has never been married and has no children. During his time in jail, Pat realized that he was tired of changing women and wants Alice to "stay put."

Pat has been working for the past 4 months as the custodian of a large department store. He is underemployed. Despite his above-average level of intelligence and his associate's degree in computer repair, his criminal record has prevented him from gaining any type of employment in his field. Although he is a self-described loner, Pat has been carefully observing his boss and fellow employees and trying to understand what makes them "tick"—this is a game he has played with himself since high school. There have been no aggressive episodes within the work environment to date. However, Pat's probation officer has mandated he participate in treatment with you. The officer meets with Pat weekly and plans to monitor Pat's progress in treatment.

There are many theoretical approaches or systems of treatment currently available for understanding Pat. Research on a variety of talk therapies has found them to be effective (Editors of Consumer Reports, 2004; Lambert, Garfield, & Bergin, 2004). So, how will you choose an approach to use with Pat? You can choose an orientation based on your personal preferences. When a client isn't appropriate for your approach, you can refer this individual to another clinician; this is a completely ethical choice. However, the outcome literature suggests that you will maximize treatment effectiveness if Pat's characteristics and presenting concerns are used to guide your choice (Hubble et al., 1999). This type of approach that "fits" the theoretical orientation to the client is referred to as integrationism or systematic eclecticism (Lambert et al., 2004).

While it is legitimate to conceptualize Pat's concerns from many different theoretical perspectives, the theory chosen will have important repercussions for treatment, including how hard it will be for Pat to understand/perceive his problems from that perspective, how unconscious or deep in the unconscious the precipitants of his problems will be, and how long treatment will take to resolve these problems (Prochaska & Norcross, 1999, 2009). For example, a behavioral approach to Pat's case would analyze his symptoms and immediate life circumstances. The focus of a treatment session might be on the immediate antecedents and consequences of a recent violent episode. The precipitants of a particular episode of violence, and the immediate consequences of it, would be in his immediate past and therefore relatively easy for Pat to recall and contemplate. In contrast, a dynamic approach to Pat's case would focus on unconscious psychological conflicts as the root cause of his violence. Pat would need to become aware of events in his distant past that resulted in his experiencing, for example, unmet needs for security and nurturance. To avoid the anxiety generated by these unmet needs, Pat may have had to develop an aggressive lifestyle, whereby through acts of violence he provided himself with a facade of security and safety. As an adult, he has perfected a violent interpersonal style that provides him with "protection" from a hostile world. Only under the influence of alcohol might Pat's anxiety be low enough for him to try to relate to women and address his need for nurturance. From this dynamic perspective, Pat would first need to develop significant insight into his unconscious conflicts before he could address his current issues with violence. Thus, Prochaska and Norcross (1999, 2009) assume that Pat would need more treatment sessions to change constructively using dynamic treatment than he would using behavioral treatment.

Developing Your Theoretical Understanding of Pat

The first step in developing a case conceptualization of Pat is to choose the theoretical viewpoint that will guide an understanding of him at the time that he enters treatment. This theoretical viewpoint will determine the types of questions you ask him and thus the type of information that is included in your case conceptualization and treatment plan.

A case conceptualization of Pat will provide a theoretical perspective for understanding who he is and why he behaves as he does. In general, conceptualizations contain case history information that is theoretically based and includes a formulation of the client's difficulties as well as strengths. Professionals prepare many other types of reports on clients that may includes this type of information, such as case histories, intakes, and assessment reports. There is no consensus across clinical settings for what constitutes each type of report. In general, case histories provide the greatest detail about the client's past history, intakes focus more on the client's present functioning, assessment reports focus on the interpretation of psychological testing, and case conceptualizations stress a theoretical understanding of the client to use in guiding treatment decisions. Comprehensive client files may include several types of reports, and what a clinician includes in the case record will be a combination of legal or funding requirements as well as what is most useful clinically (American Psychiatric Association, 2002, Section 2; American Psychological Association [APA], 2007, Guideline 2).

A treatment plan for Pat will be a theory-driven action plan for helping him change constructively. It may focus on the goals to be attained, such as "Pat will learn new methods of anger control," or on what needs to change, such as "Pat will stop assaulting others when angry." Research links positive outcome with treatment plans that are designed around a client's unique characteristics and that take advantage of the client's personal strengths and resources (Hubble et al., 1999). Treatment progress, within the first three sessions, is also related to positive outcome for 80% of clients (Haas, Hill, Lambert, & Morrell, 2002). Thus, a treatment plan that aids the clinician in conducting effective and time-efficient treatment sessions may improve client outcome.

There are no standard criteria for evaluating treatment plans beyond their need to meet legal and ethical mandates and be in a format acceptable to licensing agencies and insurance companies (American Psychiatric Association, 2002; APA, 2007). However, the research literature indicates that treatment goals stated in small and specific terms that Pat can understand and see as valuable to attain are most likely to influence him (Hubble et al., 1999). In addition, goals written in a manner that fits Pat's expectations, wishes, and values may be more motivating (Egan, 2007). Thus, this text recommends an overall strategy for writing these types of goals that also, whenever possible, take advantage of Pat's strengths and resources. The effectiveness of treatment can be documented through the step-by-step attainment of these specific goals. In addition, seeing progress documented in this way may help maintain Pat's hope; this is an important common factor in effective treatment (Hubble et al., 1999).

Key Features in Developing a Case Conceptualization

In writing conceptualizations, two key organizational features are recommended. The first feature is the premise. The premise is a succinct analysis of the client's core strengths and weaknesses, tied to the assumptions of a selected theoretical perspective. It can be organized in many ways but should always set up an organizational structure for the entire conceptualization and be theoretically sound. If *premise* is not a meaningful term to you, think of this feature as serving to provide an overview of the client, or as *preliminary* or *explanatory* statements, or as a summary of the key features of the client, or as a *proposition* on which arguments are based, or as *hypotheses*, or as a *thesis statement*, or as a *theory-driven introduction*. This series of alternative key words is provided so that you can select the words that have the clearest meaning for you.

A premise at the beginning of a case conceptualization gives the reader a concise understanding of the main issues to be covered in the conceptualization, and the topic sentence of the premise serves this same function for this introductory paragraph through setting up what is going to be discussed. The premise topic sentence could include an overview of the client demographics and reason for referral—for example, "Pat is a 25-year-old, European American male who was referred for treatment of his violent behavior by his probation officer." However, there are many other possibilities. For example, "Pat enters treatment with two major goals: to keep Alice in his life and to keep himself out of jail" or "Pat doesn't agree that he has problems with aggressive behavior, but he does agree that his current life consists of a controlling probation officer, an unstable relationship with Alice, and a boring job." After the topic sentence, the premise will go on to consider both Pat's strengths and his weaknesses, as understood through the lens of the theory that has been selected to guide treatment, and it will end with a sentence that draws a general conclusion about Pat's prognosis or ties the paragraph together in some way before transitioning to the next one.

The second organizational feature, which follows the premise, is the theoretically based *supporting material.* It can also be understood as a *detailed case analysis* that provides evidence to back up the statements made in the premise. This supportive material includes an in-depth analysis of the client's strengths (strong points, positive features, successes, coping strategies, skills, factors facilitating change) and weaknesses (concerns, issues, problems, symptoms, skill deficits, treatment barriers) considered from within the same theoretical perspective that guided the premise. Information from the client's past history, the client's present history, behavioral observations in the treatment session, and other sources may be included in the overall case conceptualization as *appropriate* to building an effective analysis of the client.

The support paragraphs should be written following a coherent organizational structure that was set up by the premise. At the end of these support paragraphs, the conceptualization should draw conclusions about the client's overall level of functioning at this time, contain broad treatment goals, include any windows of opportunity for achieving these goals, and note any barriers to goal attainment that exist at this time.

Key Features in Developing a Treatment Plan

Three organizational features will be suggested for developing an effective treatment plan. The first feature is the treatment plan overview. This is a brief paragraph, in client-friendly language, that could help increase clients' ownership of their treatment plan and responsibility for their own outcome in treatment. The overview can also be used to help a referral source understand the intent of your treatment plan and your respect for his or her role in it as appropriate.

The second feature is the development of long-term (major, large, ambitious, comprehensive, broad) goals that stem from the main concepts developed in the premise of the case conceptualization. These are goals that the client ideally will have achieved by the time treatment is terminated. The information contained in the premise, and the topic sentences of the support paragraphs, should provide the information needed to develop your long-term goals as they should reflect the most important or basic needs, issues, or goals of the client at this time.

The third organizational feature is the development of short-term (small, brief, encapsulated, specific, measurable) goals that the client and clinician will expect to see accomplished within a brief time frame to chart treatment progress, instill hope for change, and help the clinician plan treatment sessions. Early positive change is part of the trajectory toward successful treatment (Hubble et al., 1999, Chapter 14). Therefore, a plan that helps highlight for the client even small steps taken toward change is more likely to lead the client toward a positive outcome.

Every long-term goal should have a series of short-term goals that will be used to move the client toward its accomplishment. The more ambitious the long-term goal, the greater the number of short-term goals that may need to be developed. If treatment has stalled, it may be that the short-term goals were too large or difficult and need to be broken down further. It also may be that the goals were inappropriate and need to be redesigned.

Ideas for the development of short-term goals may come from the supportive detail contained in the case conceptualization. While a client's difficulties have a clear connection to treatment goals, so do strengths. For example, if Pat has strategies that help him keep his aggression under control at work, then treatment goals for expanding his use of these strategies at home and in the neighborhood would capitalize on these strengths. Additional ideas for goals will come from the theoretical model that is chosen to guide treatment. For example, in behavioral therapy, the clinician takes on the role of an educator. Therefore, treatment goals may center on the skills, or information base, that the clinician will help the client master. Taken together, the long- and short-term goals provide an action plan for helping the client change effectively.

The text exercises will guide you to develop goals that are (a) stated in specific terms that the client can understand, (b) congruent with what the client wants to achieve, and (c) viewed as attainable by the client, as such goals are the most motivating (Egan, 2007; Hubble et al., 1999). In some cases, all the long-term goals may be worked on simultaneously. In other cases, goal achievement will follow a specific order as each goal builds on what came before. The strategy for implementing the plan should be included in the treatment plan overview and clearly explained to the client since a collaborative, working relationship has been found to be critical for positive treatment outcome (Hubble et al., 1999; Lambert et al., 2004).

Developing Your Personal Writing Style

Professional writing requires a clear and specific organizational plan. Within this plan, there are many different styles for organizing an effective case conceptualization and treatment plan. Based on your prior training or style of viewing the world, it may seem at first as if professional writing requires you to abandon the style that comes most easily to you. This viewpoint often develops because the examples provided during training may follow one specific style (or use one type of organizational strategy). This text seeks to demonstrate the power and legitimacy of different writing styles by modeling the effective use of six different styles of writing conceptualizations and treatment plans; the intent is to encourage you to identify, and practice developing, your own professional writing style.

Each theoretical chapter in this book contains a complete case conceptualization and treatment plan following a particular style (see Table 1.1). At the end of this chapter, abbreviated examples of each style including premises, treatment plan overviews, and partially completed treatment plans are provided. All of these examples are based on a behavioral analysis of the case of Pat in order to highlight differences based on writing style. The labels used to describe each style have been

| Table 1.1 | Location of Case Conceptualization and Treatment Plan Examples by Domain, Chapter, Style, and Format | | |

Domain	Chapter	Style	Format
Violence	3	Historical	Problem
Gender	4	Diagnosis	Assessment
Race & Ethnicity	5	Assumption	Basic
Sexual Orientation	6	Interpersonal	Basic
Race & Ethnicity	7	Assumption	Basic
Age	8	Symptom	Basic
Socioeconomic	9	Symptom	Problem
Violence	10	Thematic	Problem

created by the author and include assumption-based, symptom-based, interpersonally based, historically based, thematically based, and diagnosis-based styles.

The assumption-based style organizes information about Pat in terms of the major assumptions of the psychological theory chosen for understanding his dynamics. The topic sentences of the premise, support paragraphs, and long-term goals are all constructed around the assumptions of the theory. To read a complete conceptualization and treatment plan using this style, see the case of John in Chapter 5 or that of Sergio in Chapter 7.

The symptom-based style organizes information about Pat in terms of the major symptoms he presents with in treatment. Therefore, the topic sentence of the premise will highlight all the symptoms that will be dealt with in the conceptualization, and each long-term goal in the treatment plan will focus on each of these symptoms in turn. To read a full conceptualization and treatment plan using this style, read the case of Alice in Chapter 8 or that of Zechariah in Chapter 9.

The interpersonally based style organizes information about Pat in terms of his relationships with significant others. The topic sentence of the premise lists the significant relationships that will be discussed in the conceptualization. Each of these relationships will have a long-term goal associated with it. Each support paragraph will discuss one of these relationships. If appropriate, another support paragraph may focus on the client's relationship with him- or herself. This can be useful in dealing with personal identity, self-esteem, one's personal view of the world, or other self-focused issues as appropriate to the theoretical orientation chosen for the conceptualization. To read a full conceptualization and treatment plan using this style, see the case of Ellen in Chapter 6.

The historically based style organizes information about Pat based on his personal history using selected time periods from past to present or vice versa. The time periods selected are individualized to the client's needs and current situation. Examples could be early childhood, elementary school, high school, college/vocational school, and adulthood. Or, for a therapeutic issue that occurred during disrupted adult development, examples could be early college years, tour of duty in war zone, return to civilian life, and divorce. If the client is a young child, it might be relevant to organize information based on such issues as physical development, cognitive development, or psychosocial development. For a complete example of the historically based style, see the case of Jeff in Chapter 3.

The thematically based style organizes information about Pat around an important theme or metaphor that epitomizes Pat's behavior or view of the world. In this style, the theme is introduced within the topic sentence of the premise. Each long-term goal utilizes the theme under the assumption that it was selected because it captures something meaningful to the client in a "nutshell." The topic sentence of each support paragraph in the conceptualization introduces an important aspect/realm of the client's life within the context of the theme. For a complete example, see the case of Jake in Chapter 10.

The diagnosis-based style organizes information about Pat around the framework of the formal diagnostic system created by the American Psychiatric Association (1994) in its *Diagnostic and Statistical Manual of Mental Disorders* (*DSM-IV-TR*). The diagnosis style is very similar to the symptom style as the *DSM-IV-TR* is primarily organized around symptoms. A diagnosis-based style is most often required within a medical setting. The premise for this style should include the major data, but not supportive details, for providing a diagnosis of the client on all five axes of the *DSM-IV-TR*. The topic sentence of the premise highlights the major symptoms of the client. Each long-term goal of the treatment plan might likewise highlight one symptom. Or, if there is only one primary symptom, each long-term goal might reflect helping improve the client's level of functioning within each of the client's primary roles such as worker, husband, and father. Each support paragraph will focus on one symptom or, when there is only one symptom, may discuss the client's current level of functioning within each of his or her primary roles. A full example of the diagnosis-based style, the case of Marie, can be found in Chapter 4.

The six styles discussed in this chapter are not intended to be all-inclusive. Other strategies could be used to effectively organize your clinical work. Professional writing allows for a great deal of flexibility in style; however, there must be a clear organizational plan that will easily communicate to other professionals your current understanding of your client and your client's treatment plan. This may be needed to support clinical supervision of your work, case reviews by accreditation boards, court-ordered evaluations, and emergency coverage of your cases by another clinician (APA, 2007, Guideline 5).

Do your conceptualization and treatment plans have to follow a parallel structure? No. An assumption-based case conceptualization does not have to be followed by treatment goals expressed in terms of the theory's assumptions. However, this can be an effective strategy in that the reader, whether it is your supervisor or a judge, can easily follow your professional reasoning. Similarly, if Pat blames his problems on the alcoholic parents who neglected him, he might be most motivated to work on treatment plan goals that are developmentally expressed. If his treatment plan meets his expectations that his problems today are not "his fault" but due to his alcoholic parents not giving him what he needed, he may be more motivated to work on them.

There is no standardized format for presenting the goals of a treatment plan. Different clinicians and different clinical settings have preferred formats. Three formats will be modeled in the examples at the end of this chapter. These have been labeled the basic format (treatment plans 1–3, 5), the problem format (treatment plan 4), and the SOAP format (treatment plan 6).

The basic format has goals stated in terms of what the client needs to achieve/learn/develop. This may be a motivating format for the client as it is stated in terms of the goals the client wants to achieve. It is also useful when the client has a very negative reaction to any indication that he or she has any "problems" or "issues." The problem format has goals stated in terms of what maladaptive behavior or issues need to be reduced. This may be most motivating for clients who are very frustrated by their own behavior and ready for change. Similarly it may be a good format for parents who are very frustrated by the maladaptive behavior of one of their children or for a probation officer who is determined to prevent recidivism in a parolee. The final format is an adaptation of the "SOAP" note that is commonly used in medical settings. This note was first developed by Lawrence L. Weed, MD. He developed it to go along with his "Problem-Oriented Medical Record (POMR)."

Dr. Weed wanted the medical record to clearly draw attention to the client's presenting problem, the current status of this problem, and the immediate plan for dealing with the problem and then conclude with why this plan was chosen. The clinician was to write a new SOAP note each day (a short-term plan) rather than come up with goals for a more long-term plan. The letter S refers to the subjective data provided by the client. The letter O refers to the clinician's objective data developed through testing or informal assessment of the client. The letter A refers to the clinician's assessment of the client based on the S and O data. The letter P refers to the clinician's immediate plan vis-à-vis the client. The uses of the S, O, and A parts of the note will be used following the procedures described by Bacigalupe (2008) and Keenan (2008) in their Web documents for training students in the use of Dr. Weed's SOAP note. For the purposes of this book, the *P* section of the SOAP note will be extended to include the long- and short-term goals described in this volume.

The three formats modeled in this text are intended to encourage you, if you have the freedom to choose, to select the format you believe will be most likely to engage the client in constructive change.

Examples of Premises and Treatment Plan Styles

All the examples provide insights concerning the case of Pat. Assume that the clinician has carried out a comprehensive intake with him as well as conferred with his probation officer. As you read each example, assume that the clinician will be monitoring Pat's potential for harm toward others whether or not this is made explicit in the treatment goals. All the examples are based on behavioral theory so that differences in writing style can be highlighted.

Behavioral theory was chosen as it has a number of strengths in considering Pat's unique characteristics at this time. It is action oriented, and he prefers a quick pace. He was recently in prison, so a highly structured approach should not seem unusual or burdensome to him. In fact, it should provide significantly less structure than he has been used to in the last 3 years. In addition, his jail term was reduced due to his learning how to be a "good inmate," and this past learning might be effectively incorporated into the treatment plan. Finally, achievement of behavioral goals is relatively quick, and this fast response may be needed to prevent Pat from being sent back to jail.

Premise 1: Assumption-Based Style

From a behavioral perspective, Pat has been taught to use aggressive strategies within all aspects of his life, and he has not been taught to use, or value, relationship-enhancing skills such as self-control or empathy. His father battered his mother on a regular basis. In addition, from Pat's perspective, both of his parents used verbal or physical violence as their only child management strategy. Pat has sought out a deviant social support network that has reinforced his aggressive behavior. Pat thus learned to be aggressive through modeling, reinforcement, and punishment. Alcohol may serve as his only mechanism for dampening his sense of personal failure in relationships and in his underemployment. His deviant social support system makes it unlikely that he received any modeling of controlled drinking. Pat may have developed a classically conditioned association of alcohol with feeling less stressed. Despite these serious issues, Pat has shown a consistent interest in observing others, which opens up the possibility of his learning from prosocial role models. He has also been able to recognize that his own violent behavior led to the negative consequence of his recent jail time. Finally, Pat is motivated to maintain his current relationship with Alice and stay out of jail. While the prognosis is guarded, treatment focused on these two issues may provide an opening for initiating changes in his destructive lifestyle.

Treatment Plan 1: Assumption-Based Style

Treatment Plan Overview. Pat is an intelligent man who wants to be in control of his own life, so treatment will focus on helping Pat learn behaviors that he may choose to use to develop a more stable relationship with Alice and stay out of jail. Relationship-building skills will be emphasized, as will how to decrease behaviors that are destructive within relationships. To decrease the likelihood of treatment having any negative impact on Pat's relationship with Alice or putting him at risk for jail time, all new relationship skills will be first practiced within the treatment relationship. Pat's probation officer meets with Pat on a weekly basis to ensure that Pat has not engaged in any violent behavior. Pat has found these meetings aversive as the focus has been exclusively on reviewing Pat's past acts of violence. Instead the officer will be asked to reinforce Pat's attempts to exert positive control in relationships within the past week as well as reviewing probation expectations. Long-Term Goals 1 and 2 will be addressed simultaneously. (This treatment plan follows the *basic format*.)

LONG-TERM GOAL 1: Provide learning experiences that enhance Pat's ability to engage in relationship-enhancing skills within his relationship with Alice when he chooses to do so.

Short-Term Goals

1. Relationship-building behaviors within the treatment relationship, such as arriving on time, coming regularly, being polite, and not making threats during discussions, will be noted and praised.
   a. Using observation, Pat will reflect on what verbal and nonverbal behaviors the clinician is using within the session to make the treatment relationship positive. Consequences of these behaviors for building trust and good feelings within a relationship will be discussed in detail.

    b. Pat will practice noticing subtle cues the clinician may be giving him to indicate approval of prosocial behavior—for example, smiles, relaxed posture, and leaning forward.

    c. Pat will practice noticing obvious cues the clinician gives, such as the use of praise or expressing appreciation for effort, that indicate approval of prosocial behavior.

    d. Pat will practice noticing his own immediate behavior within the treatment session, identify the obvious and subtle cues he is using in his interactions with the clinician, and label them as relationship building or relationship damaging.

    e. Pat will discuss what changes in his behavior were perceived, in prison, as the behavior of a "good" inmate and if any of these might enhance his relationship with Alice.

2. Pat will discuss what "good" behaviors he might direct toward Alice in terms of their potential for building a positive relationship.

    a. Subtle and obvious cues Alice might use to indicate approval of Pat's behavior will be discussed.

    b. Pat will discuss which of Alice's behaviors he likes and the subtle and obvious cues he has given her in the past to indicate approval of these behaviors.

    c. The value of providing obvious versus subtle indications of approval for increasing the strength of a relationship will be underscored within the session.

    d. Pat will practice providing obvious indications of approval to Alice within role-plays with the clinician.

3. Pat will practice effective listening skills within role-plays with the clinician to use in the future with Alice. The potential positive consequences of these skills will be stressed, and the dangers of any loss of control of his anger toward both Alice and himself (in terms of jail time) will be highlighted.

4. Pat will observe individuals that he identifies as living the good life and consider the skills they are using to sustain this good life.

5. Pat will practice positive behaviors he has observed in these successful individuals within treatment sessions.

6. At home, Pat will notice when he might use effective listening skills with Alice.

7. After Pat has achieved enough success on Long-Term Goal 2, conjoint sessions for Pat and Alice will begin where they will practice effective listening about problems they are having with other people in their lives.

    a. Pat and Alice will be coached to provide each other with positive reinforcement for sharing life concerns with each other.

    b. Pat and Alice will be coached to provide each other with positive rein-
forcement for good listening skills.

    c. Pat and Alice will be coached to provide each other with positive rein-
forcement for understanding the information the other expresses.

8. Pat and Alice will practice effective listening about problems they are
having, within their own relationship, in conjoint sessions.

9. Other goals will be developed as needed to integrate good listening with
effective problem solving from Long-Term Goal 2.

LONG-TERM GOAL 2: Provide learning experiences that will enhance
Pat's ability to use nonaggressive, conflict resolution strategies in his
interactions with Alice in order to strengthen their relationship.

LONG-TERM GOAL 3: Provide learning experiences that will enhance
Pat's ability to use nonaggressive, conflict resolution strategies in his interactions with other people, especially men, so that Pat can stay outside of
jail and have the opportunity to maintain his relationship with Alice.

Premise 2: Symptom-Based Style

Pat's most serious problems revolve around his violent behavior and
excessive drinking. From a behavioral perspective, these impulse control
difficulties may have developed because of faulty learning experiences,
including his modeling of aggressive parental behavior and lack of
explicit help in learning prosocial skills. His parents were erratically
attentive to his behavior. Sometimes they supplied no consequences in
response to his behavior; at other times, they supplied verbally or
physically abusive consequences that were not clearly tied to Pat's
behavior. Pat learned that to have control in an interpersonal relationship
he needed to be violent and that alcohol dulled the pain when he was not
in control. Pat's strengths include his ability to control his aggressive
impulses within the jail and his current work environment and to respond
positively to the reinforcement of being paid on a weekly basis. He enjoys
watching others and trying to figure out their motivations. Thus, he has
the ability to reflect on the meaning of behaviors for an individual's
character. He has also shown the ability to learn from the examples set by
others and was able to modify his behavior enough to be released early
from jail. While overall his motivation for change is low, the enjoyment he
gains from observational learning may provide an opening to begin the
treatment process.

Treatment Plan 2: Symptom-Based Style

Treatment Plan Overview. Pat's probation officer is monitoring his aggressive behavior and level of drinking. If Pat loses control of his aggressive behavior, his parole will be violated, and he will be sent back to jail. Pat will develop behavioral strategies that ensure he maintains control of his aggressive impulses. He will learn to recognize when he needs to stop drinking so he can think clearly and avoid a situation that could land him back in jail. While Pat does not agree with the probation officer that he has a problem with aggression and excessive alcohol use, he does agree with the clinician that he does not want to go back to jail. Long-Term Goals 1 and 2 will be worked on simultaneously to decrease the likelihood that Pat will come into conflict with the law. (This treatment plan follows the *basic format.*)

LONG-TERM GOAL 1: Decrease Pat's violent behavior to keep him out of jail.

Short-Term Goals

1. Pat will discuss the antecedents to the fight that resulted in his prison sentence.

2. Pat will discuss the immediate and long-term consequences (positive, negative) of the fight that resulted in his prison sentence.

3. Pat will consider what consequences he would prefer to have following his fights with other men.

4. Pat will become aware of what has happened immediately before he becomes verbally or physically aggressive (thoughts, feelings, behavior) so he can be in control of himself at all times.

   a. During the session, after warning him this is about to happen, the clinician will intentionally bring up incidents that have made Pat angry that involved treatment sessions and probationary appointments to help him develop this awareness.
   b. The clinician will follow the same procedures as in (a) but first ask Pat about a recent provocation at work.
   c. The clinician will follow the same procedure as in (a) but first ask Pat to describe a recent provocation by Alice or a neighbor.

5. Pat will become aware of what happens immediately after he has been verbally or physically aggressive (thoughts, feelings, behavior) and decide if these are positive or negative consequences.

   a. Pat will reenact with the clinician a recent act of his aggression within the treatment session to heighten his awareness of his thoughts, feelings, and behavior and whether or not he was in control of himself.

   b. Pat will reenact with the clinician a recent act of his aggression at work to heighten his awareness of his thoughts, feelings, and behavior and whether or not he was in control of himself.

   c. Pat will reenact with the clinician a recent act of his aggression at home to heighten his awareness of his thoughts, feelings, and behavior and whether or not he was in control of himself.

6. Pat will consider taking a personal time-out (taking several deep breaths, looking away, walking away, etc.) when he becomes aware that he might be verbally or physically aggressive.

   a. Pat will develop the ability to calm himself down, using strategies such as deep breathing, progressive muscle relaxation, and self-hypnosis.

   b. Pat will select the method of relaxation he prefers based on making him feel most in control of himself.

   c. Pat will try using this method when he is in a session but recalling a recent confrontation at home or at work so that he can feel in control of himself.

   d. Pat will be aware of when he becomes angry with the clinician within a session and practice taking control of his anger in the moment.

   e. Pat will try to use one of these methods when he becomes angry with Alice at home so he is in control of what he does.

   f. Other goals will be developed as appropriate to ensure Pat is in control of his actions when he feels that others are provoking him.

7. Pat will learn, within sessions, problem-solving strategies that do not involve aggressive behavior that he can use during provoking situations if he wants to.

   a. Pat will try to identify what he wanted to achieve in his most recent interpersonal conflict and whether he achieved it.

   b. Pat will learn to recognize verbally assertive, aggressive, and passive responses within conflict situations that are role-played within the session with the clinician.

   c. Pat will consider which type of response gives him what he wants without leading to a consequence that could send him to jail.

   d. Within role-plays with the clinician, Pat will practice assertive verbal responses to getting what he wants as these are least likely to get him in trouble with the law.

   e. Pat will practice using assertive responses within his next conflict with the probation officer. (The probation officer will be notified, in advance, that Pat will be practicing assertiveness within the probationary appointment so that he provides appropriate consequences for this effort.)

   f. If Pat has developed enough behavioral control, he will practice how to use assertiveness in conflicts with Alice that are reenacted within the treatment setting.

8. Other goals will be developed as it becomes safe for Pat to practice new behaviors with Alice both within sessions and later at home without harming his relationship with her or coming into conflict with the law.

9. Other goals involving men at work will be developed once it is safe for Pat to practice his new behaviors within the employment setting without being in danger of losing his employment or coming into conflict with the law.

LONG-TERM GOAL 2: Decrease the level of Pat's drinking to the point where he feels in control at all times in order to decrease the danger of his being sent back to jail.

Premise 3: Interpersonally Based Style

Whether in relation to intimate partners, coworkers, or strangers, Pat has learned that social relationships are violent and impulsive. To protect himself, he has learned to get the drop on other people before they can do it to him. With men, he is quick to accelerate from mild confrontation to physical violence, and he has never sought male friendships. With women, he allows himself to begin an intimate relationship, but at the first sign that a woman has some control over his emotions, he reacts with verbal aggression. He has learned that alcohol can effectively blot out feelings of fear and rejection. After his time in prison, in isolation from women, he has learned that he needs a woman in his life and wants to have a stable relationship with Alice. He has noticed, at the department store where he works, that other men can relate in a more relaxed way to women than he can. He admires this and may be open, at this time, to learning communication and problem-solving strategies that would allow him to have these types of exchanges with Alice. He is very intelligent and has shown himself able to analytically observe others and learn new behaviors that can get him what he wants, such as early parole from jail. This may improve his guarded prognosis for being engaged effectively in treatment.

Treatment Plan 3: Interpersonally Based Style

Treatment Plan Overview. Pat's relationships with others have been verbally and/or physically aggressive, which has brought him into conflict with the law. He is now in two relationships that he didn't seek to develop, one with his probation officer and one with the clinician. He is in one relationship that he does want to maintain, the one with Alice.

Treatment will start with using his skill at figuring out what makes other people tick, which is something he enjoys doing. He will observe men relating in a relaxed manner with women and figure out what skills they are using. He will consider using these skills in his relationship with Alice. Once this has been achieved, he will consider when using these skills with other people could help him stay out of conflict with the law and get a better job. Long-Term Goal 1 would be achieved prior to beginning Long-Term Goal 2. (The treatment plan follows the *basic format*.)

LONG-TERM GOAL 1: Help Pat sustain his relationship with Alice.

Short-Term Goals

1. Pat will observe interpersonal relationships to develop a catalog of behaviors that are verbally aggressive, physically aggressive, nonaggressive, or avoidant, and the impact of these different behaviors on the relationships will be discussed within treatment sessions.

   a. Pat will observe Alice, his neighbors, and the characters on television and keep a record of their behaviors, analyzing them into the categories of verbal aggression, physical aggression, assertive, and neutral.
   b. Pat will observe the immediate consequences (positive, negative) of the behaviors within the catalog for each person in terms of their maintaining or damaging a relationship.
   c. In the treatment session, Pat will analyze with the clinician the potential inner thoughts and feelings of the individuals he observed.
   d. Pat will observe himself and keep a record of his behaviors, analyzing them into the categories of verbal aggression, physical aggression, assertive, and neutral.

2. Pat will consider which behaviors and consequences he has observed in himself are most likely to damage versus strengthen his relationship with Alice.

3. Pat will practice, in role-plays with the clinician, behaviors he considers might strengthen his relationship with Alice.

4. When ready, Pat will use conjoint sessions to practice, with Alice, behaviors that can strengthen the relationship.

5. During a moment at home when he feels relaxed, Pat will practice behaviors that could strengthen his relationship with Alice and will catalog the consequences of this behavior.

6. Other goals will be developed as appropriate to helping Pat build a positive relationship with Alice.

LONG-TERM GOAL 2: Help Pat maintain relationships at work that will support his getting a better job.

LONG-TERM GOAL 3: Help Pat maintain relationships with strangers that will keep him out of conflict with the law.

Premise 4: Historically Based Style

As Pat developed from childhood through adolescence, his needs for physical, cognitive, and psychosocial mentoring were met with indifference or hostility. His caretakers neglected to teach him prosocial skills and modeled violence as the universal response in human interactions. As an adult survivor of a violent upbringing, Pat has developed a hostile view of the world in which all behaviors, whether neutral, positive, or negative, are viewed as threatening. His only mechanism for dealing with stress, beyond physical or verbal aggression, is through the overuse of alcohol. His maladaptive learning history has impeded his ability to develop any positive, intimate relationships. Pat's strengths lie in his ability to inhibit his aggression within the workplace despite his lack of prosocial mentoring. In addition, he is at a point in his life when he recognizes his life would improve if he could maintain a long-term relationship with an adult female, preferably Alice, the woman he is currently living with. This recognition may serve as an opening for new learning within the treatment setting.

Treatment Plan 4: Historically Based Style

Treatment Plan Overview. Due to the neglectful and violent behaviors of his parents, Pat raised himself and did not get help learning how to get what he wanted from life without the use of aggression. Pat has little motivation at this time to explore his own aggressive behavior as he does not agree that it is a problem. He is overtly angry with his parents and feels they "screwed him up." Furthermore, Pat wants to have a better relationship with Alice than his father had with his mother. Thus, he will consider learning the relationship-building skills his parents neglected to teach him. Long-Term Goal 1 will be achieved before progressing to further goals. (This treatment plan follows the *problem format.*)

PROBLEM: Pat raised himself and did not get help learning how to get what he wanted from life without the use of aggression.

LONG-TERM GOAL 1: Help Pat examine the consequences of his parents' violence involving himself and others.

Short-Term Goals

1. Pat will describe what he observed about his parents' behavior toward other adults such as neighbors and extended family members and whether they had relationships he would have called friendships.

   a. Pat will articulate how well their violent style of relating supported their getting their human needs for companionship, respect, and trust met from adult friends.
   b. Pat will reflect on whether he learned any viable friendship skills by observing his parents.
   c. Pat will reflect on how his parents' behavior influenced his choice to be a loner.

2. Pat will discuss his parents' behavior toward each other as spouses and speculate on the consequences of their behavior for each of them getting their needs for intimacy, respect, and security met.

   a. Pat will reflect on what he learned about how men and women relate to each other by observing his parents.
   b. Pat will consider the impact his violent upbringing had on his ability to relate to women in a way that would sustain a positive relationship.

3. Pat will discuss his parents' aggressive and neglectful behavior toward him as a child and the consequences of this for him receiving the care and support every child needs.

4. Pat will discuss the impact his violent upbringing had on his ability to consider other people trustworthy.

5. Pat will discuss the impact his violent upbringing had on his ability to succeed at schoolwork.

6. Other goals will be developed as appropriate to helping Pat see the impact of his past violent and neglectful learning history on his current life.

LONG-TERM GOAL 2: Help Pat examine the consequences of his own violence on himself and others now that he is a young adult.

LONG-TERM GOAL 3: Help Pat learn the nonviolent communication and problem-solving skills that his parents neglected to teach him during his childhood.

Premise 5: Thematically Based Style

"Can I ever have power in a relationship without resorting to violence?" This may be a question Pat never asked himself until his recent alliance with Alice. Faced with a history of relationship failure and in danger of losing yet another relationship, Pat may finally be open to thinking about his life and what has led him to being who he is. From a behavioral perspective, many of his difficulties can be seen as stemming from faulty learning experiences in which the use of aggression, the exertion of power, and impulsive outbursts of anger were modeled and reinforced as much as prosocial and thoughtful strategies were ignored. In his family, the young Pat was at the bottom of the power hierarchy and initially defined as the family loser. Pat only gained power as his skills at fighting back increased. Pat's strengths can be seen as his ability to reflect on, and try to learn from, his own prior experiences. He has noticed that other men can maintain male-female relationships while he currently doesn't have the power to do so. This recognition may be an opening for Pat to learn new strategies that could help him maintain his relationship with Alice. In the past, he has struggled against heavy odds to survive. This persistence has the potential to serve him well as he seeks to use his intelligence and ability to observe others in developing a different type of relationship power.

Treatment Plan 5: Thematically Based Style

Treatment Plan Overview. Pat is very interested in power. He has many questions related to power: What kind of power can he get in his current situation? How can he stop the law from having power over him? What power can he use to get what he wants out of the treatment relationship? Pat believes that without appropriate power he will be victimized as he was in his childhood. Treatment focused on his gaining power within his life will fit his values. Long-Term Goal 1 is to be completed before beginning Long-Term Goal 2. (This treatment plan follows the *basic format*.)

LONG-TERM GOAL 1: Pat will examine the role of power in interpersonal relationships.

Short-Term Goals

1. Pat will observe current interpersonal relationships in his neighborhood, work environment, and so on and explore the question "Who has power within these relationships?"

2. Pat will consider what verbal and physical behaviors provided evidence for who had power and what behaviors maintained the power.

3. Pat will observe the consequences (neutral, negative, positive) during new incidents of the use of power within these interpersonal relationships and determine who benefited and who lost in the short run and how this might influence the sustainability of the relationship in the long run.

4. Pat will consider whether he ever observed examples of the constructive use of power in which someone was influential in the relationship without causing loss to the other person.

   a. Pat will search through media, political news, work, or his neighborhood for examples of constructive power.

   b. Pat will evaluate whether the nonaggressive behaviors that supported constructive power led to stronger and more satisfying relationships in the long run.

5. Pat will make a list of behaviors he has observed that create constructive power.

6. Pat will determine what problems at home, in the neighborhood, or at work are in need of a solution and discuss with the clinician any ideas he has for solving these problems using constructive power.

7. Pat will engage in role-plays with the clinician where he uses his own ideas on how to solve problems using constructive power.

8. Pat will consider whether he would like to try to implement one of his ideas.

9. Other goals will be developed as appropriate for Pat to have power in relationships without jeopardizing his ability to keep the relationship and to keep out of jail.

LONG-TERM GOAL 2: Pat will practice strategies for beginning and maintaining interpersonal relationships using constructive rather than destructive power.

Premise 6: Diagnosis-Based Style

Pat has a lifelong history of impulsive and aggressive behavior. He appears to view the world as a hostile place in which sane people have learned to be on their guard and ready to protect themselves. He views himself as an expert in gaining the upper hand in relationships. Although he shows evidence of regretting the time he spent in prison and the loss of some past interpersonal relationships, he continues to show what appears to be an enduring tendency to externalize blame, to view other people as actively hostile, and to evidence an inability to see other people's points of view. This profile of chronic, egosyntonic, maladaptive behavior is considered most compatible with a primary *DSM-IV-TR* diagnosis of Axis II: 301.0 Paranoid Personality Disorder. Further assessment is needed to determine if an Axis I diagnosis of 305.00 Alcohol Abuse also is appropriate. In recent years, Pat's use of alcohol has increased, and there are some indications that excessive alcohol use occurred prior to his most violent outbursts. Pat's current level of physical health is excellent, so there is no diagnosis on Axis III. On Axis IV, Pat is having difficulties with the legal system, his social environment, and his primary support group, although he does have a history of constructive employment and expresses a desire for a long-term relationship with Alice. On Axis V, Pat has an estimated current Global Assessment of Functioning (GAF) of 40 and an estimated highest GAF in the past year of 50. Because of Pat's long history of maladaptive behavior, his tendency to blame others, and his difficulties in forming a trusting relationship, any positive movement in treatment must be viewed with caution as it could reflect manipulative behavior rather than adaptive change.

Treatment Plan 6: Diagnosis-Based Style

Treatment Plan Overview. Pat is motivated to stay out of jail and continue his relationship with Alice. He does not currently believe that gaining control of his alcohol use, and decreasing his aggressive behavior, is necessary to achieve these goals. The current situation will first be described from his point of view. Then, information that the clinician has garnered from other sources will be summarized. And, finally, a plan based on an integration of this information will be offered to help Pat stay out of jail and strengthen his relationship with Alice. (This treatment plan follows the adapted *SOAP format.*)

Subjective Data

> Personal history: Pat is a 25-year-old, European American male who was the only child of two alcoholic parents. He describes being treated by his parents with indifference and hostility. He states that he was often beaten for reasons he did not understand. He witnessed many acts of violence between his parents. He got into trouble in school for aggressive behavior and received poor grades beginning in elementary school. He began coming into conflict with the law as a teenager. This was also the time when he began to drink. He considers himself a loner who never had friends. He says friends are for "losers."

Relationship history: Pat has been involved in many short-term relationships with women. He met these women in bars or in his neighborhood and, after a few weeks of dating, invited them to move in with him, and then, just as suddenly, they secretly moved back out. He has observed other people having longer-term relationships than he has had, and he expresses the desire to maintain a relationship with Alice, long-term.

Legal history: Pat was recently released from prison. He was convicted of assault with intent to harm and given a prison sentence of 2–5 years. Pat was released after 3 years for good behavior. He is currently on parole. He has weekly appointments with his parole officer and is participating in treatment as a requirement of his parole. The officer wants him to decrease his alcohol use and develop nonaggressive strategies for dealing with conflict.

Work history: Pat has been gainfully employed since he graduated from high school. The only disruption of this was his time in prison. Immediately on release from prison, he set out to get a job and is now a custodian at a store.

Objective Data

Standardized intellectual testing using the Wechsler Adult Intelligence Scale-III (WAIS-III) revealed that Pat has an above-average level of intelligence. Pat denied any memory loss, cognitive disorientation, or history of head injury, so no neuropsychological testing was considered necessary at this time. Personality testing utilizing the Minnesota Multiphasic Personality Inventory-2 (MMPI-2) revealed no signs of cognitive confusion, personal turmoil or distress, or physical symptoms. Rather, his profile suggested a history of family and interpersonal discord. His relationships with others can be characterized by suspiciousness, jealousy, and hostility. His scores on items reflective of alcohol abuse are ambiguous, and thus further assessment in this area is called for. His profile suggests a pattern of behavior consistent with a diagnosis of a Paranoid Personality Disorder. As a result, Pat is not likely to view the clinician as trustworthy. The clinician must take responsibility for demonstrating trustworthiness.

Assessment

There are no signs at this time of significant emotional turmoil or distress related to his violent behavior or alcohol abuse. Pat's behavior is consistent with a diagnosis of Paranoid Personality Disorder, but his behavior is also not inconsistent with viewing Pat as an adult survivor of a traumatic upbringing. Both Pat's high level of intelligence and his ability to observe and analyze others might be utilized in making constructive change. However, safety issues must be monitored carefully as Pat is angry about the referral for treatment. While there were no signs of any loss of control of anger within the treatment session, he has a history of explosive, violent outbursts. Thus, Pat's potential for being a danger to others, including the clinician, will need to be monitored on an ongoing basis.

Plan

Long-Term Goal 1: Pat would like to maintain his relationship with Alice.

Short-Term Goal 1: Pat will read a book on relationship building and discuss with the clinician any skills within it that he finds useful.

Short-Term Goal 2: Pat will observe men and women in his neighborhood and at work and discuss with the clinician any relationship skills he sees that he thinks might be useful to him.

Short-Term Goal 3: Pat will observe TV, videos, and movies and discuss with the clinician any relationship skills he sees that he thinks might be useful to him.

Short-Term Goal 4: Pat will practice relationship skills he found useful within role-plays with the clinician.

Short-Term Goal 5: Pat will practice skills he found useful within conjoint sessions with Alice.

Short-Term Goal 6: When it is considered safe to do so, Pat and Alice will practice in the home setting the relationship skills they are learning in treatment.

Long-Term Goal 2: Pat would like to maintain constructive employment.

Long-Term Goal 3: Pat would like to remain out of jail.

Conclusions

The type of case conceptualization and treatment plan recommended within this chapter requires a great deal of critical thinking prior to actually implementing treatment. Although this is initially time-consuming, this critical thinking will serve you well in planning effective and time-efficient treatment sessions overall.

Developing new skills can create temporary chaos for the learner. As you practice these new case conceptualization and treatment planning skills, you may enter a temporary period in which your writing seems awkward, rigid, or simplistic and in which you feel confused and uncomfortable. This period of "bad" or "stressful" writing will dissipate with practice, and you will have developed a scholarly approach to writing that reflects your personal style.

Recommended Resources

American Psychological Association. (2007). Recordkeeping guidelines. *American Psychologist, 62*(9), 993–1004.

Dunn, D. S. (2004). *A short guide to writing about psychology.* New York: Pearson Education, Inc.

Pan, M. L. (2008). *Preparing literature reviews: Qualitative and quantitative approaches.* Glendale, CA: Pyrczak Publishing.

Two

The Complexity
of Human Experience

Malika is referred to you for treatment of acute anxiety attacks. Is her age, sexual orientation, gender, or racial background relevant to her treatment? What about her medical history, her religious upbringing, her socioeconomic status, her educational achievements, her history of physical or sexual abuse, or other aspects of her background? All these domains may reveal insights to help you evaluate whether Malika's anxiety is adaptive or maladaptive.

This type of discrimination is even more difficult for you to make when a client's background or identity is significantly different from your own. Then, the question becomes whether a pattern of behavior is "healthy," "different but healthy," or pathological. There is no comprehensive model of psychopathology to rely on. There is no absolute standard of mental health; all norms are influenced by the history and politics of when they were developed. As a result, professional organizations such as the American Psychological Association (2000a, 2002) and the Association for Multicultural Counseling and Development (Sue, Arredondo, & McDavis, 1992) call on clinicians to develop multicultural competencies and keep informed of new research on the complexity of human experience.

It would be overwhelming, if not impossible, to evaluate everything that makes up Malika's complex and unique identity when trying to decide if she needs treatment for anxiety; yet her behavior can be over- or underpathologized if this complexity is ignored. To make your decision, ask Malika about her identity (Hays, 2008). Supporting self-definition is important because research suggests it can be damaging to invalidate clients' self-attributions or proscribe their identities for them (Pedrotti, Edwards, & Lopez, 2008). Some aspects of Malika's identity may be very salient to her and may influence her worldview on a continuous basis. Other aspects may be more or less salient depending on time and place as she is taking on different roles or life challenges (Delphin & Rowe, 2008).

There will also be an interaction between your personal identity and Malika's; this interaction can support or inhibit the development of an effective working relationship. Hays (2008) recommends that you start each new treatment relationship by evaluating potential differences between yourself and your client on 10 critical domains of identity: (a) age and generational influences, (b) developmental disabilities, (c) disabilities acquired later in life, (d) religion and spiritual orientation, (e) ethnic and racial identity, (f) socioeconomic status, (g) sexual orientation, (h) indigenous heritage, (i) national origin, and (j) gender. Within each of these domains, you may find you differ from Malika in terms of privilege, power, and experiences with oppression. Clarifying the power differentials between yourself and Malika will be your first step in avoiding microaggressions, or the unintentional taking on of an oppressor role with her, and/or in infusing a negative bias into your conceptualization and treatment plan (Hays, 2008; Sue et al., 2007). These aggressions or invalidations may appear small to the person of greater power, but they can cause substantial psychological harm to the less powerful individual (Sue et al., 2007). By recognizing the potential for these destructive practices, you can either educate yourself in areas of deficiency and/or adapt your approach to Malika so that a positive treatment alliance can be developed.

The following sections represent introductions to the domains of age, ethnic and racial background, gender, sexual orientation, socioeconomic status, and violence history. Only an overview of information relevant to each domain is included. You can use this information to deepen your analyses of clients as you complete the integration exercises found at the end of Chapters 3 through 10. These exercises mark the beginning stage of learning how to incorporate human complexity into your work. If you are ready for a more in-depth understanding, there are recommended resources at the end of this chapter.

Domain of Age

Kevin, age 14, is struggling with self-hate and a phobia of mirrors (Chapter 3). Alice, age 9, is caught in the middle of her parents' conflicts pre- and postdivorce (Chapter 8). Each minor has been mandated into treatment by adults. How relevant are Kevin's and Alice's ages to you as their clinician? How will what constitutes adaptive behavior be different for a 9-year-old and a 14-year-old?

Children are in a continuous process of changing as they grow in terms of physical, cognitive, and psychosocial development. In addition to age, what is considered normal for a child is influenced by the child's level of intelligence, his or her caretakers' attitudes, and current social norms. The following sections provide a brief overview of the developmental periods of early childhood, late childhood, and adolescence in terms of physical, cognitive, and psychosocial development. These overviews apply only to individuals of at least average intelligence who are in good health and receiving adequate care. Issues of cognitive or physical disabilities, gender, culture, and the influence of different types of traumas on development are beyond the scope and intent of this section.

Early Childhood (Approximately Ages 4–7)

A 4-year-old looks very young and incompetent compared to a 7-year-old while, at the same time, appearing highly sophisticated and coordinated in comparison to a toddler. This is because early childhood is a time of very rapid physical development. Young children can walk, run, jump, and climb with ever-increasing speed and coordination. As they age, gross motor skills such as running and climbing are mastered more easily than fine motor skills such as how to hold a knife and fork or write with a pencil. Tasks are valued for kinesthetic pleasure rather than for goal directedness (Brems, 2008). Thus, children might play with mud endlessly without any intention of building something specific. Intrinsic motivation to master new physical skills is the norm (Berger, 2009).

While they enjoy unstructured play, young children can effectively focus their attention on challenging tasks when they are provided with appropriate, guided structure (Berger, 2009). Intense frustration may result when young children are pressured by others to master tasks they are not neurologically ready for. Physical maturity that allows for greater speed and agility builds faster than cognitive skills that help children stop and think. This results in a high rate of injuries in this group (National Center for Health Statistics, 2002).

Cognitively, young children are curious and active learners. They are in Piaget's stage of preoperational thought where the child can begin to think about something (manipulate symbols) before acting on it (Berger, 2009; Piaget, 1952). They enjoy make-believe and use symbolic play to gratify their needs and increase their understanding of the world. Preoperational thinking is egocentric, and these children have an exaggerated view of their impact on the world. They often see themselves as responsible for what has happened. This can be true of positive as well as negative events (Berger, 2009). For example, a child may think, "Dad beat my mom because I left my clothes on the floor today."

Despite this type of egocentrism, young children do have a theory of mind that allows them to recognize that other people have thoughts and feelings that are different from their own (Berger, 2009). Thus, a child can realize that another child is hurt when hit with a ball and that one teacher will be angry when a rule is broken while another will not. Young children always look to immediate events to understand cause and effect. Their views of rules are very concrete and inflexible. They master new learning best through guided participation, repetition, and scaffolding (Berger, 2009; Vygotsky, 1978). Their cognitive abilities grow the most smoothly when the challenge of the new tasks is kept within reasonable limits. In this situation, the child is intrinsically motivated to move toward mastery (Vygotsky, 1978).

In terms of language development, these children can communicate with adult-like verbal and nonverbal speech. They use complex sentences and can use speech as a tool for developing more complex thinking skills (Vygotsky, 1978). They need concrete and simple explanations that are tied to the here and now to learn new concepts (Brems, 2008). Despite these improved verbal skills, these young children still prefer learning through modeling rather than through verbal directions (Brems, 2008). Advances in their language development facilitate parents, siblings, and others in guiding the child's learning experiences. The development of private speech also plays a role in aiding self-control and guiding the child during the learning process (Berger, 2009).

Psychosocially, these children are in Erikson's stage of "initiative versus guilt." Children have a strong desire to fit in with their families and be valued as a member of the family. They model their caregivers and take in the socialized rules of their community and culture (Berger, 2009). These children can identify how they feel and can communicate this to others when helped to do so. Typically, they can be aware of one emotion at a time although they can understand a variety of emotions and have begun to learn emotional regulation skills. The ability to inhibit, moderate, and direct emotions, or emotionally regulate them, allows a child to learn to talk about being angry rather than just kicking the dog (Halberstadt & Eaton, 2003). Children without these skills may develop either internalizing problems from overcontrolling emotions or externalizing problems from undercontrolling emotions (Berger, 2009). In socializing with other children, they can begin displaying a give-and-take style in which cooperation and sharing are important. While peer influences are beginning, the approval and attention, particularly from caregivers, is still primary. Their parents, and other valued role models in the environment, can help children develop empathy or antipathy for others; mirror neurons in children's brains facilitate this emotional development (Berger, 2009).

Self-esteem develops from learning new skills and developing a sense of competency (Erikson, 1963). They begin to form a self-concept based on what they can and can't do (Berger, 2009). Their sense of pride in taking on a new task helps them concentrate and persist (Berger, 2009). They are usually optimistic that they can accomplish a new project. However, they feel guilt over their mistakes (Erikson, 1963). Connections between their mistakes or misdeeds and a punishment must be immediate and clear; otherwise the child will not learn from them (Berger, 2009).

Middle Childhood (Approximately Ages 7–12)

Children in the elementary school years master one new physical challenge after another. While gross motor skills continue to be mastered more quickly than fine motor, the overall process of physical development reflects a relatively smooth increase in coordination and competence. The ability to follow the rules of competitive games increases, and variability in success in individual and team sports provides a new arena for winners and losers. Due in part to increased myelination of the brain and increases in interconnections between areas of the brain, school-age children show a reduction in temper tantrums, impulsiveness, inattention, and insistence on rigid routines in comparison to younger children (Berger, 2009).

These children are in Piaget's concrete operational stage of thought (Piaget, 1952). They can understand logical reasoning when it is presented to them using concrete events or tools that they can experience or directly see.

This makes them much more logical and more able to use strategies for learning. In following rules and directions, these children are able to process more than one or two steps at a time, and they are able to plan ahead if the task has concrete and specific goals. Present-oriented explanations are still more effective than abstract, general discussions in helping these children understand complex life events such as divorce or death (Berger, 2009). They have begun to anticipate the consequences of their behavior (Brems, 2008). Language skills are well developed with these children having wide vocabularies and an expanded understanding of grammatical rules. They have learned to talk differently to parents than to friends (code switching). Most children master learning to read in this period, and reading skills become increasingly important for educational success.

Psychosocially, Erikson puts these children in the stage of "industry versus inferiority." These youth busily set about learning new skills, which can give them a sense of competence and a positive sense of self. However, their increased skill at social cognition makes them more aware of their social status vis-à-vis their peers. This ability to compare their skills to those of others may lead them to feel inferior resulting in a negative self-concept (Erikson, 1963).

While parents are still important, these children actively seek out others of their own age for advice and self-validation, and they model themselves after popular peers (Berger, 2009). Because social comparison is so important at this time, children show a tendency to develop friendships with peers who are similar to them in physical appearance rather than necessarily being the same age. Children who look different from the group may be left out and become lonely or unhappy. Friendships now involve more emotionally intimate sharing than in the younger years. Children begin to favor children of their own gender, and much gender role socialization occurs at this time (Berger, 2009).

Children can be popular due to positive social skills such as kindness, cooperativeness, and trustworthiness or because they are athletic, highly attractive, dominating, and arrogant. Children can be unpopular and either neglected but socially accepted, rejected due to their withdrawn behaviors, or rejected due to their aggressive behavior. Being actively rejected is a risk factor for the development of emotional problems (Berger, 2009). The overly aggressive children in kindergarten may now be the bullies in elementary school (Broidy et al., 2003). Boys are more likely to use physically aggressive behavior when bullying; female bullies rely more on relational aggression (Watson, Andreas, Fischer, &

Smith, 2005). Anxious and withdrawn children may now be the ones who are victimized at school. Effective parents can serve as buffers to help their children negotiate problems with peers (Berger, 2009).

These youth have a greater ability to modulate their emotions and express their emotions in words rather than acting them out. They can understand two emotions at the same time as long as they are either both positive or both negative. Children become more able to recognize the causes and effects behind their feelings and actions and become more self-directed. Schools demand more and more of this self-direction as these years proceed. Students who have difficulties with this, for example due to learning disabilities or attention deficit disorder, or who come from disadvantaged homes may fall behind in their schoolwork (Berger, 2009).

Adolescence (Approximately Ages 12–19)

As children progress through puberty, dramatic physical changes occur. Some teens seem to "change overnight." For others, the process is more gradual. Onset anytime between the ages of 8 and 15 is considered normal, but puberty typically starts between the ages of 10 and 13. In general, females start the process earlier than males. Self-image and identity may be influenced by early versus late development as teens prefer to mature at the same time as everyone else. Being off "the norm" can lead to additional stress; however, this is moderated by whether the home and neighborhood environments are supportive or destructive. While an earlier-maturing boy could be the football star at high school, he could also join a gang in the inner city (Berger, 2009). While hormonal fluctuations can cause more moodiness in teens, overall adolescent testiness is more a result of the higher demands placed on them by society due to their more mature appearance. Adults may make the mistake of judging maturity by height rather than brain maturation (Berger, 2009).

Cognitively, teens have sensorimotor, preoperational, concrete operational, and formal operational ways of understanding the world available to them. Which type of thinking they use will depend on their motivation, ability, and situational factors (Berger, 2009; Piaget, 1952). For example, they may use sophisticated reasoning within academic subjects in which they excel and concomitantly use more concrete, here-and-now, egocentric reasoning in areas in which they have less experience. Their lack of experience with physical injuries or sexual behavior, for example, may lead to feelings of invincibility and an underestimation of life risks

(Berger, 2009). Their limited social experiences may lead them to see themselves or their problems and strengths as being unique and therefore to consider the experiences of others to lack relevance for them.

This teenage egocentrism also results in their being preoccupied with their own behavior and having the belief that others share this preoccupation (Berger, 2009).

Brain developments may serve as a context for determining which type of reasoning skills teenagers will use in various situations. The limbic system is involved in intuitive thinking and the prefrontal cortex in logical thinking. While teens can think logically in terms of hypothetical situations involving drugs and sexual behavior, when they are emotionally excited, these feelings may well preempt logic. This may be because the limbic system is developing faster than the prefrontal cortex. The use of alcohol or drugs, "because everyone is doing it," is the type of reasoning that puts teenagers at risk of violent death and unprotected sex. Research suggests that teens do things because other teens encourage them to (social facilitation), as well as seek out others who share their interests (Berger, 2009).

Psychosocially, teens are in Erikson's stage of "identity versus role confusion." As such they focus a great deal on their own identity and may feel a great deal of anxiety if they are unsure over what they want to do with their lives. They can experiment with sexual, family, political, religious, and career identities, trying different things on for size and trying to find where they fit in the world (Erikson, 1963). While they may struggle for a sense of separateness and independence from their caregivers, they may still use, as role models, older individuals from their families or their social environment and media personalities. Most teens experience only moderate caregiver-adolescent conflicts and maintain positive relationships with their caregivers. Adolescents with serious conflicts with their caregivers have been found to come from families with chronic conflict (Berger, 2009).

At this time in their lives, peer acceptance transcends adult approval. Teens initiate and maintain effective peer group relationships without adult support. For most teens, earlier same-gender preferences now change to an interest in developing intimate relationships with an opposite-sex partner. Teens struggle as they try to understand what it means to be an adult man or woman while at the same time attempting to integrate their new sexual identity into their sense of self (Brems, 2008). Sexual minority teens may face significant challenges in developing a positive self-identity in families and/or communities that only provide support for heterosexual development (Beckstead & Israel, 2007).

Overall, the teen years are less happy than earlier school years although it is not the time of tremendous turmoil that past myths suggested. Each year teens become aware that the standards are getting more difficult, and they face increased life stress. As a result, they have the capacity to understand the full complexity of emotional reactions and to recognize that the same situation may evoke very different feelings for different people. Based on their past experiences, they can understand and empathize with the feelings of others (Brems, 2008); however, this is more likely if they have had parents or an environment that supported the learning of empathy. Teens who developed antipathy instead may already have begun victimizing others. The aggressive kindergarteners, who became the bullies in elementary school, may now be involved in both violent and nonviolent delinquency in the teen years (Broidy et al., 2003; Watson et al., 2005).

While educational achievement is stressed more and more by society, school performance declines for many teens during adolescence. They are more likely than younger children to describe school as boring and teachers as hostile, and intrinsic motivation for school success sags. The facts that (a) teachers see a student for only one period, (b) classmates change each period, and (c) rules and structure become more rigid may be important factors involved in this detachment from a positive school affiliation (Berger, 2009).

The teen years are the time when the developing person is at highest risk for suicide attempts (U.S. Department of Health and Human Services, 2001). Studies also show that sleep deprivation is a significant problem facing teens. Biologically, teens need about 2 more hours of sleep than adults. Lack of sleep is responsible for teen drowsiness, fatigue, and greater impulsivity leading to greater disciplinary problems and decreased learning at school (Carpenter, 2001).

Resilience Versus Risk

Four global factors have been found to determine whether a child will show a resilient or pathological reaction to stress during the course of development. The first factor is having formed positive connections with a confident and effective adult within the family or community. An effective parent, for example, monitors his or her child's behavior and environment to ensure safety and provides a warm and supportive atmosphere. The second factor in resilience is the child having at least average cognitive and emotional self-regulation skills to enable success in school and other social environments. The third factor is the presence of a positive view of the self. The final factor is the child having the motivation to be effective within the environment. With these factors in place, children may be protected from the negative consequences of adverse life events such as growing up in disadvantaged circumstances. The resilient youth seeks to take advantage of healthy opportunities for success, seeks connections with prosocial mentors, is less likely to associate with deviant peers, and engages in less novelty seeking (Masten, 2001).

Red Flag Developmental Guidelines

1. Assess how age appropriate the client's physical and cognitive development have been and how, and in what ways, this has influenced the client's performance and level of motivation at home, in school, or within community activities.

2. Assess how age appropriate the client's relationships with adults have been in terms of providing age-appropriate limit setting, monitoring, skill building, and emotional connection and in what ways these relationships have supported or hindered the developmental process.

3. Assess how age appropriate the client's relationships with peers have been in terms of providing age-appropriate companionship and social skill building and how, and in what ways, these relationships have supported or hindered the developmental process.

4. Assess how age appropriately the client is functioning at this time, including consideration of self-image and self-efficacy, what the client needs most to support healthy development at this time, and what, if any, barriers or facilitating factors to maturation exist at this time.

5. Consider whether your age, your stereotypes of the client's age group, or developmental biases embedded in your treatment approach might lead to negative bias, marginalization of the client's point of view, and/or the client's current situation and consider what could be done to increase the likelihood of a positive outcome.

Domain of Gender

Marie, a recent widow, gives herself no time to grieve; she feels she must focus all her attention on her children (Chapter 4). Steve, an art student, is emotionally detached from others (Chapter 7). Could their gender roles be influencing Marie's and Steve's psychological well-being? Does and should gender influence how you understand their cases or how you plan their treatment?

On the 2000 Census, individuals were presented with the categories male and female and self-identified as one or the other (U.S. Census Bureau 2000, 2001). Based on this, women represented 50.9% of the population of the United States, and men represented 49.1%. More baby boys were born than baby girls, with this disparity lasting through age 24. In older groups, women have slowly overtaken men. By age 85, there were twice as many women as men (U.S. Census Bureau 2000, 2001). One result has been that many older, heterosexual women must face older age without their male partner. Another result should be that women begin to dominate positions of authority in later years, as they come to represent a larger and larger majority; however, this hasn't happened. While the 21st century has seen the emergence of some powerful female political leaders, such as Senator Dianne Feinstein taking office in 1992, Nancy Pelosi becoming Speaker of the House in 2007, and Hillary Clinton becoming Secretary of State in 2009, women represented only 14% of the House and 13% of the Senate in 2008. This has been the result of a hierarchy of power within the United States that gives males more power than females and inculcates them with the idea that men's accomplishments are more valuable and deserve more respect than females' in order to preserve the power status quo (Kimmel, 2008).

Biological differences between males and females are a constant. However, what it means to be female or male has been socially constructed and varies across cultural groups, historical time periods, and political climates. Worell and Remer (2003, p. 15) defined gender roles as "patterns of culturally approved behaviors that are regarded as more desirable for either females or males in a particular culture." Despite the large body of research documenting greater heterogeneity of abilities within genders than across them, gender stereotypes have still been used to define, and limit, the roles males and females take on in their personal and social identities (Worell & Remer, 2003). Masculinity and femininity have been defined in opposition to each other (Kimmel, 2008).

The following discussion of the impact of gender roles on males and females has been based on research derived from primarily White, Western, middle-class, Christian samples within the United States. The generalizations presented may have less or limited validity for other populations as gender constructions vary across socially identifiable groups. However, culturally different youth, as they attempt to assimilate into dominant society, have been found to incorporate the gender stereotypes of the dominant population into their own experiences (American Psychological Association [APA], Joint Task Force, 2006; Mazure, Keita, & Blehar, 2002; Worell & Remer, 2003).

How are men supposed to behave? Traditional stereotypes have encouraged them to be self-reliant, tough, aggressive, dominant, and emotionally controlled (Addis & Mahalik, 2003). Boys' peer groups have supported teamwork and competition, and boys and men who are assertive in expressing their opinions may be viewed as leaders (Worell & Remer, 2003). However, males have also been discouraged from experiencing a full range of emotions. They have been socialized to view their emotions as something to act on rather than to experience. "What American men have been taught for centuries when they are upset and angry," according to Kimmel (2008, p. 122), is that "men don't get mad; they get even." As a result they might have "alexithymia," or an inability to articulate their emotions (Feder, Levant, & Dean, 2007). Men have been allowed to be angry, but males who cry or show other vulnerable emotions have been perceived as weak, emasculated, and in need of toughening up. As a result, some men have had their emotional awareness truncated. Help-seeking behavior has also been discouraged in males. As a result, they have been less likely to access either health or mental health services than women; if men feel that asking for help jeopardizes their autonomy, they have avoided it (Addis & Mahalik, 2003). The male standard of health has required them to "prove" their masculinity through success at work and in sports, dominance with women, and a heterosexual and married lifestyle (Kimmel, 2008).

Societal messages exhorting men to seek dominance and prove their masculinity might be directly responsible for their higher rates of violent behavior as teens and young adults. While acts of violence have been referred to as "teen violence," "drug violence," "school violence," and "terrorist hijacker violence," in fact the perpetrators were almost always males (Kimmel, 2008). Society has pressured all males to think, feel, and behave in similar ways despite their heterogeneity. The external pressure for them to be emotionally stoic and self-reliant at all times may have resulted in role stress. Books written by women and goals achieved by women have been analyzed for their "gendered" influences. However, the parallel process has not occurred for males; this has left issues of masculinity invisible. Thus, the challenges faced by male scientists, who also wanted to be good fathers, have never been discussed (Kimmel, 2008). Men have been oppressed by cultural norms that limit their individuality and jeopardize their physical and mental health by setting unrealistic standards of behavior, yet these issues have been socially ignored (Kimmel, 2008; Worell & Remer, 2003).

How are women supposed to behave? Traditional stereotypes of women have included their being submissive, passive, nurturing, emotionally attuned in relationships, and dependent on others (APA, Joint Task Force, 2006; Papp, 2008). Women who acted assertively have been viewed as "bitchy," not leaders (Worell & Remer, 2003). Women have been encouraged to tune into their emotions and talk problems through. Girls' peer groups have supported the development of emotionally intimate relationships. This might be why women reported experiencing greater emotional intensity than men in terms of both positive and negative emotions (Brannon, 2002). Women have also been encouraged to make relationships with others, both friends and romantic partners, central to their view of themselves (Nolen-Hoeksema, 2000).

Societal messages have encouraged women to believe that sexual attractiveness is the key to success in relationships with men. When problems have arisen in these relationships, women have been encouraged to internalize or deny anger (APA, Joint Task Force, 2006). Despite this emphasis on sexual attractiveness, society has left women confused about themselves as sexual people. Language has trapped women with derogatory sexual labels such as "bitch," "frigid," and "ho." This has left them insecure as to how to behave as a sexual person (Worell & Remer, 2003). In addition, women and girls have been deluged with unrealistic media images and social norms of attractiveness. To feel feminine, by these images, has required a cult of thinness. Women have been encouraged to focus a great deal of time on grooming and grooming products, and the inability to meet these unrealistic images has led many women to have low self-esteem and to be more vulnerable to depression, anxiety, and eating disorders than men (APA, Joint Task Force, 2006; Mazure et al., 2002). A female who expressed anger rather than depression might have felt guilty about it or been disapproved of by others. Thus, in many ways, the physical and mental health of women has been limited by gender role stereotypes (Worell & Remer, 2003).

The 21st-century family has been taking longer to develop as men and women are remaining single longer, marrying later, and having fewer children (Worell & Remer, 2003). Fifty-two percent of households contain married couples with about two thirds of all children living in these married households. Once married, men and women have been divorcing at high rates and then remarrying. Thus, families might consist of two parents, single parents, or stepfamilies (U.S. Census Bureau 2000, 2004b). Men and women have faced the need to adapt to changing family structures and increased role strain (Worell & Remer, 2003). Marriage has moderated life stress in men but not in women (APA, Joint Task Force, 2006). Family dissolution has led to financial strain. This has been especially true for children living with mothers; children have been 5 times more likely to be living in poverty when living with a single mother than with married parents (U.S. Census Bureau 2000, 2003). In terms of parenting skills, when single men have been confronted with the need to actively parent, they have taken on similar behaviors and attitudes to women who parent (Kimmel, 2003).

What happens to men and women at home? The traditional mother role has been to take responsibility for raising the children and caring for the home. Women's reproductive capacities and abilities to nurse have been equated with meaning that women are born to be mothers. Good mothering has been treated as a natural ability rather than consisting of difficult skills that need to be learned (Goodrich, 2008). Although mothers have been idealized for being loving and caring and for sacrificing their own needs for their children, they also have been blamed for any types of psychopathology found in their children (Papp, 2008). Women have been criticized for mothering too much or too little, as well as for working outside the home too much or too little; this puts women in a double bind (Papp, 2008). Being unable to have healthy children, while painful for both parents, may be particularly problematic for women due to the coupling of femininity with motherhood. On the other hand, the greater availability of birth control and fertility options has given women more freedom to choose if and when they will become mothers (APA, Joint Task Force, 2006).

The traditional father role has been to provide financial support for the family. Fathers typically have played a comparatively minor role in the management of their home, the development of their children, the caring for other dependents, and the maintaining of social networks (Papp, 2008). While fathers today are more likely than fathers in the past to express the attitude that they should be involved in child rearing and household responsibilities, they overestimate their time doing these tasks. Social norms in the United States continue to support the idea that men's work is more demanding and significant and a man's leisure time is more necessary for him than for his wife. This has led to inequities in the home where women have taken on more domestic responsibilities than men even while they were likely to be working outside the home (Brannon, 2002). Husbands and wives often accepted the power imbalances and privileges within the home. These are interpreted as reflecting differences between masculinity and femininity rather than cultural expectations that men "deserve" more power and privileges than women (Goodrich, 2008; Papp, 2008). Thus, male oppression within the home could be conscious, with men refusing to share household chores or take care of children as this is "women's" work. However, men have been found to gain a greater sense of confidence in themselves, as parents, when they spend more time with their children (Barnett & Hyde, 2001). Male oppression might also occur at the unconscious level, with a husband getting very angry if his wife made a decision against his advice (McIntosh, 2008).

What did children learn about their genders? Starting at birth, males and females have been socialized differently and inculcated with the political beliefs that males deserve more power than females; differential sex role socialization served to maintain this power differential (Kimmel, 2008). Parents have often modeled a relationship in which the father was dominant. Children have seen their mothers being more expressive and loving and their father being more detached, in control, and dominant (Worell & Remer, 2003). At early ages young children have already begun to identify some professions as being for males rather than females. In the school system, most teachers have been female, and most males have been the principals and superintendents; this has reinforced gender stereotypes and gender-based power differentials (Worell & Remer, 2003). At school, boys have been found to receive more mentoring and encouragement. Girls have been more likely to be victimized by discriminatory testing and counseling by school officials that discourage their achievement (APA, Joint Task Force, 2006). As boys and girls slowly change into old men and women, their views of masculinity and femininity change also. For example, what represents femininity for a prepubescent female has been found to be different from that for postmenopausal women (Kimmel, 2008).

What happened to men and women at the office? Women were more likely to be underemployed than men, feeling trapped in jobs that underutilized their abilities. They also earned less than men with equal qualifications (U.S. Census Bureau 2000, 2001). However, when given equal opportunities, powerful women exhibited the same work behaviors as powerful men—using language to exert power and authority—while subordinate men exhibited the same behavior as subordinate women such as providing ego strokes to the boss and being sensitive to this person's moods (Kimmel, 2008). Most men expected to dedicate themselves to this worker role while most women expected that they would be trying to balance family and work roles (Brannon, 2002). In 2009, the U.S. Bureau of Labor Statistics' *Monthly Labor Review* revealed that 70% of working women had children at home in the mid-1990s. Even when women started out in high-status jobs, they frequently faced slower rates of advancement than men because of their need to take pregnancy leave. Once a woman took this leave, the company prejudice that women were not as dedicated to their work as their male counterparts was reinforced (Goodrich, 2008).

It has been true that working women have, of necessity, divided loyalties. Since they continued to be disproportionately responsible for the parenting role, they were subject to disadvantages in the workplace. For example, when a child got sick, it was the mother who was most likely to rush out from work to take the child to the doctor (Goodrich, 2008). While taking on multiple roles could lead to greater life stress, success in one role has also been found to buffer the effects of problems within another (Barnett & Hyde, 2001). Society has encouraged men to evaluate their success based exclusively on their earning capacity and employment status. Thus, unemployment or underemployment might have a greater negative effect on their physical and mental health, sense of identity, and general outlook on life than it does for women (Papp, 2008).

Women have not been as welcome in the workplace as men. They have often faced sexual or general harassment at work. They might not mention small slights at work to coworkers or supervisors for fear of being considered "too sensitive." Over time, these slights have created hostile environments that leave women feeling less appreciated and more devalued than men (Goodrich, 2008). Currently, men working full-time earn one dollar for every 73 cents women earn. Men earn more money at every job classification. Whatever the job, work has been treated with more respect if a man did it than if a woman did (Goodrich, 2008). Women, due to their decreased earning power, have more limited economic resources to use during times of need (APA, Joint Task Force, 2006).

How might gender influence psychological health? Women have access to fewer occupational and educational resources than men. This may lead them to be more vulnerable to psychological stressors. Men, on the other hand, have been less likely than women to seek out help for physical or emotional problems (Addis & Mahalik, 2003). Overall, men have been diagnosed more often with substance abuse and antisocial personality disorder, and women have been diagnosed more frequently with depression, anxiety, and eating disorders. Currently, women compared with men have higher levels of poverty and victimization, which have been linked with greater vulnerability to stress-related disorders (APA, Joint Task Force, 2006; Mazure et al., 2002). Men and women have also been found to use different coping mechanisms when faced with stress. Men frequently socialize within the context of physical activities and use these activities to distract themselves from their problems. While this strategy has provided an immediate feeling of relief from stress, it could also lead to minimizing, rather than solving, the problems behind the stress (Mazure et al., 2002). Women have been more likely to seek out companionship within which to discuss problems, and they may take on a ruminative response set in which they spend more time thinking about their problems. This greater attention to problems could lead to problem solving. However, it could also lead to increased feelings of failure and hopelessness (Nolen-Hoeksema, 2000).

Society trains boys and girls to believe that males have been given more power than females in society because of innate differences in their abilities; in fact these differences are created by unequal treatment and supported by the devaluation of women's roles over men's (Kimmel, 2008). As adults, men have been given the most culturally respected roles both at home and at work, and female contributions to society have been minimized. Men have been treated as the "norm" or the "neutral point" against which women have been measured and found deficient. For example, female scientists have been expected to act like male scientists while the effect of men's masculinity on their work as scientists has remained invisible (Kimmel, 2008). While as a group males have more power, authority, and resources than females, they often haven't been as interpersonally connected, and their mental and physical health has been jeopardized by sex roles that portray getting help as being weak (Papp, 2008). Thus, in differing ways, men and women have had their unique potentials limited by rigid gender role stereotypes that ignore the reality that there are more differences within sexes than between them (APA, Joint Task Force, 2006; Kimmel, 2008). Flexible expectations and standards for behavior that allow each individual to fully explore his or her own interests and abilities would increase the well-being of both men and women (Kimmel, 2008; Worell & Remer, 2003).

Red Flag Gender Guidelines

1. Assess the personal costs or benefits to the client's current gender role in terms of self-image, emotional life, expectations, perceptions, behavior, and access to personal resources.

2. Assess the social costs or benefits to the client's current gender role in terms of family relationships, social relationships, educational or work relationships, and access to social resources.

3. Overall, how much have the client's view of masculinity and femininity, society's definition that they are opposites of each other, unrealistic societal expectations for males and females, and the devaluation of women and their values influenced the client's mental or physical health, and how aware is the client of this?

4. Overall, how much power and choice does the client have to live life as a nongendered individual with unique needs and goals, and how strong are counterpressures on the client to be a gendered individual?

5. Consider whether the gender role you have taken on, your stereotypes of the client's gender role, or gender biases within your treatment approach might lead to marginalization of the client's point of view and/or the client's current situation and consider what could be done to increase the likelihood of a positive treatment outcome.

Domain of Race and Ethnicity

John, a middle-aged European American male, the chief executive officer of an international company, finds his wife has abandoned him (Chapter 5). Sergio is a Mexican American high school student who is struggling with racial prejudice, poverty, and a drug conviction (Chapter 7). Tanisha and Marcus are a financially successful African American couple who enter treatment due to unresolved grief (Chapter 8). Kayla, an internationally renowned Native American writer, enters treatment with complaints of malaise and acculturation conflicts (Chapter 10). To what degree, and in what ways, might their racial or ethnic backgrounds influence your treatment decisions?

There are 281,420,906 people residing within the United States based on the 2000 Census (U.S. Census Bureau 2000, 2006a). You may be one of them. Are you African American? American Indian? Hispanic or Latino American? European American? Can you be biracial? Multiracial? Who has the right to decide your race or ethnicity? Only you. Who has the right to decide for clients? Only them. An important thing to remember, as you read this section, is that you should not assume you know an individual's race or ethnicity based on his or her appearance. It is important to ask clients to self-identify (Hays, 2008; Rodriguez, 2008). In the year 2000, individuals were finally allowed to indicate all of their ancestries or ethnic group affiliations on the Census rather than being forced to select only one affiliation from the six major Census categories of White, Black or African American, American Indian or Alaska Native, Hawaiian or other Pacific Islander, and "Some Other Race" (U.S. Census Bureau 2000, 2004a).

Based on this ancestry data, four ethnic groups represent the majority of individuals in the United States. German ancestry or ethnicity represents the largest group in the United States, containing 42.8 million people and representing 15.2% of the population. The next largest group is individuals of Irish ancestry. They represent 30.5 million individuals, or 10.8% of the population. African American ancestry follows with 24.9 million individuals, or 8.8% of the population. The last group contains individuals with English ancestry, who represent 24.5 million people, or 9% of the total population. While three European ethnicities remain within the top four largest groups, their populations have been decreasing while African American, Latin American, and Asian American populations have been increasing (U.S. Census Bureau 2000, 2004a).

How well a racial or an ethnic group fares economically is influenced by its standing in comparison to the dominant group. This is because the dominant cultural group has its values infused into all of the institutions of society such as the school system and the court system. Dominant group members see their institutions as neutral and objective when in fact they are culturally influenced and put nondominant groups at a disadvantage (Sue & Sue, 2008).

Day-to-day microaggressions, perpetrated by dominant group members and institutions, have been found to cause substantial psychological harm to groups that differ substantially from the dominant society (Solorzano, Ceja, & Yosso, 2000; Sue et al., 2007). These negative events occur most often for individuals whose skin is not perceived as white. The "color line" (Du Bois, 1903/1997; Ignatiev, 1995) has been found to play a substantial role in facilitating or inhibiting the acculturation of groups into dominant society; dark-skinned immigrants are the most disadvantaged when trying to immigrate and assimilate. New immigrants quickly come to see how skin color, hair texture, and facial structure can add to or decrease an individual's status and power in U.S. society. They also learn that they can better their own status if they can ally themselves with the White race and against the Black race (Rodriguez, 2008).

As a result, you must actively consider when a "culturally different" client's presenting problems might reflect assimilation conflicts, or oppression, rather than be caused by internal or family-based problems. Sue and Sue (2008) discuss three major barriers to clinicians correctly understanding the needs of their clients: class-based values as clients from nondominant groups are often lower class while clinicians are often middle or upper class, language biases that lead to misunderstandings as these groups may speak dialects or have another language as their first language and clinicians expect a high facility in the English language, and clashes in cultural values where the clinician assumes that the clients implicitly understand and agree with the White values embedded within most treatment approaches.

It is important that you collaborate with your clients through making explicit your expectations, modifying them to suit your clients' needs, and accurately assessing the role of realistic life constraints in your clients' presenting concerns. While presenting problems can have their major determinants in individual or family-based problems, research has shown that individuals from groups with the least power are more aware of when their problems are actually a result of acts of injustice and discrimination than members of the dominant group are (Sue et al., 2007). Therefore, if you are from the dominant group and your clients are not, they may be more accurate than you in determining whether oppression has a role in their presenting concerns. In addition, the White culture considers race an important category of identity while many other cultural groups consider their national origin to be more important. In addition, they may see continuums of racial affiliation that change with context rather than clear categories that are immutable aspects of their identity and that have been developed by Whites, without regard for their collaboration (Rodriguez, 2008).

The following sections will include broad-brush descriptions of the heritage of African Americans, American Indians and Alaska Natives, Latinos and Latinas, and European Americans with white skin. Why were these groups included and not others? Hard decisions had to be made keeping in mind the main goals of the text, the limitations of the author's expertise, and practical constraints set by page limitations for the text. There is no intent to demean or devalue the important contributions of other racial and ethnic groups to the United States by their exclusion from this text.

African Americans

In the Census of 2000, 36.2 million individuals indicated they were African American or Black when given a choice among the six major Census categories; this represented 12.9% of the population of the United States (U.S. Census Bureau 2000, 2005). Out of this population, 2.6 million were foreign born, and 51% entered the country starting in the 1990s. Individuals from Latin America were 66% of these immigrants, and individuals from Africa were 30% (U.S. Census Bureau, 2007). This was a relatively young group with an average age of 31.2 years in comparison to 40.1 years for non-Hispanic Whites and with 31% of this population being minors (U.S. Census Bureau, 2007).

From an educational standpoint, 74% of African Americans or Blacks have attained at least a high school diploma; this is in comparison to 81% of the general population. In terms of a bachelor's degree, 16% of African American women have achieved this degree, as have 13% of African American men. While African American adults value education, their children have experienced significant problems within the current public school system. Tutwiler (2007) summarized how schools jeopardize school success, particularly of African American boys, by treating them in a racist and classist manner. When youngsters tried to resist negative stereotypes and assert their self-worth, school personnel often misunderstood and either punished the youth or further intensified an already hostile environment. Statistics have indicated that African American children are 2 to 5 times more likely to be suspended from school than their White peers (Monroe, 2005), and they may have disconnected their self-esteem from their academic performance during middle school and high school (Caughy, O'Campo, & Muntaner, 2004). Racist environments within the school system are partially responsible for this. In addition, some students intentionally underachieve as a form of resistance to an oppressive school system (Ogbu, 2003). Children from families that attend church regularly are less likely to exhibit problems in school (Christian & Barbarin, 2001).

In terms of vocations, one quarter of all African American workers are employed within management and professional occupations while 22%

are employed in service jobs. African American men make $100 for each $85 made by African American women. Finally, African American men and women earn less than their counterparts in the general population (U.S. Census Bureau, 2005). Economically, the median household income is $31,969, which is significantly less than the median income of the general population, which is $44,334. Twenty percent of this population is living below the poverty line in comparison to 12.7% of the general population. This represents 1 in 4 Black families and more than one third (36%) of African American children living in poverty (U.S. Census Bureau, 2005).

The poor have been more likely to end up in the criminal justice system. Thus, the high rate of poverty within the Black population has led to Black citizens having a 16% chance of being incarcerated at some point in their lives; this is in comparison to a 5% risk for the general population. A Black male infant has a 1-in-6 chance of being incarcerated in his lifetime (U.S. Department of Justice [DOJ], 2006b).

While these statistics are grim, much of the data collected on African Americans has been drawn from predominately lower socioeconomic groups and thus might not be representative of the experiences of middle- and upper-class individuals (Ford, 1997; Holmes & Morin, 2006). Many specialty organizations have been developed to support these more economically advantaged people continue to experience economic success. For example, Black Entertainment Television offers a free membership in "Black America Saves," and the Consumer Federation of America offers services to aid in the accumulation of wealth. In addition, the National Urban League (www.nul.org), the Coalition of Black Investors, the Investment Company Institute (www.ici.crg), and New York Life Insurance Company (2008) provide seminars to aid effective investment.

Families come in many different constellations. While most African American or Black individuals have chosen to live in family households, their marriage rates have been lower than those of many other groups, and their families are more likely to be headed by women. For example, in 2005 only 34% of individuals within a Black household were married in comparison to 57% of non-Hispanic Whites (U.S. Census Bureau, 2005). African American women head the household 30% of the time in comparison to 9% for non-Hispanic White women. In a 2007 survey, 42.3% of all Black women had never been married, and 70% of professional women had never been married (Nelson, 2008). While fewer women were marrying, they were still having children. Of Black women who had a child in the last year, 60% were unmarried in comparison to a rate of 20% for non-Hispanic White women (U.S. Census Bureau, 2007). Finally, when grandparents were living in the household, 52% of the time they were responsible for the care of their grandchildren.

The category African American or Black is very heterogeneous. Therefore, the following more detailed information has been based on the African Americans who were descendants of the slaves who were forced to emigrate to the United States and endure 200 years of slavery. These slaves were stolen predominately from sub-Saharan, middle African coast communities where polygamy was a common part of clan life (Comer & Hill, 1985; Du Bois, 1903/1997). The traditions of these communities emphasized family and kinship ties as being more important to self-identification than an individualized self.

The leaders of the clan, the chief and the priest, were separated from their people during the enslavement process. Furthermore, plantation-based slavery actively worked to subvert the formation of committed relationships (Du Bois, 1903/1997). Masters would pressure their slaves to form bonds; in order to give birth to more slaves, couples might be forcibly separated, and one might be sold into slavery on another plantation where he or she might be pressured to find a new partner. Two hundred years of this cruel practice caused deterioration of the traditional family practices of the African people.

Some of the major political events that shaped African American life following slavery and the Civil War included the development of the Freedmen's Bureau in 1866 and a series of amendments to the U.S. constitution. The 13th amendment abolished slavery, the 14th defined the rights of citizenship, and the 15th gave African Americans the right to vote. Despite these legislative advances, oppression and racism continued. Overly harsh and discriminatory practices within the school systems, legal systems, housing authorities, land authorities, and so forth eventually led to the civil rights legislation that was passed in 1964 and 1965. According to Du Bois (1903/1997), the "color-line" kept African-Americans from integrating into the dominant culture of society. They struggled with the integration of two identities, that of being an "American" and that of being "African American" (Du Bois, 1903/1997).

Affirmative action programs, beginning in the 1970s, were designed to make reparation to these people for their years of oppression. The goal was to increase the numbers of qualified African Americans in higher education and employment. Clear economic gains were made by people who benefited from these affirmative action programs. However, a backlash began in the 1980s. The 14th amendment's equal protection clause, as well as Title VII of the Civil Rights Act of 1964, began to be used to make the argument that affirmative action was "reverse discrimination." Polls suggest that a misperception exists that many White males have been harmed by affirmative action. Research data suggest that discrimination against White males has been rare (5% or less) while a much larger percentage of people of color and women have been harmed by a lack of affirmative action (Pincus, 2001/2002).

Research suggests that African American families have been more likely to emphasize interconnection and interdependence among members and take on a holistic perspective to life, in comparison to the dominant culture's emphasis on individual achievement and a linear view of events (Hall & Greene, 2008). To deal effectively with the hostile and oppressive historical and political realities, African American families have developed four major strengths (LaRue & Majidi-Ahi, 1998). The first was to use their religious beliefs and their affiliations with the church as a starting point for their social and civic activity. The majority of African Americans are Protestants who attend Baptist churches, Methodist churches, and Churches of God; many of these churches are part of the fundamentalist movement. However, the Black Muslims and the more liberal Protestant churches have been gaining in membership in recent years (LaRue & Majidi-Ahi, 1998). Many important African American leaders have come out of religious careers—for example, the Reverend Martin Luther King, Jr., the Reverend Jesse Jackson, and the Reverend Al Sharpton.

A second major strength of the African American family has been its inclusion of extended family and a kinship network in its definition of family (LaRue & Majidi-Ahi, 1998; Sue & Sue, 2008). The sharing of money, resources, and emotional support has been critical to the survival of many poor families within the African American community. However, this has also meant that money was often spread too thinly across family members (Greene, 1997).

A third strength has been the willingness of the African American family to care for extended family members who were in trouble. For example, adolescents in need of a change in environment or those in highly conflicted relationships with their immediate family members might be sent to live with other relatives (LaRue & Majidi-Ahi, 1998).

A final African American family strength has been the willingness of the adults within a household to take on flexible roles (LaRue & Majidi-Ahi,

1998). Family members divide up tasks based on what would be most functional within each person's work or school schedule, rather than adopting the European American custom of dividing tasks by sex (LaRue & Majidi-Ahi, 1998). Thus, African American men are often involved in child-rearing responsibilities (Sue & Sue, 2008). Economic realities have fueled this more androgynous lifestyle, as African American women have always needed to work, and this work has often been within low-pay and low-prestige settings. Thus, these families were dual-income families by necessity, not choice (Greene, 1997). In addition, a racist society has offered more employment opportunities to women than to men. While some women experienced guilt over this, the community as a whole recognized that many employers actively discriminate against African American men (Greene, 1997). Many African American women have become frustrated and overwhelmed when they have had to take on the stereotypical role of the strong woman in the family—the one who always keeps the family going. This role has led to a neglect of their needs as individuals. African American men are harmed by stereotypes labeling them as irresponsible, incompetent, and violent (Hall & Greene, 2008).

African American parents have been found to actively support the development of assertiveness and self-esteem in their children (Sue & Sue, 2008). Within an atmosphere of warmth and support, African American parents were more likely to use physical discipline than their European American counterparts. While this physical punishment correlates with negative outcomes in European American populations, it has not with African American populations (Pinderhughes, Dodge, Bates, Pettit, & Zelli, 2000). African American families who directly taught their children how to deal with racism and oppression had children with lower levels of anxiety when confronted with injustice (Neal-Barnett & Crowther, 2000). Children struggling with poor self-esteem have been helped by programs that teach them about African American culture (Belgrave, Chase-Vaughn, Gray, Addison, & Cherry, 2000).

The African American community continues to have a realistic lack of trust for dominant culture institutions based on past and continuing acts of direct and indirect oppression (Sue & Sue, 2008). As an example, 61% of African American families felt that quicker and more effective help would have been given to victims of Hurricane Katrina in New Orleans if more of these victims had been European Americans (Washington, 2005). In addition, more subtle forms of domination continue, such as children's toys most often featuring White faces, powerful characters in television shows being predominately White, and powerful people such as policemen and politicians being predominately White (McIntosh, 2008).

However, many powerful African Americans have arisen on the political scene in the 21st century including Secretary of State Colin Powell who took office in 2001, Secretary of State Condoleezza Rice who took office in 2005, and President Barack Obama who took office in 2009. These leaders make visible the contributions of African Americans to the prosperity of the United States.

African Americans coming into treatment may experience a disconnection between what is offered and what they are seeking. This disconnection may result from (a) the client coming from the lower class while the clinician is often from the middle class; (b) use of a Black dialect and an emphasis on nonverbal behavior rather than standard English; (c) a people orientation including an emphasis on extended family versus an individualistic one that relies on a nuclear family structure; (d) emphasis on immediate, short-range, and concrete goals rather than long-range goals with a focus on personal exploration; or (e) a social viewpoint in which oppression plays a pivotal role versus a belief in a just world (Sue & Sue, 2008).

American Indians and Alaska Natives

According to the 2000 Census, American Indians and Alaska Natives represent the indigenous population of North America. Included in this population are any people who originated in North, South, or Central America and maintain tribal affiliation or community attachment. As of 2006, 4.5 million people were classified within this population, representing 1.5% of the total population of the United States. There were 561 federally recognized tribes. There were more than 100 other tribes that were recognized at the state level as well as other tribes that were not recognized by the Bureau of Indian Affairs (BIA) (U.S. Department of Health and Human Services [HHS], The Office of Minority Health [OMH], 2006a). Only recognized tribal members were covered by the Indian Health Service (IHS). This organization is part of the Department of Health and Human Services. Most individuals served by the IHS live on reservations or in rural communities.

The median family income for American Indians and Alaska Natives is $33,627, which is substantially below the general population income of $44,334. One fourth of all American Indians are living below the poverty line, and they have an infant mortality rate that is double that of the White population (HHS, OMH, 2006a; U.S. Census Bureau 2000, 2006a). Along with this high poverty rate comes a high crime rate.

Department of Justice statistics have revealed that Native people between the ages of 25 and 34 are 2.5 times more likely to be victimized by violent crime than the general population. Males, 12 and older, have a 1-in-10 chance of being victimized by violent crime, and historically the perpetrator was often a White individual under the influence of alcohol. The rate for female victimization is lower; however, Native females are twice as likely to be victimized than females in the general population. Native women who have been assaulted or raped and assaulted are most likely to be attacked by someone outside the family while non-Native women are most often attacked by an intimate partner (APA, Task Force, 2006; DOJ, 2002). Thus, American Indians and Alaska Natives may have a realistic fear for their safety around White people.

American Indians are less likely to graduate from high school than other cultural groups, although they start out very successfully in the earlier school years. In terms of education, 74% of Indians received at least a high school diploma, which was significantly lower than the 81% of the general population who did so. A hostile environment or a sense of social stigmatization seems to increase in the early teen years as Indians come to see they were marginalized and treated unfairly (Sue, 2005). The U.S. government has frequently sent underqualified teachers, and even teachers with criminal records, to staff schools on Indian reservations (French, 1997). While intentional oppression does exist in the schools, teachers trained in dominant society values can also unintentionally create an uncomfortable environment. For example, being singled out at school to receive an award will make an American Indian child uncomfortable unless the child sees that the whole group will benefit from this achievement. The nonverbal communication patterns of these youth may also be incongruent with dominant culture expectations. For example, to show respect, direct eye contact with an elder is to be avoided. Teachers at school could view this behavior as disrespectful and see these children as passive or uninvolved in schools that often value competition between students (French, 1997). In addition, Indians tend not to ask direct questions, so teachers may not know when they need help (Sue & Sue, 2008). Despite these difficulties, 14% of Native people go on to achieve a bachelor's degree, and some go further to attain advanced professional degrees.

Seventy-three percent of American Indians and Alaska Natives prefer to live in family households compared with only 68% of the general population. However, more than twice as many Native families as general population families are female-headed households without a husband present. More marriages are intact among families residing on tribal lands than among those living within the dominant culture (U.S. Census Bureau 2000, 2006b).

Catastrophic historical and political events enveloped Native people when European American immigration began. Europeans spread infectious diseases such as measles, diphtheria, cholera, smallpox, and tuberculosis for which Indians had no immunity. These diseases depopulated the land. Indigenous cultures were extensively damaged by this massive population loss, which allowed Europeans to literally take North America away from them. European immigrants moved into the homes and property that were abandoned due to death or people fleeing infection (Mann, 2005).

Once the U.S. government was formed, it used military force to continue the process of stealing Indian land away from those who had survived the pandemics. Policies of the government included acts of genocide by U.S. troops, forcible relocation of survivors away from their traditional lands, and repeated force of Native populations into political treaties that were to their disservice. These treaties were later violated by the U.S. government; examples of this are the Fort Laramie treaties of 1851 and 1868.

In addition to this physical decimation, a malignant social agenda was carried out on the surviving American Indians in an attempt to wipe out their cultures. Children were forcibly abducted and raised in boarding schools as Christians with European values. At these schools, children were punished if they spoke in their native language or tried to participate in any spiritual rituals or cultural practices. American Indian children and youth were systematically abused by non-Indians— notably those employed by the federal government to be their teachers. As a result, politicians, lawyers, teachers, and social agencies of the dominant society were not perceived as trustworthy based on a pattern of oppression, injustice, and victimization; many Indians have a justifiable distrust and hatred of the institutions supported by the U.S. government (French, 1997).

The grouping "American Indians and Alaska Natives" represents highly diverse people. Therefore, for the purposes of providing more specific cultural information, the Lakota Sioux will be used as a reference group. The Sioux Nation is itself highly diverse, containing three major subdivisions: the Lakota, which has seven bands; the Dakota or Santee with four bands; and the Nakota or Yankton with three bands (Snow Owl, 2004). The people who originally made up the Sioux were mound builders who lived within the woods (French, 1997). They survived using hunting, gathering, and horticulture. Historic migrations led to the development of the three basic groups. These groups met episodically but were not united as a coordinated Sioux Nation until White persecution began.

To many citizens of the United States, the Plains Sioux fulfilled the characteristics of the stereotypical Indian. They were nomadic, lived in teepees, and hunted buffalo. They were a warrior-oriented society whose warriors wore feather headdresses as they raided other tribes.

These people have a complex belief system that has at its center the "Great Mystery" or Wakan Tanka, which also has the name of "Chief God, Great Spirit, Creator, and Executive" (French, 1997, p. 114). This Great Mystery has a complex and sometimes contradictory nature and was the amalgamation of 16 Sioux superior and subordinate gods and godlike beings. The numbers 4 and 7 are very important to the Sioux and are tied to nature (such as the four directions), to animals (crawling, flying, two-legged, four-legged), and to the Sioux virtues (bravery, fortitude, generosity, and wisdom). Every summer, the "Seven Council Fires" powwow occurred, at which the most important ceremony—the Sun Dance—took place. This ceremony focuses on the warrior's fulfillment of important vows. The Sioux viewed all power as coming from Wakan Tanka. Thus, the warrior turned to this supernatural power to draw strength. The warrior also sought visions to aid in this process of gaining strength from the creator. There are six other sacred ceremonies in addition to the Sun Dance including Purification, Vision Seeking, Ball Throwing, Making a Buffalo Woman, Making as Brothers, and Owning a Ghost. Integral to Sioux spirituality is the use of the sacred pipe, which represents the universe. Smoking this pipe is part of making the connection with Wakan Tanka (French, 1997).

Historically, chiefs were not rulers who told their people what to do; it was an honorary title. They were men who had fought well during wars and whose actions and opinions were respected by the tribe (French, 1997). Important decisions resulted from the unanimous vote of a Council of Chiefs (Snow Owl, 2004). Some important chiefs in history were Sitting Bull, Big Foot, and Crazy Horse. More recent leaders known for fighting for justice for the Indian people come from groups such as the American

Indian Movement, the National Congress of American Indians, and the National Indian Youth Council.

The Sioux moral code is grounded in the beliefs that good is stronger than evil and that good is a result of harmony within the group. Mind, body, and spirit are considered interconnected and inseparable (French, 1997). A lack of harmony between them may cause physical or psychological difficulties (Sue & Sue, 2008). The tribe is very important to the Indian and is an extension of him- or herself. The value of each person is contained in his or her usefulness to the tribe. The tribal land or reservation is also critical to the identity of an American Indian. When an individual leaves ancestral land to pursue economic prosperity, the individual's sense of identity may be damaged (Sue & Sue, 2008). Indians tend to live in the present rather than planning for the future. Thus, Indians might keep a job only long enough to pay basic expenses so that they can dedicate themselves to spiritual rituals; unfortunately this may serve to perpetuate poverty (Sue & Sue, 2008).

Males and females are to show the four Sioux virtues, and their status in the tribe comes from how well they demonstrate these virtues. While men and women take on defined sex roles, with men as warriors and women as bearers of children, both sexes are to show the virtue of bravery and its related virtue, fortitude. Bravery requires self-sacrifice. For a warrior, this could be shown through acts of bravery such as counting coup (a nonviolent act of bravery where an enemy is touched briefly with a hand or a stick and then the warrior runs away), dog soldiering (being an elite warrior who would fight to the death in defense of the tribe), and participating in the Sun Dance (a public demonstration of bravery and self-discipline). Fortitude, the second virtue, describes how men and women would demonstrate bravery. In public, both males and females are socialized to show self-discipline and emotional self-control both in confronting fear and pain and in terms of positive experiences. Affection and physical intimacy are private behaviors, and it is taboo to engage in public displays of affection.

Generosity, or sharing food and possessions, is the third virtue. It illustrates the profound difference between the Sioux ethic and that of the early White immigrants. These European immigrants gained respect from each other by making money and owning individual property. Amongst the Sioux, respect came from participating in the "giveaway" (French, 1997, p. 118). Individuals who could give away their possessions, to be distributed amongst the tribe, particularly toward the neediest in the tribe, were those who earned prestige and respect. Those who gave away the most achieved the highest status.

A combination of age and life accomplishments is used to determine status within the tribe. The final virtue, wisdom, comes from accumulating knowledge. Elders in the tribe are valued for their opinions based on life experience and are often used to help bring conflicts to an acceptable conclusion (French, 1997). The Sioux strongly endorse the concept of harmony and have traditions that are designed to keep conflicts down. They do not interfere in other people's business. They are taught to observe and consider carefully rather than act impulsively.

Children are prized and treated indulgently. Even when misbehaving, they are not physically punished as tribal harmony includes that the children need to be happy. The most severe punishment given to children was for angry parents to dump a bucket of cold water over the child (History Learning Site, 2008). Young people are encouraged to be sensitive to the feelings of others and not seek competition as this leads to discord (French, 1997).

Today, many American Indian tribes have lost contact with their traditional ways. A Pan-Indian movement has developed to try and rectify this. Sioux ceremonies and spiritual songs are being incorporated into the traditional healing ceremonies of other Indian groups; indeed, Sioux leaders are training healers from many different tribes (French, 1997). The dominant culture of the United States continues to suppress traditional Sioux ways, and this has led to reciprocal anger and hostility between American Indians and their White neighbors. Thus, while unemployment, substance abuse, suicide, posttraumatic stress disorder, and victimization are high base rate problems for American Indians and they need help, these people are unlikely to trust non-Indian clinicians (DOJ, 2002; French, 1997; Sue & Sue, 2008). Many culturally specific treatments have been developed to empower them in the recovery process such as bibliotherapy for traumatized children and youth, Cherokee cultural therapy, the traditional healing practices of the Sioux, and the Navajo Beauty Way perspective. Each of these treatments seeks to revitalize cultural connection and pride and promote religious freedom (French, 1997). At the present time, American Indians range from living totally within their Native culture to being completely assimilated within the dominant culture of the United States. Many Native people might benefit from help achieving a balance between their cultural and personal identities (Sue & Sue, 2008).

The American Indian culture does not fit well with the expectations of treatment orientations that stem from White, middle-class culture. Areas of conflict may include (a) that its tribal dialects and nonverbal communication patterns are very different from those used in English and within the White culture, (b) emphasis on cooperation over competition, (c) focus on present needs and immediate short-range goals over a future orientation and long-term goals, and (d) its family structure relying on active participation from extended family over a nuclear family (Sue & Sue, 2008).

Hispanic or Latino and Latina Americans

According to the 2006 Census estimate, there are roughly 44.3 million Hispanics living in the United States (HHS, OMH, 2006b). "Hispanic" is a category created by the Census that defines people by their country of origin rather than by their racial group (U.S. Census Bureau 2000, 2004d). It consists of people from Mexico, Puerto Rico, Cuba, El Salvador, Nicaragua, and other Central and South American countries as well as Spain (U.S. Census Bureau 2000, 2004d). These people often have an ethnic and racial heritage that could include full Aztec Indian or other Indian heritage, along with biracial or multiracial heritage involving Indian, African, Spanish, and White ancestors (Comas-Diaz, 2008).

Hispanics consider racial mixtures and multiple identifications as typical. There is a great variability in skin color amongst these groups that may lead people who are not Latino to misidentify them as White when they don't view themselves as White, to misidentify them as Black when they don't view themselves as Black, and so forth. They may be highly offended by others selecting a racial identification for them rather than asking them to self-identify. Latinos identify themselves more by national origin than through racial categorization. In fact, their self-identification of race is more fluid. They tend to see race as more of a social construction influenced by context than a biological reality. For example, some contexts may lead to a national origin self-designation, some to a Latino designation, some to an Afro Latino designation, some to a Black Cuban designation, and so forth (Rodriguez, 2008).

Mexican Americans are the largest subgroup within the Hispanic population, representing 18.4 million people. Central and South Americans are the next largest group followed in order by Puerto Ricans and Cubans. Immigration from Latin America has been steadily increasing. In fact, 40% of the Hispanic population is foreign born. Almost 50% of those foreign-born people entered the United States between 1990 and 2000 (U.S. Census Bureau 2000, 2004d).

The median household income for Hispanics is $34,397 in comparison to $44,334 for the general population (U.S. Census Bureau 2000, 2004d, 2006a). While male Hispanics earn less than the general population of men, they earn more than Hispanic women. Seventy percent of Hispanic males and 53% of Hispanic females are in the workforce. Hispanic females are most likely to be employed in sales and office work while Hispanic males are most likely involved in construction- and production-related employment. A total of 22.6% of Hispanics are living below the poverty line compared with 12.7% for the general population. One in four Hispanic children is living in poverty (U.S. Census Bureau 2000, 2004d, 2006a). Higher poverty rates are accompanied by higher crime rates. The Hispanic population has an incarceration rate of 9% in comparison to the 5% rate for the general population (DOJ, 2006b).

The educational attainment of Hispanics has been lower than that of the general population. Only 52% of Hispanic individuals over the age of 25 have a high school diploma, which is substantially below the general population figure of 81%. However, 1 in 10 Hispanics has earned a bachelor's degree. Educational background varies considerably amongst Hispanic groups with Spanish and South Americans showing the highest educational attainment and Mexican and Central Americans having the lowest. Only 31% of individuals who were born in Mexico have at least a high school education (HHS, OMH, 2006b; U.S. Census Bureau 2000, 2004d). Due to tremendous diversity within the Hispanic population, the more in-depth analysis that follows is focused on Mexican Americans.

Mexicans originally became citizens of the United States through acts of conquest and purchase. The largest changeover in citizenry occurred at the conclusion of the Mexican-American War in 1849 when Mexico lost 45% of its national territory to the United States. In this Southwestern territory, citizenship was granted to all Mexican and Spanish people. Later, an ambivalent and destructive cycle began wherein Mexicans were encouraged to emigrate to the United States when their labor was needed and then were expected to return to Mexico when it was not. For example, during the 1930s depression years, 300,000 Mexicans and Mexican Americans were repatriated or deported. During World War II, the *Bracero* agreement encouraged Mexicans to work for short periods of time within the United States. When the war ended, politicians enacted legislation to again restrict immigration of Mexican workers into the United States (Bernal & Enchautegui-de-Jesus, 1994). Despite the ambivalent and sometimes actively hostile attitude of the U.S. government, many Mexicans continued to emigrate to the United States in search of economic opportunities. Mexico, which has approximately 92 million people, has 40 million living in poverty. Political and economic instability in Mexico has also encouraged emigration (Santana & Santana, 2001). The legal status of an individual as "documented" or "undocumented" has a huge influence on his or her ability to attain any rights within the employment, educational, medical, or social structures within the United States. Fear of disclosure may prevent undocumented workers from seeking the services they need (Atkinson, Morten, & Sue, 1979). However, they remain in the United States because of shortages of paid work in Mexico. In their turn, many agricultural communities in the United States are dependent on Mexican workers (Santana & Santana, 2001).

There is considerable heterogeneity across Mexican American families due to family dynamics and patterns of acculturation to the dominant culture of the United States; however, some common important Latino and Latina values include the importance of family membership and pride in the family. The term *familismo* refers to the importance placed on family needs over the individual family member. Family includes an extended network of relatives, some of whom are tied by customs of obligation and feeling rather than blood; family unity and honor are emphasized (Atkinson et al., 1979). For example, even families three or more generations removed from Mexico may maintain extended kinship ties back home. Mexican families may also rely on *compadres* (godparents) for financial, emotional, and social support (Ramirez, 1998). Coming from a collectivist culture, Mexican Americans draw their personal identities from the sociopolitical and historical context in which they have developed as well as their ancestral histories (Comas-Diaz, 2008). Family histories may include multigenerational dislocations and disruptions including traumas that have not been processed. Deep family ties and cross-generational influences may have resulted in the continued transmission of racial and gender oppression from past injustices. Elders pass down family history through stories so that past trauma continues to have an impact on younger family members (Comas-Diaz, 2008). Spanish continues to be spoken in most Mexican American homes. In addition, according to the Census, 2 in 5 Mexican American adults don't speak English "very well" (U.S. Census Bureau 2000, 2004d, p. 10).

Latinos and Latinas have a strong sense of hierarchy and deference for authority and may consider it impolite to disagree with an authority figure. This may inhibit them from asserting their rights (Ramirez, 1998; Santana & Santana, 2001). Traditionally, men have assumed the role of provider and final decision maker. They are to have *machismo* by being strong, being loyal, and doing everything possible to ensure the happiness of family members. In fact, even if suffering from severe pain, the man is expected to stoically bear this while continuing to support his family. A man is expected to take pride in his role of husband, father, and son and put the well-being of his family first (Santana & Santana, 2001). The concept of *machismo* has sometimes taken on sexist and authoritarian elements. Men may be considered the superior of women and exert unjust power over them. Rather than being protective, they may be restrictive of their girlfriends or wives due to jealousy.

The tradition of the eldest male in the household holding the most dominant role in the family may be changing because of economic realities that push women to work outside the home to provide financial support to the family. Immigrant women using their sewing, cleaning, and cooking skills may find it easier to gain employment than their men using their agricultural skills (Santana & Santana, 2001). This has led to a shifting toward more egalitarian households (Ramirez, 1998). For some families, these shifting roles cause stress and turmoil (Santana & Santana, 2001).

Traditional women take on the role of homemaker and caretaker of children. They are to show *marianismo*. The word stems from the belief in the Virgin Mary as the ultimate example of motherhood. *Marianismo* includes being warm and supportive to family members literally as a sacred duty. Women are to work to bring pleasure to others while not seeking pleasure for themselves even to the level of martyrdom. They are also to show *hembriso*, or devotion to the home. The family home is expected to be the center of the family, and women are to put family loyalty first. Mothers, while appearing very submissive, actually have a great deal of power within the home as their skills at caring for others are considered even more important than skills at providing financial support. Mother love is considered stronger than romantic love. The role of parents is considered primary over the role of being a spouse. While motherhood and a mother's authority to run the household are highly respected, paradoxically, the father is given the most authority in making final family decisions (Santana & Santana, 2001).

Mexican Americans are generally very accepting of the individual needs and qualities of their children. They are less likely to push their children through developmental stages. Young children are indulged and dealt with affectionately by both parents. The father takes on a very playful role while children are young and is a disciplinarian when they are older. The mother continues throughout development to take on a very loving role with her children and serve as an intermediary when needed to reduce conflicts between her children and her husband. Having proper *respeto* for authority is emphasized within the home. Children are to listen to and obey parents, and younger children are to obey and model the behavior of older siblings. As children enter the later elementary school years, they are expected to take on more and more family responsibilities (Ramirez, 1998). Self-worth is defined in terms of children's inner qualities of uniqueness, goodness, and integrity that give self-respect and dignity and earn for them the respect of others.

Family members are expected to be dependent on rather than independent of each other. Young people are to work hard to improve themselves beyond what was achieved by their parents' generation. Rebellion against parental authority is unacceptable within traditional families. In general, teenage girls are traditionally afforded less freedom than boys and are channeled into homemaker activities while boys are encouraged to socialize with their male peers. Adolescents who push for freedom, due to greater levels of acculturation, may cause crises within the home and may struggle trying to bridge the identities they develop within each culture (Santana & Santana, 2001). Young adults are expected to live with their parents until marriage, and when parents become frail it is assumed they will move in with one of their adult children (Santana & Santana, 2001). Girls are to be chaste before marriage and not to show interest in their sexuality. In fact, women who do so may be considered "bad" women (Santana & Santana, 2001). Families who are just beginning to acculturate to the dominant culture within the United States may be forced to use their children as interpreters at times. This may disrupt the traditional family hierarchy of authority and cause stress. In addition, it may result in the clinician gaining inaccurate information (Sue & Sue, 2008).

Mexican Americans emphasize friendliness and warmth in their interactions with others. They value *personalismo*, or the individualized and personal manner of interacting with others, rather than the more professional or distant method of interacting often favored in dominant culture institutions. When Mexican Americans interact with individuals who behave in a distant and impersonal manner, they feel disrespected and uncomfortable.

The church is integral to family life, and priests are highly respected and officiate in important religious rituals as well as weddings and the *quinceañera* where 15-year-old girls cross into adult roles (Santana & Santana, 2001). The majority of Mexican Americans are Catholics (80%–90%) with a strong belief in divine providence. While beliefs are diverse, the *Virgen de Guadalupe* is an important spiritual mother for many Mexican women. She is considered a Black Virgin Mary (Comas-Diaz, 2008; Santana & Santana, 2001). Guadalupe stems from the Catholic Church but has also been used within more indigenous belief systems. She is believed to provide nurturance, warmth, and acceptance to the oppressed. She has been used as a symbol of hope in political struggles both within Mexico and within the United States (Comas-Diaz, 2008).

Overall, the Mexican American population is younger, less educated, and poorer than the general population of the United States. This population continues to grow due to its high birth rate and the continuing growth of undocumented workers (Ramirez, 1998; U.S. Census Bureau 2000, 2004d). Intergenerational history plays an important role in how family members interact with each other and with society (Comas-Diaz, 2008). Family context is so important to identity that immediate and extended families try to live close to each other (Santana & Santana, 2001).

Current treatment practices may come into conflict with Latino expectations and competencies in many ways including (a) an emphasis on Spanish rather than English within the home, which may reduce facility with communicating in English; (b) a family rather than an individualistic orientation; (c) a style of being silent and compliant with an authority figure; (d) an expectation that communication will be unidirectional from the clinician within a highly structured approach; and (e) an expectation that treatment will be action oriented and focused on short-range goals that are concrete and specific (Sue & Sue, 2003).

White Americans/European Americans

The classification "White American" is a category that was created by the U.S. Census Bureau at its inception. "White" is a heterogeneous group that includes individuals of European American descent who are perceived to have white skin, as well as individuals who are perceived to have white skin whose ancestors were not from Europe. Currently, "White" Americans represent the dominant group within the United States. They represent 80.1% of the population when Hispanic people are included as "White" and 66.4% of the population when Hispanics are not included (U.S. Census Bureau, 2000a).

The median household income of non-Hispanic Whites is $52,423. This is significantly higher than the median income of the population at large, which is $44,334. The percentage of this population living below the poverty level is 8% in comparison to 12.7% for the general population (HHS, OMH, 2006b; U.S. Census Bureau 2000, 2006a). Only 11% of non-Hispanic White children live in poverty (U.S. Census Bureau, 2007); this represents the lowest poverty rate of any racial or ethnic group within the United States. As economic welfare is related to crime rates, White individuals have only a 2% chance of spending time in prison; this is a significantly lower rate than the 9% for the general population (DOJ, 2006a).

From an educational perspective, 85% of the White population have graduated from high school, and 24.6% have attained a bachelor's degree or more (HHS, OMH, 2008). Vocationally, the greatest percentage of White workers are in the management, professional, and related occupations category (37.6%) followed by those who have sales and office occupations (26.9%) or are in service occupations (13.7%). Only 11.7% of White workers have classified themselves as working within production, transportation, and material moving occupations; 9.6% consider themselves to be in construction, extraction, and maintenance occupations; and 0.5% have classified themselves as working in farming, fishing, and forestry occupations (U.S. Census Bureau, 2007).

The first politically powerful or "privileged" population within the United States comprised White Protestants. Only Protestant males had the right to vote. They were also the head of the household in their families. They used the values from their belief system to create the institutions and rules of society. More recently emigrated and less financially successful groups needed to adhere to these already created institutions. Early in the nation's history, many Caucasian populations were actively discriminated against and were not considered White. A case in point was the treatment of early Irish American immigrants. They were treated with the same type of discrimination and oppression as

African Americans and were part of a highly exploited working class in the 19th century. They were referred to as "white Negros" (Ignatiev, 1995, p. 34). Before the Civil War, the Irish played an active role in the abolitionist movement. Southern slaveholders came to realize that to maintain their power, they needed support amongst the Northern working class. They funneled money into political battles to give the Irish citizenry the right to vote in exchange for their support against the abolitionists. Over time, the Irish came to see their white skin as their ticket out of marginalization, and they took it (Ignatiev, 1995).

During the World War II era, other formerly marginalized groups from so-called inferior races/Euro-ethnics became accepted as White once they earned enough money to enter the middle class and gain some political clout. Despite quotas that tried to keep them out, they were able to pursue higher education for their children. These more educated offspring had learned skills that were needed in the workforce (Brodkin, 2001). This type of entry into Whiteness was further accelerated after World War II. The new industrial complex had a need for skilled labor, and this employment boom spread economic prosperity amongst white-skinned groups.

Similarly, as a result of the 1944 Servicemen's Readjustment Act and loans from the Federal Housing Administration, White male service members gained loans that allowed them to buy homes for the first time; this further set the stage for economic prosperity; it was their white skin and their male gender that gave them these privileges (McIntosh, 2008). These same benefits were systematically denied to women and minority veterans who had similar military service and economic stability. Brodkin (2001) considered the GI Bill the largest affirmative action movement in U.S. history; it provided privileges that allowed white-skinned Catholic and Jewish men to enter the middle class. Being a member of the White race conferred privileges beyond access to better housing. It carried with it the cache of social respectability where you were assumed to be a good employee, a good citizen, and a safe neighbor (McIntosh, 2008; Sue & Sue, 2008).

However, "true" Whiteness came at the expense of separating from allegiance to country of origin. If a family continued, for example, to speak Italian in the home, then it was considered White but of "such and such descent" and thus an inferior type of White (Frankenberg, 2008, p. 83). A racial and cultural hierarchy developed where skin color, hair texture, facial features, and language were used as criteria for where one fit in the hierarchy. A carryover from colonialism, the view that non-White cultures were less sophisticated, less civilized, or deviant pervaded this hierarchy. White was made equivalent to being "average" or "typical" and a quality of the true American. White was what everybody else who was "normal" was, and true Whites only spoke English (Frankenberg, 2008).

The "Protestant Ethic," a term coined by Weber (1904–1905/1958), is thought to epitomize what has come to be called White culture. This ethic incorporated aspects of aesthetic Protestantism, which values hard work, self-reliance, self-denial, emotional control, and guilt as a mechanism of control (Albee, 1977). These values were intermixed with the qualities needed by the newly developing capitalist system, as conceived by wealthy Protestant businessmen. They wanted loyal workers who would find more satisfaction in their job success than in their relationships with family and friends. Workers who would sacrifice their time with their families to support company growth were rewarded with financial success (Weber, 1904–1905/1958) A more individualistic orientation was fostered in which success was measured by accumulating wealth and social status rather than fulfilling societal obligations (Albee, 1977). Capitalism and industrialization were powerful forces transforming the values of White groups to consider the production and consumption of goods as their primary goals (Frankenberg, 2008).

This new cultural ethic redefined the concept of breadwinner for men. Now, they were to be the major financial support of their families, rather than an active participant in day-to-day family life. Family members were to support the breadwinner in his single-minded pursuit of advancement in the workplace. Having children was delayed so that the breadwinner could become more educated and upwardly mobile. Smaller families were encouraged so that each individual child could be given the education and financial support needed to be upwardly mobile (Albee, 1977). Breadwinners were expected to have self-discipline so they would pursue long-term goals, not hedonistic short-term ones. They needed a sense of agency, within the context of independent thinking, rather than within the context of interdependence with others (Weber, 1904–1905/1958). These pressures brought on by capitalism actively worked to homogenize Whites to have the same values and to speak English (Frankenberg, 2008). Legal and educational institutions were developed to fit in with the specific schedules and lifestyles that were congruent with the new capitalism. Social reform moments and developments within the school system served to further socialize white-skinned immigrants to take on these values and behaviors (Frankenberg, 2008; Ignatiev, 1995). Time, and partitioning time into segments that were useful for business, became the norm. "Wasting time" became a serious offense. This new ethic selectively disadvantaged employees from cultures that had a different sense of time and that encouraged active involvement in family life (Weber, 1904–1905/1958). All cultural groups were measured in terms of how similar they were to the "norms" set by the White culture; the more different they were, the more they were excluded and considered inferior or deviant (Frankenberg, 2008).

A social myth of the United States as a meritocracy was created; success was assumed to come to all who had merit and who worked hard. People were assumed to be the masters of their own destiny. A malignant corollary was that individuals who were financially successful were morally superior to individuals who had less money and possessions. Thus, the idea of "agency" came to be intermixed with the idea that only the morally weak or lazy would be poor or disadvantaged (Quinn & Crocker, 1999). In addition, the active exclusion of non-White groups from employment opportunities, and how this served as a serious barrier to success, was ignored (Zweig, 2008).

Parenting practices were changed to support the ideals of White cultural success. Parents trained their sons to focus on long-range goals, be sensitive to signs of success, and actively pursue it. Parents might promote the view that short-term failure was acceptable, as long as the son learned important lessons that would support success in the long run (Ng, Pomerantz, and Lam, 2007). This fostered the view that the healthy male was independent and competitive. To build a self-confident and independent son, White parents have been found to provide positive feedback for successes while downplaying situations involving failure. As some segments of society have become more androgynous, these parenting practices have also been applied to girls. Middle-class, White parents may use reasoning strategies, within their disciplinary practices, in order to encourage their children to take the initiative and behave independently. A side effect may be that this results in adolescents who have less respect for authority figures during decision making (Dixon, Graber, & Brooks-Gunn, 2008). Overall, White adolescents have been found to consider autonomy from parents as a high priority (Fuligni, 1998).

White people are a heterogeneous group composed of people from different ethnicities and religions. What they have in common is the privilege that comes with being White in the United States. As a result, white-skinned immigrants automatically have an advantage when they are trying to integrate into the society of the United States. They have the implicit privilege of considering their racial category as nonexistent or "unmarked," their values and behaviors as natural or the norm in society, and their cultural values as the reference point for all other cultures (Frankenberg, 2008, p. 81; Smith, Constantine, Graham, & Diz, 2008). White parents assume they can keep their children out of situations where they will be mistreated, and White children turn on the television and can see members of their race portrayed as the "good guys" (McIntosh, 2008).

D. W. Sue and D. Sue (2008) call these "unearned privileges" because they haven't come as the result of any positive action on the part of the individual. Members of the White culture have more social and political power than other races/ethnic groups, and they maintain this greater power through carrying out explicit and implicit policies that maintain a society of racial inequality (Frankenberg, 2008). Whites can continue to believe they live in a meritocracy and be blird to their unearned power (McIntosh, 2008).

The people in power in the United States are primarily White. However, many Whites do not have access to power and have worked in sweatshops and experienced financial oppression (Frankenberg, 2008). However, the fact they have White skin has given them the ability to assimilate, while other groups have been actively excluded from assimilation. It has allowed these individuals to live in any neighborhood where they can afford the cost, to vote without facing impediments on Election Day, to take it as a given that the school system and judicial system will be responsive to their needs, and to have the right to fight against injustice (Frankenberg, 2008; Sue & Sue, 2008). Many White individuals perceive themselves as "color-blind" and judging people only by their own unique qualities; while they may acknowledge the existence of racism, they vastly underestimate its prevalence and impact. These types of beliefs support the racism of today, which consists of microaggressions carrying a highly negative impact on people of color (Smith et al., 2008; Sue et al., 2007). Whites are unaware of the privileges their skin gives them. For example, in missing a college class, a White student may feel comfortable asking the professor, who is probably White, for extra help. In addition, this student may feel comfortable asking to copy the notes of anyone else in class, most of whom are likely to be White. In contrast, an African American student may not feel comfortable approaching a White professor, having experienced many directly racist acts, as well as many microaggressions, in school in the past. In addition, this student may only feel comfortable asking another African American student for notes, and there may not be another African American student to ask. This might lead the student to fall behind in class while the White student is able to catch up (McIntosh, 2008).

The current domination of White culture within the United States, and the domination of the United States in world affairs, serves as implicit justification of the superiority of White culture and the justice of it imposing its values on other cultural groups (Frankenberg, 2008). Economics is inextricably linked to race. The middle and upper class formed the attitudes and behaviors now assumed to be from White culture. Lack of money brings with it crowded housing, little privacy, and jobs that involve intense, physical labor. These factors keep non-White cultural groups from living in the ways that Whites consider "traditional," "normal," and "healthy" (Frankenberg, 2008).

Two general forms of White privilege exist within society. One is the privilege to be treated with respect and to have fair access to education, housing, and so forth. This type of privilege should be extended to all racial and ethnic groups. The second type of privilege is the malignant kind; it confers the power to dominate others. This type of privilege needs to be eradicated (McIntosh, 2008).

The values of White middle-class culture have been infused into the treatment strategies used by clinicians, and thus most White clients will feel more comfortable than non-White clients within the treatment setting. These embedded values include (a) an individualistic orientation, (b) an emphasis on verbal expressiveness and thus its reliance on a facility with English, (c) an emphasis on active participation of the client in communicating needs and solving problems, (d) an emphasis on emotional expressiveness as key to health, and (e) a future orientation with an emphasis on long-term goals (Sue & Sue, 2008).

Red Flag Racial and Ethnic Guidelines

1. Assess the role of clients' self-identified racial and ethnic group(s) in their lives in terms of the strengths, resources, and power it (they) may be bringing to them within personal, family, social, vocational, and political spheres.

2. Consider how current or historical events have influenced the clients' identified racial and ethnic group(s) and assess if any of their current

problem(s) could be a result of direct or indirect oppression or trauma, their responses to this oppression, assimilation stress, and/or a mismatch in values with the dominant society and its institutions.

3. Assess how well the clients are functioning at this time, including a comparison of their functioning through the lens of their racial and ethnic heritage with that of the lens of the dominant cultural group. Consider if there are realistic constraints influencing the clients' functioning at this time, and discuss if any of their behavior within the dominant society might represent a healthy adaptation to injustice that would be supported by their racial and ethnic community.

4. Assess the clients' personal worldview and the role of their racial and ethnic group(s) within it; consider if there are any culturally specific resources, treatment strategies, or helpers they would value at this time; and consider how these might be used within your treatment plan.

5. Assess whether any aspects of your identity and cultural conditioning, or implicit bias within your treatment approach, could lead to communication problems, values conflict, difficulty understanding the clients' lifestyle or experiences, or invalidation of their strengths, and consider how treatment could be modified to increase the likelihood of a positive outcome.

Domain of Sexual Orientation

Sixteen-year-old Eric is struggling to come to terms with his sexual identity amid family chaos (Chapter 4). Ellen is lonely and trying to improve her relationships with her family now that she has come out as a lesbian (Chapter 6). Should their sexual orientations influence their treatment, and if so, how?

Sexual orientation can be "defined in terms of the sex, or sexes, of the people to whom individuals are sexually and affectionately attracted and toward whom they experience feelings of love and/or sexual arousal" (Schneider, Brown, & Glassgold, 2002, p. 266). Sexual orientation is different from a person's gender identity, which refers to the individual's adherence to socially defined roles of what a male or female is prescribed to assume within a specific culture. It is also different from the sexual activities the person engages in because some individuals engage in sexual behavior with an opposite-sex partner or a same-sex partner for convenience's sake. In addition, while sexual orientation is considered to be stable and enduring, an individual's sexual identity is considered more fluid. Sexual identity refers to the feelings, perceptions, and meanings that the individual draws from his or her sexual behavior. This is highly influenced by social context and stage of development of the individual (Savin-Williams, 2001).

Recent ethical guidelines of the American Psychological Association (2000b, 2002), the American Psychiatric Association (2000), and the Association for Lesbian, Gay, Bisexual, and Transgender Issues in Counseling (n.d.) stressed the importance of recognizing sexual minorities as following a different but normal developmental pathway. These guidelines also stressed that providers must learn how to respond in affirming and constructive ways with these clients. In a policy statement on lesbian and gay issues, the American Psychological Association Committee on Lesbian and Gay Concerns (1991, p. 1) stated that "homosexuality per se implies no impairment in judgment, stability, reliability or general social and vocational capabilities" and went on to indicate that practitioners had an obligation to educate the public about this. This type of advocacy was needed; a poll as recent as the year 2000 showed that close to 50% of the general public still considered homosexuality a sin (Newsweek, 2000).

At that time, sexual minority group members sought out more treatment than heterosexuals. This was due to the stresses of stigma, discrimination, and victimization (Cochran, 2001). Discrimination might include easily definable actions such as being denied a job or bank loan. It might also include subtler negative actions that leave the individual feeling disrespectfully treated. At the present time, federal laws do not protect sexual minorities from discrimination in housing or in the workplace (Human Rights Campaign, 2000). Therefore, the ability to "come out" may at times rest on whether it is economically viable to do so. While there are realistic risks to the "coming out" process, there are also clear benefits. Individuals have cited gaining a sense of personal freedom to be who they are as an individual. This freedom also has allowed them to develop deeper relationships with others that were based on self-affirming behavior rather than social facades (Riggle, Whitman, Olson, Rostosky, & Strong, 2008).

Recognition that one is a member of a sexual minority group often emerges during adolescence. Biologically timed changes in physical development bring with them a budding interest in sexuality for all teens. Research has indicated that teens are well able to recognize stable patterns of sexual attraction and romantic feelings toward same-sex partners when they are allowed to participate in the same type of normal sexual exploration that is typically allowed for heterosexual teens (Schneider et al., 2002). It is typical for teenagers to struggle with understanding their sexual feelings and knowing how to function as an adult male or female (Berger, 2009). Sexual minority youth are often struggling to do this while living within a "heterosexist" or "homonegative" context (Beckstead & Israel, 2007, p. 222). This is because cultural messages about sexuality, as expressed by parents, religious leaders, the media, and other influential socialization agents, are likely to be exclusively heterosexual and homonegative—that is, suggesting that homosexual development is inherently less healthy than heterosexual development (Savin-Williams, 2001).

When heterosexual youth are confused about their identity, they can try out new roles and behaviors they see modeled by other overtly heterosexual individuals. They will receive at least some parental acceptance for this exploratory behavior. These same types of exploratory opportunities may not exist for homosexuals and bisexuals. If they do find potential partners, they usually do not receive validation from family, peers, or the media that exploring their feelings is acceptable. Instead, they often face prejudice and disapproval from adult peers, violence at home, and hate crimes in their communities (Schneider et al., 2002). These dangers might begin as early as junior high (American Psychological Association, Commission on Violence and Youth, 1993; D'Augelli & Dark, 1994). Youth who have been, or are in danger of, physical violence or persistent verbal abuse will need help learning to cope with a hostile environment in addition to help with understanding their sexuality (Hershberger & D'Augelli, 2000).

Some heterosexual parents, while not overtly rejecting their minority teens, might still not be fully accepting. Parents assume their children will be heterosexual and may be unprepared for the truth. They might invalidate their teens' growing sexual awareness by saying their children are too young to decide and by encouraging them not to rush into making any decisions (Schneider et al., 2002). Sexual minority teens have sometimes given in to psychological pressure to ignore their sexual feelings so that they could fit within religious and cultural norms (Haldeman, 2000). Overall, 25%–84% of sexual minority youth did not come out to their families out of fear of losing either financial or emotional support (Savin-Williams, 2001).

The "coming out" process for teens may be a complex one. The first step might involve an increasing personal awareness and ability to label their sexual identity; the next step might be making the first disclosure to someone else and then proceeding to tell "important" others, although many people don't go through such a linear process and there may be many different trajectories to development rather than one stage model (Savin-Williams, 2001). There also might be a multiplicity of reasons to not "come out" fully or to decide to stay fully "closeted" until the youth is ready to be independent from the family (Hershberger & D'Augelli, 2000). Some sexual minority teens have felt their family relationships would be jeopardized if they came out while others find this leads to improved relationships. Youth don't have control of the neighborhoods they live in or the schools they attend. This might result in few opportunities for exploring their identity without the risk of being outed by peers (Hershberger & D'Augelli, 2000). For some, this results in dating within bars and clubs. These environments have been designed for adults and may have a highly sexualized atmosphere. Thus, sexual minority youth may need strategies for navigating through these shoals and selecting safe and appropriate partners for dating (Hershberger & D'Augelli, 2000). Teens of all sexual orientations face most of the same challenges in growing up, and they all have more or less accepting families.

Even in adulthood, society pressures sexual minorities to change to a heterosexual identity (Beckstead & Israel, 2007). Human beings have unique personalities and backgrounds and want to participate within a broad spectrum of social groups (Bartoli & Gillem, 2008). However, sexual minorities frequently feel forced to choose between their sexual identity and another aspect of their identity such as their religious or ethnic beliefs to gain acceptance within an important group (Beckstead & Israel, 2007). As a result, a period of questioning their sexuality might occur, which could last for years as individuals try to make peace among diverse aspects of themselves. These ambivalent struggles with "who am I" are a common part of the "coming out" process and are likely to lead eventually to a healthy and sexually integrated identity. However, some ambivalent individuals have participated in conversion therapies; 66% of them do this to fit in with their religious beliefs. Conversion therapy has a negative impact for most individuals including an increased level of homophobia and self-loathing because of an inability to change, hatred for parents whose parenting mistakes are blamed for a nonheterosexual orientation, feelings of depression and loneliness, the loss of support from sexual minority communities, misinformation about the causes of sexual minority desires, and fear of being or becoming a child abuser (Shidlo & Schroeder, 2002).

Sexual minority members often become parents. Sometimes this has occurred because the individual was living a heterosexual lifestyle. However, some cohorts, such as lesbians in the 1980s, began using reproductive technology to become parents within same-sex unions. In addition, sexual minority members became foster parents and adoptive parents around this same time due to the needs of the child welfare system (Cooper & Cates, 2006). Research has found that they are just as likely as heterosexual parents to provide appropriate parenting. No significant differences have been found between the developmental pattern, or psychological adjustment, of children raised by lesbians and that of children raised by heterosexuals (Cooper & Cates, 2006). In addition, young children have been found to be highly accepting of their sexual minority parents. This dynamic might change during puberty. Teens might go through a period where they are embarrassed by their parents' same-sex attractions and partners.

Sexual minority parents may have realistic fears of losing custody of their children during divorce proceedings (American Civil Liberties Union, 1998). If their same-sex families break up, the legal precedents are still scant and unstable. Individual judges have significant power in interpreting the custody statute of "best interest of the child," and there have been significant levels of discrimination documented in states such as Alabama, Mississippi, North Carolina, and Virginia (Cooper & Cates, 2006; DeAngelis, 2002).

Clinicians are ethically mandated to advocate for the full human rights of sexual minorities. The media have also been a driving force in support of these human rights. While motivated by profit rather than ethics, the media have provided a growing stream of sexual minority role models within movies and television. Stars, such as Ellen DeGeneres, have been able to maintain their popularity after coming out to the public. Political leaders who are openly gay or lesbian have been able to be elected, such as Gerry Studds in Massachusetts. Same-sex marriage, while not legal at the federal level, did become legal in Massachusetts in 2004, followed by California and Connecticut in 2008 and by Vermont and Iowa in 2009, although with the passage of Proposition 8 and the state Supreme Court decision to uphold it, California has since overturned the decision. The

Internet provides a private forum where individuals can gain a wealth of information on sexuality. Agencies such as PFLAG (Parents, Families and Friends of Lesbians and Gays) and GLSEN (The Gay, Lesbian, Straight Education Network) support the healthy development of sexual minorities, and COLAGE (Children of Lesbians and Gays Everywhere) provides education and support for children of sexual minority parents. Thus, while negative stereotyping, discrimination, and hate crimes are still forces to contend with, many positive forces also exist that provide a background of normality to individuals as they explore their sexual identities.

Red Flag Sexual Orientation Guidelines

1. Assess where clients are in the process of identifying their sexual orientation in terms of desires, fantasies, attitudes, emotions, and behavior related to sexuality and whether their sexual identification is stable, ambivalent, questioning, or shifting.

2. Assess the past and present environments that are influencing clients' comfort with their sexual identification including strengths or barriers within the work or school environment, family relationships, social relationships, and level of access to information and resources.

3. Assess the potential benefits there are, or would be, if clients come out at this time and which aspects of their world might benefit the most from coming out at this time considering their personal identity, family relationships, peer relationships, and educational or vocational relationships.

4. Assess the potential costs there are, or would be, if clients come out at this time and which aspects of their world might carry the most risk in the "coming out" process at this time considering their personal identity, family relationships, peer relationships, and educational or vocational relationships.

5. Assess whether clients need to find a common ground between their sexual identity and other aspects of their identity such as religious or racial and ethnic identifications and consider how to connect them with resources and decrease barriers to this process.

6. Assess whether any aspect of your identity, or your treatment approach, might lead to negative bias, marginalization, or invalidation of clients' sexual identity or minimize the potential negative impact of societal homophobia on clients' well-being and consider what can be done to increase the likelihood of a positive outcome.

Domain of Socioeconomic Status

Sharon, a 34-year-old European American woman, raised as a member of the working poor, is struggling to parent her children as a new member of the upper class (Chapter 5). Zechariah, an 18-year-old African American male, the first member of his family to enter college, is accused of being a danger to others (Chapter 9). What role, if any, might their income level play in their current dilemmas? Socioeconomic status (SES) is an index that attempts to represent someone's income as well as access to resources in health care, housing, and education.

For an individual, SES could enhance or limit opportunities within a person's public and private life. The three major class distinctions in the United States could be made on the basis of how much power, independence in decision making, and quality of life a group has (Zweig, 2008). As a group, the capitalists (2% of the labor force) have the power to dominate in the workplace and in the political arena. Even amongst this top group, there is considerable diversity of power. Those individuals who are in charge of the largest corporations (less than two tenths of 1%) control not only their own money but the wealth of the nation. These predominately White men, along with the top political leaders of the federal government, could be said to constitute a "ruling class" within the United States (Zweig, 2008, p. 132).

Middle-class individuals have significantly less power than the capitalists, but they have stable jobs, own homes and cars, and take paid vacations. This class contains professionals (lawyers, doctors, professors, etc.) and small-business owners, as well as supervisors in industry; this group represents 36% of the population. They may have some political clout through lobbying from their professional associations. The border between this group and the capitalists may be unclear as some high-level corporate attorneys and accountants, for example, may make salaries commensurate with those of some capitalists. They have considerable authority over what they do but they are not final decision makers, and it is the power to control decisions that sets the capitalists apart from the middle class.

Similarly, while some members of the working class may, through overtime, make as much money as middle-class workers, they don't have the power to control their work tasks or work calendar and do not receive the same respect for their work as middle-class workers do. Their jobs are regimented, they have limited autonomy in how they conduct their work and in the pace of their work, and they don't have authority to make decisions. This class (62% of the labor force) has little power except as represented by the unions they may belong to, which do lobby for their membership (Zweig, 2008).

In the United States, the median household income within the general population is $44,334; this is far behind the $677,900 of the wealthiest households (U.S. Census Bureau 2000, 2006a). Statistics indicate a clear chasm growing between the most and least financially successful populations within the United States. Data from the Center on Budget and Policy Priorities show that after-tax income for the poor has dropped by $100 in recent years from $10,900 to $10,800. Within the same time interval, the wealthiest households had their income increase by 36% from $263,700 to $677,900. The middle fifth of households had their income rise by 10%. Thus, the gap between the poor and the middle class has broadened, and the middle class has been left far behind by the rich. Tax legislation, promoted by President G. W. Bush, favored the upper class and further accelerated the disparities between the classes during his two presidencies (Shapiro, Greenstein, & Primus, 2001).

Currently 12.7% of the general population is living in poverty, and another child enters this deprived life every 33 seconds. A child who is Black or Latino is 3 times more likely to be part of this population than a White child. One million of these are children born into homeless families. Seventy percent of poor families contain a parent who is working; a killing combination of low wages, high living costs, and high medical and other critical resource costs combines to keep these families living below the poverty line (Children's Defense Fund [CDF], 2008). The poverty rate is highest in families where the mother is the head of the household. In 40% of these families, children are being raised in poverty (U.S. Census Bureau 2000, 2004b).

The United States spends more of its gross domestic product on health care than any other country, yet it ranks only 37th out of 191 countries in quality of health care according to the World Health Report. This low ranking is caused by the large percentage of the population that is uninsured as well as the significant discrepancy that exists between the quality of health care given to the poor and that given to the rich (World Health Organization [WHO], 2000). When a family member becomes seriously ill, it represents a crisis for poor families. Illness leads them into greater indebtedness as they try to pay for services they can't afford. Lack of access to quality care may result in family members dying or being left with disabilities that were preventable (WHO, 2000). Within the United States 8.9 million children have no health insurance, and this problem is much more severe for children of color than for White children (CDF, 2008).

Economic welfare is highly dependent on educational achievement. As schools are funded by property taxes, there are serious disparities among the quality of schools available to wealthy children, that available to middle-class children, and that available to poor children. If a neighborhood school begins to deteriorate, middle- and upper-income households may be able to move out of these neighborhoods and into areas with better schools. This leaves an even smaller income base to support the schools, and so a further decline in quality occurs. The children left behind go to schools that are run down, poorly equipped, crowded, and often dangerous (Books, 2007). Head Start, which helps children learn to be successful in school, only receives enough funding to enroll one half to two thirds of income-eligible children (CDF, 2008). In the 25-and-older group, 80.4% are high school graduates, and 24.4% went on to achieve either a bachelor's degree or a higher professional degree. Almost 25% of children live in a home with someone with at least a bachelor's degree (U.S. Census Bureau 2000, 2004b).

Schools are more effective when parents are actively involved, but poor, working parents have no time to do this. National surveys show that 60% of parents living above the poverty line are involved in school activities on a regular basis. In contrast, only 36% of poor parents are similarly involved (HHS, 1999). This further increases poor children's lack of identification with their school, which has also been found to lower educational success (Evans, 2004). Current statistics reveal that two thirds of fourth graders educated in public schools can't read or do math at grade level. This deficiency is higher in minority children than White children (CDF, 2008). A new type of educational risk factor that limits the educational attainment of poor children is their lack of access to the Internet. Ninety-four percent of poor children have no access to the Internet; this lack of access occurs for only 57% of more affluent youth (Evans, 2004).

Living in poverty brings many negative experiences to family life. This includes that, due to having jobs with low wages, parents must work long hours to pay the bills. This leaves them little time to spend with their children. Thus, 40%–58% of families above the poverty line read to their preschool children, while only 38% of low-income families do (HHS,

Federal Interagency Forum on Child and Family Statistics 2000, 2008). Poor parents are more likely to allow their children to watch television more and read less.

The longer a family remains in poverty, the more family life deteriorates with husbands and wives fighting more, parents behaving less responsively to their children, and parents engaging in harsher disciplinary practices (Evans, 2004). The rates of depression are also higher amongst the poor, and depressed parents provide poorer-quality care to their children (Mazure et al., 2002). Poor children are also more likely to be separated from their families through foster care and other out-of-home placements than more well-off children (Evans, 2004).

Poor families are also more likely to live in dangerous neighborhoods where children are exposed to personal risk and trauma including exposure to street violence and involvement in traffic accidents. In addition, they may live in neighborhoods that are closer to toxic waste dumps and other environmental hazards, placing young children at risk for lead and carbon monoxide exposure. Thus, 35% of poor toddlers are exposed to six or more environmental risk factors during development while this occurs for only 5% of middle-income toddlers (Evans, 2004).

Who are the poor? Statistics on poverty vary by racial and ethnic group and gender of the adult in charge of the household. White, married families have the lowest poverty rates. When children are living with both parents, statistics indicate they are most economically well off (U.S. Census Bureau 2000, 2004b). White children living only with their mothers had a 28.1% poverty rate in comparison to 14.1% for those who live only with their fathers. The ethnic or racial group with the highest poverty rate is American Indians and Alaska Natives. Relative to the general population, they are more than twice as likely to live in poverty (U.S. Census Bureau 2000, 2006b). While these statistics may lead to the perception that the "average" poor person is from a minority group, in fact, the average poor person is White, female, and young. These women are not on welfare. They are the working poor who take jobs most people do not want (Jackson, 2000). Whether it is the school system, the health system, employment, or housing, the poor are dehumanized and treated disrespectfully. The services and resources available to them are often deficient or significantly lower in quality than those provided to more advantaged groups. This results in many poor individuals having a realistic distrust of the institutions of society (Lott, 2002).

Historical and political contexts can influence society's openness to helping less advantaged people within one's country and the world (Delphin & Rowe, 2008). When the general population is faced with what they consider to be clear and convincing evidence of financial need, they give freely to help others. For example, money poured in to help the victims of the 2001 attack on the World Trade Center. The RAND Corporation (Dixon & Stern, 2004) estimated that charitable donations reached $2.7 billion. What concerned citizens were not aware of was how a concerted series of political policies treated the poor as invisible and expendable. The disaster following Hurricane Katrina is a dramatic example. That a disaster was coming had been well predicted. However, 40 years of low-budget governmental policies left the levees in disarray. The Federal Emergency Management Agency (FEMA) had been cut by the Bush presidency and its monetary resources transferred to the war on terror. The poor, encompassing 27% of households, had no way to evacuate and nowhere to go when the hurricane struck as the only evacuation plan was for individuals to drive themselves out (Ignatieff, 2005). This left the poor to drown. This initial disaster was followed by political conservatives, in a Republican-dominated congress, blocking a plan to allow the hurricane victims to gain health care using Medicaid (Krugman, 2005). The poor of New Orleans were further exploited by reconstructive efforts. The Davis-Bacon Act, which ensures a decent wage on all federal contracts, was suspended, and political cronies of President Bush and Vice President Cheney got preferential access in gaining contracts to rebuild (Lipton & Nixon, 2005); they exploited the poor further by giving work to those who would accept the smallest wages.

How can such exploitation continue? Often there is no day-to-day evidence of need because structurally middle-class, lower-class, and upper-class families live in different neighborhoods, attend different schools, and are insulated from each other's day-to-day experiences. This leads to ignorance of each other's challenges and strengths and often leads to cognitive distancing where the suffering of the poor is underestimated (Lott, 2002). Middle- and upper-class families can give their children access to the Internet, higher-quality schools, and safer home and neighborhood conditions. Wealthier adults attain higher levels of education and gain greater occupational success. They have the ability to pay for services such as housekeeping, child care, and more comprehensive medical care. Thus, in times of trouble, wealthier individuals have many more resources they can turn to for help than do poor individuals.

Red Flag Socioeconomic Guidelines

1. Assess clients' economic and social class and consider how this has influenced their access to resources within the family such as time to give and get attention from other family members and resources for daily living, safe housing, privacy, and recreation.

2. Assess clients' economic and social class and consider how this has influenced their access to resources within the community such as medical care, educational choices, social choices, vocational choices, legal resources, and social/political power.

3. Considering 1 and 2 above, assess the impact of clients' economic and social class on their self-esteem and personal welfare; family welfare; ability to make independent decisions at home, at school, and/or within a work setting; and ability to influence their own life circumstances versus their lives being under the control of others within the work, social, or political spheres.

4. Considering 1–3 above, consider if SES is serving more to constrain clients' life or to support it, how SES might be the cause of or be related to their strengths and/or weaknesses at this time, and how SES might inhibit or facilitate any lifestyle changes for them at this time.

5. Assess the role that your economic and social class might have on your expectations and perceptions of clients, as well as how classist values might be implicitly embedded within your treatment orientation, and consider what might be done to increase the likelihood of a positive treatment outcome.

Domain of Violence

Jeff is mandated into treatment after assaulting a woman in a parking lot (Chapter 3). Nicole is abused by her father and brothers and fears emotional intimacy with her boyfriend (Chapter 6). Josephina, a victim of domestic violence, has begun abusing her infant son (Chapter 9). Finally, Jake, while terrorizing his son, wants to be a good father (Chapter 10). What impact will their violent histories have on their ability to develop a treatment relationship with you? What impact will their violent histories have on your treatment plan?

Both women and men report being victimized by an intimate partner. Estimates worldwide are that from 10% to 69% of women report abuse by their intimate partner. In the United States, 1.5 million women and 800,000 men report being abused by a partner (Centers for Disease Control & Prevention [CDC], 1998; Gondolf & Jones, 2002; WHO, 2001, 2002).

Violence may begin with one partner, but this often serves to elicit violence from the other either for self-defense or for revenge (Archer, 2002; Graham-Kevan & Archer, 2005). Violence may include physical assaults, sexual assaults, threats of physical or sexual assaults, and emotional abuse (CDC, 2006). Assaults between partners can range from temporary injuries due to slaps and scratches to fatal injury as a result of repeated punching, kicking, use of weapons, and so forth. Emotional abuse includes acts such as name-calling, deliberate public embarrassment of the victim, isolating the victim from family and friends, controlling finances, and so forth (CDC, 2006).

Nonlethal injury can result in acute medical conditions and/or chronic consequences. While legal statutes label all partner abuse as "battery," men's attacks often show a higher level of lethality than those initiated by women (Samuelson & Campbell, 2005; Stuart, 2005). Partner violence is often a family secret. Many reasons for this have been posited including beliefs that the victimization is one's own fault, that victimization is a universal family experience, or that it would be dangerous to the self or family to reveal its existence (Stuart, 2005).

Violent couples may fit roughly into two broad categories. The first, common or situational couple violence, occurs in a broad range of couples including gay and straight, married and cohabitating (Frieze, 2005). For these couples, violence is mutual and occurs in reaction to negative experiences within the day-to-day life of the family. These individuals consider violence an acceptable reaction to stress (Johnson & Leone, 2005).

The other type of couple violence, "intimate terrorism," occurs less frequently and involves the most extreme behavior. The perpetrator uses violence and fear to maintain absolute control over the partner who experiences severe emotional reactions to the victimization (Johnson,

1995; Koss, Bailey, Yuan, Herrera, & Lichter, 2003). The perpetrator also uses intense psychological abuse as another mechanism of control (Dye & Davis, 2003).

There are no simple explanations for the occurrence of intimate partner violence. A complex model that examines predisposing factors, potentiating factors, and eliciting factors may have the most potential for use in preventing and treating violence (Stuart, 2005). Predisposing factors include biological and cultural variables that together explain the individual's mental capacity and worldview. Potentiating factors include internal and situational variables that together encompass the individual's potential for volatility and the couple's relationship dynamics. Eliciting factors include internal and situational events that lower self-restraint and increase vulnerability in the immediacy of the situation.

Not all violent individuals are equally amenable to treatment. One typology classifies individuals as predatory abusers, affectively motivated abusers, and instrumental abusers (Stuart, 2005). The abusers who are least motivated to change, and most dangerous to their victims, are the predatory abusers. They engage in frequent and recurrent violence that is instigated for their own idiosyncratic purposes and unrelated to their partner's behavior. Prior to the assault, they may be calm, and they find the violent episode arousing. They severely injure their victims both physically and emotionally yet after the incident show a lack of empathy or regret for what they have done to the victim.

The instrumental abuser engages in violence in order to gain something from the partner and incidences of violence are rare. These individuals are calm before the assault and mildly aroused upon gaining whatever it is they wanted from the partner. They have limited motivation to change because their desire for personal gain is more important to them than their concern for the victim. The injuries inflicted are incidental to the perpetrator trying to get what he or she wants from the victim.

The perpetrator most amenable to change is the affectively motivated assailant. This individual has actually been provoked by the victim or at least interprets the behavior of the victim as provoking. Violent behavior occurs only occasionally. The perpetrator is highly aroused before the assault and calms down afterward. The violent acts occur impulsively, may involve relatively less severe actions, and may result in only mild consequences to the victim in comparison to the acts of other abusers. The acts may have the greatest impact on the victim's self-esteem, and the perpetrator may show empathy for the victim's injuries and regret for having caused them.

Victims of partner violence are heterogeneous and come from all socioeconomic levels, ethnic or racial groups, educational backgrounds, sexual orientations, and so forth (CDC, 2006). A commonality among victims is that they view the violent experience as a betrayal of their relationship with the perpetrator; even those who are not physically injured experience significant emotional sequelae, losing self-confidence and feeling worthless. Victims may also show fearfulness and be vigilant for signs of danger from the partner (Stuart, 2005).

Violent relationships that fall within the domain of common couple violence or that stem from an affectively motivated abuser may be most open to change (Frieze, 2005; Stuart, 2005). Motivation for change may come from dynamics such as regret over harming the partner, the wish to be a good parent, the desire to protect children from harm, or a future orientation (CDC, 2006).

When partners engage in violence, an estimated 3 million children witness it (Fantuzzo & Mohr, 1999). Children may see or hear the violent acts of the adults in their lives or witness the sequelae later. These acts may involve physical as well as sexual assaults (Kantor & Little, 2003; Wolak & Finkelhor, 1998). In addition to the negative psychological impact of secondhand violence, the assaultive parent may force the child to participate in the assaults, require the child to spy on the victimized parent, and indoctrinate the child with the message that the victim was responsible for the assault (Kantor & Little, 2003).

Boys and girls exposed to prolonged domestic violence may take on the beliefs that men are superior to women, that the use of violence against women is justifiable, and that violence is an appropriate problem-solving tool (Bancroft & Silverman, 2002). Male batterers may use destructive parenting practices. They may choose favorites among their children and ridicule their children for showing an attachment to their mother (Bancroft & Silverman, 2004/2005). They may unintentionally undermine the mother's authority in parenting children by modeling contempt for her abilities. They may also deliberately overrule her decisions. For example, if she forbids an activity, the batterer may help the child engage in it. He may also reward his children for defying their mother. Overall, boys may be socialized to become victimizers while girls may be indoctrinated to tolerate abuse (Jaffe & Geffner, 1998).

Domestic violence and child abuse overlap; studies report 30%–60% co-occurrence. Men are 3 times more likely than women to assault both their partners and their children (Administration for Children and Families, 2006). If mothers try to protect their children from maltreatment, the father may respond by assaulting her or intensifying his attack on the children, thereby teaching her it is better not to interfere (Bancroft & Silverman, 2004/2005). Women who do not intervene are sometimes prosecuted by authorities for failing to protect their children (Kantor & Little, 2003).

The abuse and neglect of children also occurs in the absence of domestic violence. An estimated 3.3 million reports of child maltreatment were investigated in 2006. Within founded cases of maltreatment, neglect was most common (64.1%), followed by physical abuse (16%), sexual abuse (8.8%), and emotional maltreatment (6.6%). The vast majority of perpetrators were parents (79.4%) or a biological relative of the victim (Administration for Children and Families, 2006). Parents from maltreating households use harsh physical discipline when children make mistakes or misbehave (Consortium for Longitudinal Studies of Child Abuse and Neglect, 2006). The impact of maltreatment is to put children at higher risk for lower cognitive and academic functioning as well as to increase their risk of exhibiting behavioral problems that involve aggression, anxiety, and/or depression.

When they go to school, maltreated children are at increased risk of being bullied by other children or taking on an aggressor role themselves. Maltreated children with uninhibited temperaments are likely to act aggressively. They develop maladaptive cognitive schemas for processing social information and attribute hostile intentions to others, who are often engaging in neutral behavior. These children respond impulsively and get angry quickly. They have learned a repertoire of aggressive retaliatory behavior at home, they view aggression as morally acceptable, and their parents are tolerant of their aggressive behavior toward peers (Dodge, Pettit, Bates, & Valente, 1995: Watson et al., 2005).

In contrast, children who are behaviorally inhibited may be more likely to respond with internalizing symptoms to victimization at school. However, they can become aggressive over time in certain circumstances or within certain family contexts (Watson et al., 2005).

The inhibited child who becomes aggressive may be the one who engages in aggressive fantasies in response to his or her own victimization. Victimized children who are raised in cold and high-conflict families may also become aggressors over time in response to sustained bullying in school (Watson et al., 2005). Once aggressive behavior begins, it is likely to be maintained.

Longitudinal studies show that children who are physically aggressive at age 5 often continue to be aggressive throughout the elementary years and even into adolescence (Broidy et al., 2003; Watson et al., 2005). Teens who have been abused as children are more likely to be arrested for both violent and nonviolent offenses; they are also more likely to engage in violence in their dating relationships and more likely to have externalizing behavior problems. They are also at greater risk for the nonviolent events of dropping out of high school, being fired from employment, and having a higher risk of teen parenthood (Lansford et al., 2007).

The likelihood of youth violence increases as several risk factors increase. These risks include presence of substance abuse in the home, easy access to weapons, a child needing to move back and forth between different family households, exposure to violence in the community, participation in deviant peer groups, and living in poverty (Garbarino, 1999; Hanson et al., 2006; Surgeon General. 2001; Watson et al., 2005). Gender is also a major risk factor for committing acts of violence especially during the teen and early adult years (Kimmel, 2008). Starting in kindergarten, boys show greater levels of aggression than girls at all levels of aggressiveness (Watson et al., 2005), and young men are 10 times more likely to commit murder than young women (Garbarino, 1999).

Many children exposed to violence in the home or school do not become violent themselves. A caregiver who provides social and emotional support to the child may moderate the negative impact of violence exposure. Practical support in coping with the violence is critical to this process rather than just supplying emotional support (Consortium for Longitudinal Studies of Child Abuse and Neglect, 2006). Other protective factors include a positive attachment to adults who do not tolerate violent or deviant behavior and a commitment to school success (Surgeon General, 2001).

The clinician faces many challenges in dealing safely with violent clients. They often have a negative view of the world, including the intent of treatment. The perpetrator of violence may have a hostile bias that influences the interpretation of the clinician's behavior and the behavior of others. Clinicians need to assess carefully the level of dangerousness within the home, school, neighborhood, and treatment session itself within the immediate, short, and long term. The victim's experiences need validation, but at the same time the clinician must clarify that the abusive behavior is illegal and causing the victim both physical and psychological damage; damage to child witnesses should also be underscored, and this may enhance motivation for change in some parents. Reducing risk factors for violence is the first priority in treatment, and a safety plan should be in place that encompasses reducing as many risk factors for continued violence as possible. A careful lethality assessment is critical before escalation occurs that could be fatal to the victim (Samuelson & Campbell, 2005). Once safety has been adequately addressed, goals that will increase the number or quality of protective factors should be undertaken such as skill building that aids emotional regulation, nonviolent problem solving, building of positive emotional bonds with nonviolent others, and school and/or occupational success.

Red Flag Violence Guidelines

1. Assess the risk factors for engaging in violence and the protective factors discouraging violence that are currently in place for clients, considering:
   a. The *internal* factors within them such as the ability to control impulses, set limits on their own behavior, regulate emotions, engage in reflective problem solving, and understand the emotions and behaviors of others.
   b. The *long-term* social network and environment during clients' childhood and whether they supported or constrained violence such as the existence of traumatic, ambivalent, or nonexistent emotional bonds; positive emotional bonds; family violence; level of family toleration for violence as a problem-solving strategy; positive or negative school or neighborhood experience; and religious background.
   c. The *current* environmental supports or constraints on violence from family relationships, peer relationships, educational attainment, vocation, current neighborhood, and current religious beliefs.
   d. Any *immediate* eliciting or triggering factors that might serve to justify and/or make a violent or prosocial response more likely such as presence or absence of a weapon, level of alcohol or drug use, level of frustration/anger, and encouragement or discouragement of violence from others.

e. Their worldview including a consideration of whether violence plays a generalized or circumscribed role in it and whether they are currently generating/promoting violence or generating/promoting prosocial behavior.

2. Assess clients' safety and that of others within their environment at this time and if, and how, safety could be enhanced both in the immediate and the longer term including careful consideration of the *characteristics* of the perpetrator of the violence in their life.

3. Assess the overall psychological and physical impact of violence on clients and others, whether there are more forces supporting violence or supporting nonviolence, and the prognosis for clients living a life free of violence at this time.

4. Assess whether your past experiences with violence, your stereotypes of clients' violent lifestyle, or biases embedded in your treatment approach might lead to negative bias, marginalization of clients' point of view, or an increase in danger to clients and others and consider what you might do to modify your approach to increase the likelihood of a positive outcome.

Conclusions

A theoretical perspective, such as behaviorism, may be helpful in acquiring an understanding of *who clients are* and *why they do what they do*. Will it be worthwhile to further investigate the client's individuality by considering the impact of gender, sexual orientation, violence history, or other domains of complexity? The exercises in Chapters 3 through 10 are first steps in answering these questions and in providing a framework for practicing skills at integrating human complexity into your clinical work. As your comfort with complexity increases, expand your readings on the domains introduced within this text, as well as study the many important domains that have not been covered, such as religion and developmental disabilities.

Table 2.1 provides a quick reference guide to locating the domains of human complexity highlighted in client interviews by chapter, presenting problem, referral source, and treatment setting. Table 2.2 provides a quick reference to how theories and areas of complexity are compared within Exercise 6 in Chapters 3–10.

Table 2.1   Location of Domains Highlighted in Client Interviews

Domain	Chapter	Presenting Problem	Referral Source	Treatment Setting
Age				
Kevin	3	Self-hate, phobia	School	School
Alice	8	Immaturity, divorce war	School	Outpatient
Sexual Orientation				
Eric	4	Sexual confusion, neglect	School	School
Ellen	6	Divorce, sexual intimacy	Self	Outpatient
Gender				
Marie	4	Bereavement, single parenting	Self	Outpatient
Steve	7	Intimacy	Self	School
Race & Ethnicity				
John	5	Marital crisis	Self	Outpatient
Sergio	7	Drug conviction	Court	Outpatient
Tanisha, Marcus	8	Bereavement	Self	Outpatient
Kayla	10	Malaise, intimacy	Self	Outpatient
Socioeconomic				
Sharon	5	Marital, parenting	Self	Outpatient
Zechariah	9	Racism, adjustment	School	School
Violence				
Jeff	3	Assault, rage	Court	Outpatient
Nicole	6	Physical abuse, intimacy	School	Outpatient
Josephina	9	Child abuse, violence	Court	Outpatient
Jake	10	Child abuse, parenting	Court	Outpatient

Table 2.2	Comparisons of Theories and Areas of Human Complexity Within Exercise 6

Chapter	Theory	Client	Theory Comparison	Complexity Comparison
3	Behavioral	Kevin	Cog-Behavioral	Age; Violence
4	Cognitive	Eric	Cog-Behavioral	Sexuality; Violence
5	Feminist	Sharon	Cognitive	SES; Gender
6	Emotion Focused	Nicole	Feminist	Violence; Age
7	Dynamic	Steve	Emotion Focused	Gender; SES
8	Family	Tanisha & Marcus	Feminist	Race; Gender
9	Constructivist	Josephina	Family Systems	Violence; Race
10	Transtheoretical	Kayla	Constructivist	Race; Sexuality

Recommended Resources

Domain of Age

American Academy of Pediatrics. (n.d.). *Children's health topics: Developmental stages.* Retrieved May 29, 2009, from http://www.aap.org/healthtopics/stages.cfm

American Psychological Association. (2007). *Parenting: Communication tips for parents.* Retrieved May 29, 2009, from http://www.apahelpcenter.org/articles/article.php?id=48

Brems, C. (2008). *A comprehensive guide to child psychotherapy and counseling* (3rd ed.). Long Grove, IL: Waveland Press, Inc.

Child Development Institute. (1998–2008). *Development.* Retrieved June 8, 2009, from http://www.childdevelopmentinfo.com/development/normaldevelopment.shtml

Domain of Race and Ethnicity

Hays, P. (2008). *Addressing cultural complexities in practice: Assessment, diagnosis, and therapy* (2nd ed.). Washington, DC: American Psychological Association.

National Alliance for Hispanic Health (NAHH). http://www.hispanichealth.org/

National Black Child Development Institute (NBCDI). http://www.nbcdi.org/

National Indian Child Welfare Association (NICWA). http://www.nicwa.org/

Society for the Teaching of Psychology. (n.d.). *OTRP teaching resources: Presidential Task Force on Diversity Education*. Retrieved May 29, 2009, from http://teachpsych.org/diversity/ptde/index.php

Domain of Gender

U.S. Department of Labor, Women's Bureau. http://www.dol.gov/wb/
Worell, J., & Remer, P. (2003). *Feminist perspectives in therapy: Empowering diverse Women*. New York: John Wiley & Sons, Inc.

Domain of Sexual Orientation

Biescheke, K. J., Perez, R. M., & DeBord, K. (2007). *Handbook of counseling and psychotherapy with lesbian, gay, bisexual, and transgender clients* (2nd ed.). Washington, DC: American Psychological Association.
Children of Lesbians and Gays Everywhere. http://www.colage.org
Parents, Families and Friends of Lesbians and Gays. http://www.PFLAG.org

Domain of Socioeconomic Status

Books, S. (2007). *Invisible children in the society and its schools* (3rd ed., pp. 1–22). Mahwah, NJ: Lawrence Erlbaum & Associates.
Centers for Disease Control and Prevention. http://www.cdc.gov
Children's Defense Fund. http://www.childrensdefense.org/
Institute for Research on Poverty. http://www.irp.wisc.edu/

Domain of Violence

American Psychological Association. (2007). *Warning signs of youth violence*. Retrieved May 29, 2009, from http://apahelpcenter.org/featuredtopics/feature.php?id=38&ch=3
Child Welfare Information Gateway. http://www.childwelfare.gov/
Myers, J. E. B., Berliner, L., Briere, J., Hendrix, C. T., Jenny, C., & Reid, T. A. (2002). *The APSAC handbook on child maltreatment* (2nd ed.). Thousand Oaks, CA: Sage.
National Council on Child Abuse and Family Violence. http://www.nccafv.org/
Stop It Now! http://www.stopitnow.org
Zorza, J. (2006). *Violence against women Volume III: Victims and abusers*. Kingston, NJ: Civic Research Institute.

Three

Behavioral Case Conceptualizations and Treatment Plans

Introduction to Behavioral Theory

You have just received a phone referral from the probation department. Jeff is a 22-year-old White male. He dropped out of high school at the age of 16. He has been working since that time as a cook at a fast food restaurant. He has recently begun pursuing a GED. He has been married to Karen, who is 21 years old, for 2 years. They have a son, John (3 years), and Karen is 4 months pregnant. Jeff was convicted of assaulting a 50-year-old woman and was sentenced to 100 hours of community service and the same number of hours of treatment focusing on anger management.

You are a behaviorist and assume that all behavior is learned. How did Jeff learn to be violent? Your model assumes that this occurred according to the principles of classical conditioning, operant conditioning, and/or social learning (Bandura, 1986; Pavlov, 1927; Skinner, 1938). How would treatment proceed? The focus would be on a behavioral analysis of Jeff's overt adaptive and maladaptive behaviors and the specific circumstances in which they occur (Ingram, 2006). Within sessions, Jeff will actively participate in learning experiences to modify or extinguish maladaptive behavior patterns as well as teach or increase the frequency of adaptive behavior. If Jeff's overt behavior changes, it is assumed that related cognitive and affective changes will follow. However, there are times when conditioned emotional responses, or mediating cognitions, might be the focus of change (Ingram, 2006).

If Jeff has learned violent responses through classical conditioning, it was unintentional learning (Pavlov, 1927). Classical conditioning involves reflexive, elicited behavior that occurs outside the person's conscious control. For example, as Jeff was growing up, an initially neutral stimulus (a door slamming) was present at the same time as an unconditioned stimulus (Jeff receiving a physical blow from his father). Over time, Jeff developed an unlearned, reflexive response (respondent) to this unconditioned stimulus of a fear reaction (increase in blood pressure, heart rate, body temperature). Through repeated association between the neutral stimulus (a door slamming) and the unconditioned stimulus (receiving a physical blow from his father), Jeff learned to show the respondent (fear reaction) when the neutral stimulus occurred even though it was no longer paired with the unconditioned stimulus.

A door slamming has now become a conditioned (learned) stimulus for Jeff. The fear response to this conditioned stimulus is now considered a conditioned (learned) response. Unlearning of a classically conditioned response requires a break in association between the conditioned stimulus (door slamming) and the unconditioned stimulus (physical blow). Throughout the course of his childhood, Jeff may have learned to generalize his fear response to any sudden loud noise when his father was present. However, if he learned to discriminate loud noises where his father was present from loud noises where his father was absent, Jeff's fear response may play a functional role in his life. However, if Jeff has generalized his fear reaction to loud noises in any circumstances, his fear may be immobilizing him or leading him to take dysfunctional actions.

If Jeff has learned violent responses through operant conditioning, then he learned by intentionally doing something (operating on his environment) and experiencing the consequences (Skinner, 1938). If there is a positive consequence, the behavior increases in frequency. If there is a negative consequence, the behavior decreases in frequency. Positive consequences can consist of receiving positive reinforcement (getting something you want) or receiving negative reinforcement (having something you don't want removed). For example, if Jeff yelled at his wife that he was hungry and she rushed to get him food, then her giving him food served as positive reinforcement that would increase his yelling.

Similarly, if he hated being asked questions, her being quiet the moment he raised his voice could increase his yelling through negative reinforcement. What serves as reinforcement is specific to the individual.

Jeff's behavior can also be modified by either positive or negative punishment. If a young Jeff yelled at his father and his father punched him, the punch would serve as positive punishment to discourage his yelling. If his father wouldn't let Jeff watch TV if Jeff yelled at him, this would be using negative punishment to discourage yelling. Positive punishment involves getting something you don't want, while negative punishment involves something you want being taken away. Across environments, Jeff could learn to discriminate when yelling would result in punishment and when it would lead to reinforcement.

One incident of a reinforcement or punishment does not usually cause a lasting impact on an individual. It is Jeff's overall history of reinforcements and punishments that produced his current behavioral repertoire. Jeff may need to be taught new behaviors that would be functional in his life. In this case, he should be reinforced for taking small steps toward development of this new competency. If he needs skills in an area where he is unlikely to spontaneously take a "step in the right direction," prompts or shaping will need to be used. Prompts are antecedent events (cues, instructions, gestures) that can initiate a behavior so that it is then possible to reinforce it. Shaping refers to reinforcing successive approximations of the response that is wanted. Unlearning (operant extinction) occurs when a previously reinforced behavior ceases to produce positive consequences.

Jeff may have learned violent behavior and its consequences through observing a model or models (Bandura, 1986). Whether this learned behavior is later performed depends on the consequences that are associated with it. Jeff will be more likely to learn from a model that he perceives as similar to himself or a model he considers high in prestige, status, or expertise. Jeff's father, who had total power within the family, may have served as a powerful role model for teaching violent behavior. Jeff may have received vicarious reinforcement for his own dominating behaviors from seeing his mother acquiesce to his father's verbally and physically controlling behavior. The extinction of an observationally learned response can be through direct or observed (vicarious) punishing consequences.

While behaviors are the primary focus of attention, it is possible for cognitions or emotions to be "learned behaviors." For example, through classical conditioning, Jeff could have been taught to associate anger and feelings of hostility with women. Therefore, in any interaction involving women, he may have a conditioned emotional response that leads him toward maladaptive behavior. Similarly, he may have learned the belief, from his father, that any attempt to ask a question is, in fact, an attempt to dominate him. Therefore, whenever anyone asks him a question today, he may have automatic thoughts such as "This person is trying to control me. I must show who's boss, or I'll be this person's slave." These types of thoughts might fuel Jeff's aggressive behavior in situations that most people would find neutral or benign (Ingram, 2006).

Role of the Clinician

How will you help Jeff? You will be a teacher, trainer, and contingency manager who actively guides treatment. First, you assess Jeff's behavior and define his current problems in behavioral terms, including the dimensions of frequency, intensity, duration, form or quality, and appropriateness to context. Jeff's behavioral strengths also will be noted in a similar manner. This information may be collected through self-report inventories, interviews with Jeff and significant others, behavioral observations, and other methods. Concomitant with this process, you will analyze the conditions maintaining Jeff's problems in terms of the antecedents (triggers, where, when, whom) and consequences (reinforcements, punishments) and the environmental supports or barriers to the change process. After making these determinations, you will plan sessions to provide Jeff with the learning experiences that he needs in order to change. Jeff may need to initiate, increase in frequency, or modify certain behaviors. Similarly, he may need to terminate, decrease, or alter others. You will take an active and directive role in structuring the learning environment to support these changes.

An active search for adaptive behavior will also be part of this behavioral analysis as modifying potentially adaptive behavior, increasing already present adaptive behavior, and teaching new skills are integral to achieving treatment success. While Jeff's problems with violent behavior should not be underestimated, there may be many areas in which true behavioral strengths can be found. For example, Jeff has shown the ability to discriminate situations in which it is and isn't safe to yell at others; this demonstrates that even when angry, he has some self-control. Jeff is motivated and has a finely tuned ability to observe others. He may learn most effectively if given the opportunity to use these skills. For example, he might more quickly recognize antecedents and consequences to aggressive behavior if he was given a homework assignment that dealt with observing his "buddies" after work rather than one where he was to self-reflect on his own behavior. As a final example, behavioral treatment is very action-oriented, rather than insight-focused. Jeff may find concretely described homework assignments that involve him "doing something" more congruent with his personal style than activities that involve purely self-reflection.

You might introduce many types of learning experiences, including relaxation training, anger management training, and social skills training, in trying to help Jeff. Historically, behavior therapy did not focus attention on cognitions or emotions (Skinner, 1938). However, many current behaviorists consider that "cognitions" and "emotions" can be conditioned and thus serve as appropriate targets for intervention (Ingram, 2006).

How will Jeff's progress be measured and monitored? Goals will be set that are specific, clear, functional, and attainable, and they may involve modifying or decreasing maladaptive behaviors, as well as modifying, enhancing, or teaching adaptive behaviors. Interventions targeted at providing environments that will support constructive change may be initiated. His wife will be involved in changing the behavioral consequences she gives Jeff for his behavior at home if it is safe for her to do so. An effective teaching environment will not occur within the treatment sessions if Jeff and you do not develop a trusting, and mutually respectful, working relationship in which you design individualized learning experiences and Jeff actively participates in them.

Case Application:
Integrating the Domain of Violence

Jeff's case will now be examined in detail. There are many domains of complexity that might provide insights into his behavior. The Domain of Violence has been selected to consider within a behavioral case conceptualization and treatment plan. Assume that during a brief intake, Jeff got very angry in response to mental status questions about harm to others. However, he signed release forms to the court and his probation officer. He did this to prove that he had a laid-back personality. When asked if he had any preferences about who was assigned as his clinician, he said he would take anyone who was available, as he wished to get treatment over as soon as possible; as an afterthought, he said he preferred a clinician who was "not an idiot."

Interview With Jeff (J) From a Behavioral Perspective

C: I understand that you are coming here as a condition of your probation. Why are you on probation?

J: (tensely) Because this woman stole my parking space and I wouldn't put up with it.

C: How did she steal your parking space?

J: (angrily) I was running late for work because my wife Karen was having a hysterical fit. When I got to work, the whole lot was full. I circled and circled until a space opened up. I put on my turn signal to back up for the space when this woman pulled into it. Well, I got out and banged on her car window and told her to move. She ignored me. I pretended to walk away. She got out of the car, and I was on her in a second. I told her to get back in the car and move out of my space. She tried to push past me. So, I gave her a shake.

C: How badly was she hurt?

J: (emphatically) She wasn't hurt. Someone in the parking lot ran into the restaurant and called the police. The police jerked me around and sent her to the hospital. She didn't need a Band-Aid!

C: What did the police do?

J: (angrily) They took me to court. The judge asked me why I lost control. I told him I had just had a bad fight with my wife and was running late for work. Then I told the judge my wife was pregnant and I would lose my job if I went to jail; Karen was sitting there crying. I got probation.

C: Karen being there helped to get you probation?

J: (angrily) The whole stupid mess was her fault to begin with. She made me late to work. My boss was furious about the fight. It frightened off some customers. He said one more false step and I'm out!

C: Is this job important to you?

J: (rigidly) I will qualify for a management training program at the restaurant when I have finished the GED. Then I can earn enough money for the kids Karen keeps producing.

C: You are working hard to support your family. Can you stay in control at work and keep your job?

J: (glaring at C, tensely) I won't hit my boss, if that's what you mean.

C: When your boss pressures you, you can control your anger. Why didn't you control your anger with that woman?

J: (firmly) Women don't step on me. If she had backed down when I threatened her, I would have backed off. It was HER fault. I felt relaxed once I had put her in her place. I didn't stay calm long because the police began jerking me around.

C: Did you explode again?

J: (dismissively) No, I had to control it.

C: You could control your anger with the police.

J: (irritably) I didn't want to go to jail—but I felt jumpy.

C: What does it mean to feel jumpy?

J: (tensely) At first, I just have trouble concentrating. After a while, if I still can't let the tension out I begin to feel hot. If I get too hot I go onto autopilot—I fight until I win.

C: Is that what happened with that woman?

J: (angrily) I had been jumpy in the car, it got worse as I circled, and then when she tried to push by—that was it.

C: What helped to get rid of the tension after you went to court?

J: (matter-of-factly) I went to work, and I overcooked the food. The burning smell always gives me some satisfaction.

C: What about at home—how do you release tension?

J: (intently) When I get home, Karen better have everything the way I want it.

C: If it's not?

J: (hostilely) Then, I'm all over her.

C: What do you do?

J: (matter-of-factly) It depends how mad she has made me. Maybe I just shove her around a little. Maybe I have to get more physical.

C: Has Karen ever needed medical attention after a fight?

J: (slowly and emphatically) Noooo. I don't hit her that hard.

C: Could you give me a recent example?

J: (tensely) The day I got into the fight, she wanted to know when I would be home so she could take the car to the store. I shoved her away from me, just hard enough to make the point that she had better not try to control me.

C: On a scale from 1 to 10, how hard a shove was it?

J: (irritably) Don't fret over Karen; she can handle it. She whines a lot when she is pregnant, but she got a dozen whacks from her parents for every one I give her!

C: How many times a day do you hit or kick her?

J: (highly frustrated) KAREN IS OK. The push I gave didn't stop her mouth at all. She grabbed my arm as I was opening the door. I kicked her, hard. She let go of me and I was able to get out the door, but it left me all worked up.

C: Why didn't kicking Karen leave you feeling relaxed?

J: (intently) I didn't get relief because I hadn't made her back down. When she backs down, I end up in a pretty good mood.

C: What do you do when you are in a good mood?

J: (matter-of-factly) I'm ready for sex. (pause) I may insist on it.

C: You feel sexually aroused after a physical fight with your wife?

J: (calmly) Only after a big blowout because then all my frustration gets released. That fight right before I went to work didn't do it for me; I was still furious as I left.

C: What happens after you have sex?

J: (smugly) I feel really relaxed.

C: Do you have any other way to handle being angry besides physically fighting?

J: (smugly) I'm pretty good with my mouth too. Often, a few threats will go a long way.

C: Can anything stop you from fighting once you are mad?

J: (tensely) If the person backs down, I still feel edgy, but I can let it go. If I haven't got hot yet, I can walk away if it's a work situation. I must control myself. I hate it.

C: Having to control yourself?

J: (angrily) I hate feeling edgy and having to wait to get rid of it.

C: If you get hot?

J: (emphatically) As I said, I'm on autopilot. But, I'm in control most of the time. In fact, I'm always razzed by everyone for being an "underachiever" and taking things too easily.

C: Who is "everyone"?

J: (dismissively) My mom and dad. They only did three things: complain that I was lazy and wouldn't ever get anywhere, beat on me, and ignore me.

C: What would happen when you were growing up?

J: (reflectively) If my dad was home and he noticed me, he would find a reason to hit me for being lazy. If he wasn't hitting or kicking me it was because he was too busy to notice me. Now my mom would wait for me to "screw up," like getting an F from school or being truant. Then she would pounce. My only break was when my parents were too busy fighting each other to notice me.

C: Did you ever need medical attention after a beating?

J: (dismissively) My arm was broken a few times.

C: Did any medical personnel or other adults recognize you were being abused?

J: (calmly) No one cared. Even when I showed up at school with loads of bruises no one seemed to see them. The teachers thought I was lazy. By about 14, I had learned to disappear if my dad was around. I'd learned to keep my mom in her place.

C: How did you learn that?

J: (intently) From listening to my dad and watching TV day and night.

C: What did you watch?

J: (intently) I always liked to watch action shows about police, spies, war. That's still what I watch.

C: What do you like about the action shows?

J: (intently) The quick action, the rage. I have gotten some good tips from these shows, how to use intimidation as well as my fists. My parents think I'm an idiot. But, I can learn fast when I want to.

C: What are you interested in learning right now?

J: (emphatically) As long as no one tries to push me, I will get the GED.

C: If I don't push you, are you willing to learn to express your anger and feel relaxed with ways that don't risk jail time? (J looks hesitant) I know a lot of ways to help people relax.

J: (challengingly) You think you can teach me more than I already know about sex?

C: I am talking about nonsexual and nonviolent ways to relax.

J: (sarcastically) We're going to drink together?

C: No. (pause) Does drinking help you relax?

J: (matter-of-factly) No, but I like the taste.

C: How much alcohol and drugs do you consume a day?

J: (irritably) I don't take drugs. I drink a couple of beers after work with the guys.

C: At home?

J: (intently) Maybe, if I'm watching football.

C: Do you ever get drunk? (J shakes head no) Does drinking make you more or less edgy?

J: (angrily) If I'm edgy, I'm edgy whether I'm drinking or not.

C: There is no connection between when you lose control and when you drink?

J: (frustratedly) I've told you. I'm an easygoing guy most of the time.

C: What do you do for fun?

J: (reflectively) Watching TV is OK. I also like to swap stories with the guys at work about "situations" we've handled.

C: Do you ever get into physical fights with these guys?

J: (intently) No, I don't fight that much. The guys—maybe we push and shove a little at a bar after work just to get some material for a story session at work the next day.

C: Have you ever physically fought with your son? (J: No.) Is he scared of you? (J: No.) Is there anything that he does that makes you angry?

J: (emphatically) NO. He is only 3. Karen takes care of him.

C: What does he do when you and Karen are fighting?

J: (reflectively) He always runs into his room. Sometimes he seems to know, before the first blow, that a fight is going to start, and he goes off to watch TV.

C: Smart kid—he knows what triggers a fight. You are slumped pretty low in that chair. Are you feeling edgy or tense now?

J: (angrily) I'm in control. This is how I usually am.

C: Are you angry now?

J: (dismissively) No. (pause) Why would you ask?

C: Well, you were pushed into coming, and I have asked you a lot of questions. You have told me it makes you mad when people push you.

J: (frustratedly) It was this or jail; the choice was clear.

C: We need to talk very specifically about what things are making you feel tense and lose control. We need to develop nonaggressive ways to help you feel relaxed. Is it going to be safe for me to help you with this?

J: (challengingly) Safe?

C: If I make you feel tense and edgy, will you be able to tell me, or will you move in to shake me up?

J: (emphatically) I don't want to end up in jail.

C: You think you can control it here. (long pause during which J shakes his head yes) If I make you edgy, will you go home and shake Karen?

J: (irritably) I don't know. I don't plan to shake Karen up. If it happens, it's her fault.

C: Do you recognize when the tension is building?

J: (dismissively) Sometimes I do.

C: If you feel that in here, will you tell me?

J: (angrily) My probation officer says if I beat anyone up while I am on probation, I go straight to jail.

C: I'll come up with a plan to show you next week. If you want to follow it, you will gain control over your edgy, tense feelings. I will make sure to include skills that can help you stay out of jail and be an effective manager. I need to remind you that if I think Karen, or anyone else, is in danger, I'll have to call them and the police.

J: (intently) I'm not going to hit Karen or anyone else. I don't want to go to jail.

Behavioral Case Conceptualization of Jeff: Historically Based Style

As a developing person, Jeff had needs for physical, cognitive, and psychosocial mentoring that were met with verbal intimidation and physical aggression by his parents and with neglect from other adults such as teachers and medical personnel. No one actively taught him prosocial or nurturant life skills. Jeff became an active self-learner, concentrating on mastering violent responses that he could use to get his survival needs met. He did not recognize the need or perceive the value of learning prosocial competencies. As an adult, Jeff is quick to perceive and respond aggressively to any sign of attention from others. Neutral, positive, or negative behaviors by others are experienced as negative or threatening consequences, and his most common response is aggression. Jeff's current behavioral assets are his ability to learn quickly when motivated and his present motivation to stay out of jail and support his family through gainful employment.

As a young child, Jeff learned that adults were aggressive. His parents had many violent interchanges with each other, thereby serving as role models for the use of aggression in intimate relationships, the use of aggression in communicating about problems, and the use of aggression to solve problems. This emphasis on aggression "to teach people how to behave" or "as punishment for misdeeds" was further entrenched by its use as the sole active parenting strategy used to influence Jeff's behavior. Both parents were supportive of each other's physical abuse of Jeff. When not providing violent consequences, Jeff's parents may have ignored his behavior. Jeff had the ability to learn nonviolent skills, but he wasn't provided with an environment that supported this type of skill development.

As Jeff entered the school years, he perceived teachers as providing only negative consequences to his behavior, such as calling him lazy and ignoring obvious signs of abuse. These learning experiences further reinforced Jeff's negative identifications with his parents. Jeff turned to TV for company and for learning how to negotiate through a hostile world. The shows that he selected to watch confirmed his prior learning that the world was a hostile place and that self-esteem and security were gained through mastery of verbal and physical aggression. He developed a positive identification with the characters in the action shows who earned respect through their use of physical violence and lack of toleration for bending to the authority of others. He was highly attentive to these role models and began to actively learn through observing them.

As a teenager, Jeff had developed the physical strength and had mastered enough violent techniques to learn how to use verbal and physical intimidation with his mother. He had begun using the skills he had learned observing his father and his TV role models. She provided reinforcement for this by acquiescing to his demands and not beating him anymore. Jeff used physical avoidance to protect himself from his father. Thus, Jeff had learned how to keep himself safe at home. The quality and extent of his peer interactions as he was developing are unclear. His teachers continued ignoring obvious signs he was a victim of abuse, such as a broken arm, and he didn't receive any consequences from them that he found reinforcing. As a result, he did not consider them role models. He did not actively try to learn nonviolent ways of relating to others from observing them, and he did not learn to find academic success rewarding; he dropped out of high school.

As an adult, Jeff continues to have his violent view of the world reinforced by the environmental experiences he selects. He socializes exclusively with other violent men. These peer activities focus on demonstrating who is most expert at the use of verbal and physical aggression. Women (his wife, his mother) have reinforced his verbal and physical aggression by acquiescing to his demands. Jeff's knowledge of Karen's abuse by her parents, as well as his memories of his mother's abuse by his father, further underscores to him the acceptability and usefulness of violence against women. A further positive reinforcer for Jeff's violence is the feeling of relaxation he gains after physically dominating a woman. Classical learning also may play a role in the autonomic symptoms he describes as being immediately antecedent to his losses of control. Jeff was a repeated victim and witness of violence within his home. It is possible that many neutral stimuli within his home environment became conditioned stimuli as they were unintentionally paired with physical assaults. Jeff may enter these loss-of-control states only with women. He has learned to control the level of his anger in situations in which he might lose a fight (with his dad, other men) or in which his income or personal freedom are at stake (with his boss, the probation officer). While his life is full of rage, he maintains gainful employment and is committed to supporting his wife, son, and future children. He also plans to improve his employment opportunities through completing a GED and attending management training; thus, he has a willingness to learn new skills when the consequences for doing so are clear and motivating to him. At the present time, Jeff's violent behavior is determined in complex ways. He has his violent responses consistently reinforced. He is exposed daily to violent role models. He may respond violently when exposed to certain classically conditioned stimuli. Yet, there is more to Jeff than his propensity for violence. As a child, he developed a facility for learning through observation despite receiving little if any help from others to do so. As an adult, he is showing a willingness to work hard and learn new skills in order to better support his family. At this point in his learning history, Jeff has come into conflict with the legal system. Prior to being sentenced to probation, Jeff did not receive any consequences for his violent behavior that he found negative. Thus, he had no motivation to change. The knowledge that he could go to jail if he commits another violent offense has provided him with an incentive to increase his self-control. This probationary period is a window of opportunity for engaging Jeff in learning experiences that could increase his range of nonviolent responses to anger, frustration, and tension and increase, modify, or teach him prosocial interpersonal skills.

Behavioral Treatment Plan: Historically Based Style

Treatment Plan Overview. Jeff's present goals are to stay out of jail by attending anger management training and to attain a GED so that he can become promoted at work. These goals may provide enough incentive to engage Jeff in treatment at this time. The clinician and probation officer will need to collaborate and evaluate Jeff for dangerousness on a session-by-session basis. Karen and other women are at most risk should he lose control. Long-Term Goals 1 and 2 will be worked on simultaneously, followed later by Goals 3 and 4. The treatment plan follows the *problem format.*

PROBLEM: Jeff raised himself and did not get help learning how to get what he needed or wanted from life without the use of aggression. The clinician and probation officer will need to take on the educational role (not taken by his parents) of inhibiting his aggression and encouraging the development of his adaptive competencies. For each goal, either the probation officer or the clinician will underscore the consequence of negative behavior (going to jail) and the consequences of positive behavior (success as a manager, staying out of jail, developing intimacy).

LONG-TERM GOAL 1: Jeff will receive the learning experiences his parents and teachers did not provide him with on how to use environmental controls to inhibit his aggressive behavior so that he will stay out of jail.

Short-Term Goals

1. Jeff will attend weekly probation appointments and receive positive social consequences for arriving on time, being polite, and not making threats.

2. Jeff will attend weekly treatment appointments and receive positive social support for arriving on time, being polite, and not making threats.

3. Jeff will avoid bars and socializing outside of work with violent individuals to decrease triggers to aggressive behavior that could lead to jail time.

4. Jeff will seek out opportunities, within GED study sessions and management training sessions, to observe how others manage to keep their arousal level low in social situations, and he will consider the value of copying this behavior himself.

5. Other goals will be developed as appropriate.

LONG-TERM GOAL 2: Jeff will receive the learning experiences that his parents and teachers did not provide him with on how to use anger control and stress reduction strategies so that he can control his edgy feelings.

Short-Term Goals

1. Jeff will be given introductions to a number of relaxation and anger control strategies so that he can select the ones he wants to learn.

2. Jeff will learn to identify, within sessions, the physical signs that he is becoming angry or tense.

3. Jeff will practice using his preferred relaxation strategies to prevent himself from getting "hot" during role-plays of conflict situations.

4. Jeff will use avoidance to remove himself from out-of-session situations, as soon as he begins to feel angry or tense, to keep himself out of jail.

5. Jeff will begin to use strategies he has learned in sessions to prevent himself from getting "hot" outside of sessions.

6. Other goals will be developed as appropriate.

LONG-TERM GOAL 3: Adult Jeff will learn new nonaggressive communication and problem-solving strategies he was not taught in childhood so that he can gain positive reinforcement from his boss, his probation officer, his clinician, and so forth for showing self-control in conflictual situations and be prepared to be a manager.

Short-Term Goals

1. Jeff will be introduced to alternative strategies for effective listening, assertive communication and problem solving so that he can select the ones he would like to learn.

2. Jeff will practice effective listening strategies first within treatment sessions, then within probation sessions, then at work, and finally at home.

3. Once he has mastered listening skills, Jeff will practice (in-session) assertive responses to conflict situations involving others; if he gets angry he will stop the role-play and help himself relax.

4. Jeff will practice assertive responses to conflict outside of the session; if he gets angry he will remove himself from the situation and help himself relax.

5. Other goals will be developed as appropriate.

LONG-TERM GOAL 4: Jeff will learn strategies for developing emotional intimacy that he was not taught in childhood.

Short-Term Goals

1. Jeff and the clinician will discuss what emotionally intimate behavior refers to and the concrete rewards that can follow this type of behavior.

2. Jeff will observe others and develop a list of the positive, neutral, and negative consequences that he has seen following emotionally intimate behavior.

   a. Jeff will observe nurturing behavior occurring between Karen and his son John and then discuss his observations with the clinician.

   b. Jeff will observe nurturing behavior occurring between coworkers or customers and then discuss his observations with the clinician.

3. Jeff will practice play skills with the clinician and then will join Karen and John in emotionally intimate play first within sessions and then outside of sessions.

4. Other goals will be developed as appropriate.

Practice Case for Student Conceptualization: Integrating the Domain of Age

It is time to do a behavioral analysis of Kevin There are many domains of complexity that might provide insights into his behavior. You are asked to integrate the Domain of Age into your behavioral case conceptualization and treatment plan.

Information Received From Brief Intake

Kevin is a 14-year-old White male going to high school in a rural area. He has a long history of high scholastic achievement and plans to attend college after finishing high school. He is living with his biological parents and two older sisters. His father is a self-employed farmer. At the age of 7, Kevin was diagnosed with an inoperable brain tumor. Extended chemotherapy arrested the tumor growth but resulted in Kevin temporarily losing his hair. Because of this tumor, Kevin had extended school absences in the first and second grades. Kevin's high school counselor referred him for treatment; Kevin had told the counselor that he couldn't look in mirrors and hated himself. His parents disapproved of him coming for this appointment but did not prevent it.

During a brief mental status exam, there were no indications of suicidal or homicidal ideation or severe psychopathology. Kevin was asked to sign release forms for consultations with school personnel and his family. Kevin was only willing to sign these forms for the school system. When asked if he had any preferences for whom he saw in treatment, Kevin indicated he would take the first appointment available.

Interview With Kevin (K) From a Behavioral Perspective

C: Kevin, I understand that you consider yourself to be phobic of mirrors. Can you tell me exactly what you mean by this?

K: (openly) I can't look in mirrors. If I try, I break out into a sweat and begin to feel dizzy.

C: Can you remember a time when you could look in mirrors?

K: (reflectively) Before I had chemotherapy and my hair fell out, I looked in mirrors all the time. After my hair fell out, I looked like a freak—it was scary. I can still remember the day I came home from the hospital and the way my older sisters ran when they saw how I looked.

C: You were frightened by losing your hair or by their reaction to it?

K: (intently) Both. After they ran away, I rushed into the bathroom and stared at myself for a while. Until that moment, I was so glad to get out of the hospital that I hadn't thought about my looks. I came to realize I was a freak.

C: A freak?

K: (angrily) That's what all of the kids at school called me after I returned to school.

C: All of the kids, even your friends?

K: (angrily) I had no friends from the time I left the hospital. No one wanted to associate with a freak. (long pause) I was alone.

C: Did anyone associate with you?

K: (thoughtfully) Some of the teachers. They were repulsed by me, but they were nice and always gave me additional assignments.

C: How, specifically, did they react toward you?

K: (sadly) They looked other kids in the face but not me.

C: What did the doctors tell you?

K: (intently) They saved my life. (long pause) What more could I expect?

C: Has there ever been a time, since your operation, that you could look into mirrors?

K: (anxiously) No, every time I try, I break into a sweat, and my heart feels like it will burst open. It's a real phobia.

C: What have your parents done to help you?

K: (matter-of-factly) I'm on my own. They took me to the hospital when I was sick but never visited. (long pause, scornfully) Surprise, I didn't die. They had to bring me home.

C: Didn't they want you home?

K: (calmly) Sure, it was spring planting time. They needed my help.

C: Did they ever try to help you with your phobia?

K: (anxiously) My father tried to make me get over it in the third grade by forcing me to look in a mirror; I passed out.

C: What happened exactly?

K: (anxiety rising) I was getting ready to catch the school bus. My father said that I had forgotten to comb my hair. I disagreed. We argued about it for a while, and then he dragged me into the bathroom to look in the mirror. When I came to, my mother handed me a comb and told me to hurry or I would miss the bus.

C: What brought you in to see me now?

K: (sweating profusely) Other boys in my class have started to grow beards. How will I shave if I can't look into a mirror? If I don't shave, I'll look even more like a freak. (desperately) Can you help me?

C: Yes, phobias can be cured. Together we will work out a plan to overcome yours.

K: (intently) Other people may be able to stop being afraid, but can a freak like me?

C: You sweat and feel like your heart will burst when you go near a mirror, but you are not a freak. I know that you have the brains and skills to combat your problems just by the way you have come forward today.

K: (hopefully) What do you mean?

C: Most people are afraid when they come here and don't want to talk. Most people can describe having trouble breathing or feeling faint but don't know the term *phobia*. That's a professional description of your problem. You already have an insight and expertise into your problem that few adults have. You also show an open-mindedness to seeking out help.

K: (excitedly) What's next?

C: I need to ask a few more questions. Is there anything that makes the phobia worse?

K: (reflectively) After the kids or someone in my family has taunted me, I can't even go near a room that has a mirror in it without feeling panicky.

C: Does someone have to taunt you about your appearance to bring on this reaction, or can someone taunt you about something else, like calling you an idiot?

K: (painfully) No one sees me as anything but a freak, except for some of my teachers. They've always encouraged me and thought I could make it to college.

C: How is your physical health now?

K: (dismissively) I haven't needed any medical exams for years. My mom still tries popping pills or vitamins into my mouth.

C: Your mom seems worried about your health, but it's not necessary?

K: (irritably) I'm fine; the doctors don't even follow up with me anymore. My mother doesn't get what the real problem is—I'm an outcast. My father only cares about problems that relate to our farm.

C: Is there anything besides mirrors that triggers your fear?

K: (thoughtfully) Anything that is really shiny so that it reflects an image. At school there's a corridor where one side is all windows. The hallway is lit in a strange way. I have to look down at the floor or I can see my reflection in the windows.

C: What happens if you see your reflection?

K: (anxiously) I have to run out of there as fast as I can or else I'll be sick.

C: How often have you had to do this?

K: (intently) Maybe once a month, I get distracted by something, and I forget to keep my eyes on the floor.

C: Have any of your teachers or peers noticed?

K: (calmly) No teacher has ever said anything to me. The kids know better by now. I learned early on that the only way to stop their mouths was to kick ass. At first, it was my ass that got kicked, but now, I know how to handle things. They may think I'm a freak, but they keep their distance if they know what's good for them.

C: What happens before you kick ass?

K: (reflectively) It could be anything from a direct statement, to someone shoving me in the hall, to giving me a nasty look. I don't always beat kids up; sometimes I just give them my LOOK, and if they back off, I leave them alone. When I was little, I always had to fight. Since I reached 6 feet tall, my look has gone a long way.

C: What happens after you kick ass?

K: (proudly) No one bugs me for a long time. Sometimes the teachers tell me to cool off. I think my school counselor, the one who sent me here, thinks that I need more self-control. He doesn't know what it's like to be a freak.

C: What have you tried to do to help yourself with this problem?

K: (nervously) Once in a while I try to get myself to look in mirrors. I usually try the mirror in the basement bathroom at home because no one else in the family likes to go down there. I start walking down the basement stairs telling myself to be cool—I can handle the mirror. As I get to the bottom of the stairs, my heart starts to pound. Usually, I cannot get into the bathroom. I have also tried rushing down the stairs trying not to think. Once, I actually got the door open before I panicked.

C: What helped make this time work better?

K: (reflectively) I was going down to the basement to get something for my mom, so I hadn't planned in advance to try to look into a mirror.

C: Have you tried anything else?

K: (furiously) DON'T YOU THINK I'VE DONE ENOUGH?

C: I think you are a very strong person. I'm impressed with the efforts you have made. I just want to make sure I understand everything you have tried.

K: (apologetically) I'm sorry I lost my cool. I know you are here to help.

C: It's been a tough hour for you. I am going to spend the time between now and our next session working out our battle plan. I'll share my ideas with you next week, and you can make any suggestions you think might make it work better.

K: (anxiously) Can anything be done?

C: If it wasn't hard, you'd have handled it by yourself years ago—you've got guts. But it's hard. You did the right thing to come for help. I would like you to keep a record this week of each time your anxiety about mirrors begins to build. Try to describe how anxious you are each time, on a scale of 1 to 10. Then, indicate what happened right before the anxiety started. Try to do something to help yourself chill out. Then, write down what you did and, on a scale of 1 to (Kevin interrupts)

K: 10, write down how successful I was.

C: Absolutely right! I know you can do it.

Exercises for Developing a Case Conceptualization of Kevin

Exercise 1 (4-page maximum)

GOAL: To verify that you have a clear understanding of behavioral theory.

STYLE: An integrative essay addressing Parts A–C.

NEED HELP? Review this chapter (pages 95–100).

  A. Develop a concise overview of the assumptions of behavioral theory (the theory's hypotheses about key dimensions in understanding a client's behavior; think broadly, abstractly).

  B. Develop a thorough description of how each of these assumptions is used to understand a client's learning history (for each assumption provide specific examples).

C. Describe the role of the clinician in developing learning experiences for the client (consultant, doctor, educator, helper; basic treatment approach; technique examples).

Exercise 2 (3-page maximum)

GOAL:　　　　　To aid application of behavioral theory to Kevin.

STYLE:　　　　　A separate sentence outline for each section, A–C.

NEED HELP?　Review this chapter (pages 95–99).

A. Create a list of Kevin's behavioral deficits/excesses and behavioral assets/skills and for each provide:

1. An operational definition; frequency, duration, and intensity of behavior; what, if anything, decreases its frequency or intensity; what, if anything, increases its frequency or intensity; and the antecedents and consequences of behavior.

2. A discussion of the type(s) of learning that might be involved: operant, classical, and/or social learning.

3. A discussion of the environmental factors that exist that would support change in the problematic behavior and/or would enhance more adaptive behaviors as replacements as well as those that might provide barriers to change.

B. Discuss the strategies Kevin has used to adapt to his environment in the past, his preferred manner of learning, and his present attitude toward new learning.

C. Discuss how adaptively Kevin is functioning within his environment at this time.

Exercise 3 (3-page maximum)

GOAL:　　　　　To develop an understanding of the potential role of development in Kevin's life.

STYLE:　　　　　A separate sentence outline for each section, A–E.

NEED HELP?　Review Chapter 2 (pages 32–39).

A. Assess how age appropriate Kevin's physical development and cognitive development have been and how, and in what ways, they have influenced his performance and level of motivation at home, in school, or within community activities both at age 8 and at age 14.

B. Assess how age appropriate Kevin's relationships to adults have been in terms of their providing limit setting, monitoring, skill building, and emotional connection and in what ways these relationships have supported or hindered the developmental process both at age 8 and at age 14.

C. Assess how age appropriate Kevin's relationships to peers have been in providing casual social skill building and friendship and in what ways these relationships have supported or hindered the developmental process at ages 8 and 14.

D. Assess how age appropriately Kevin is functioning overall at this time; include consideration of his self-image and self-efficacy, what he needs most to support his healthy development as a teen, and what, if any, barriers or facilitating factors there are to his maturation at this time.

E. Consider whether your age, your stereotypes of teenagers, or developmental biases embedded within your treatment approach might lead to marginalization of Kevin's point of view and/or Kevin's current situation and consider what could be done to increase the likelihood of a positive treatment outcome (be thoughtful and detailed).

Exercise 4 (5-page maximum)

GOAL: To help you integrate your knowledge of behavioral theory and development into an in-depth conceptualization of Kevin (who he is and why he does what he does).

STYLE: An integrated essay consisting of a premise, supportive details, and conclusions following a carefully planned organizational style.

NEED HELP? Review Chapter 2 (pages 32–39) and Chapter 1 (pages 7–28).

STEP 1: Consider what style you should use for organizing your behavioral understanding of Kevin that (a) would support you in providing a comprehensive and clear understanding of his learning history and how this influences him at this time and (b) would support language that he'd find persuasive as a teenager.

STEP 2: Develop your concise premise (overview, preliminary or explanatory statements, summary of key features, proposition, hypotheses, thesis statement, theory-driven introduction) that explains Kevin's strengths and weaknesses as a teenager who has a mirror phobia and has often been in charge of his own learning. If you're having trouble with Step 2, remember it should be an integration of the key ideas of Exercises 2 and 3 that (a) might provide a basis for Kevin's long-term goals, (b) are grounded in behavioral theory and include a developmental context for understanding his past and current behavior, and (c) highlight the strengths he might bring to behavioral treatment.

STEP 3: Develop your supporting material or detailed case analysis of strengths and weaknesses from a behavioral perspective that integrates within each paragraph a deep understanding of Kevin as a socially rejected teen. If you are having trouble with Step 3, consider the information you'll need to (a) support the development of short-term goals, (b) be grounded in behavioral treatment that is sensitive to development, and (c) integrate an understanding of Kevin's strengths in the learning process whenever possible.

STEP 4: Develop your conclusions and broad treatment recommendations including (a) Kevin's overall level of functioning, (b) anything facilitating or serving as a barrier to his learning new skills at this time, and (c) his most basic needs as a learner at this time, being careful to consider what you said in Part E of Exercise 3 (be concise and general).

Exercise 5 (3-page maximum)

GOAL: To develop an individualized, theory-driven action plan for Kevin that considers his strengths and is age appropriate.

STYLE: A sentence outline consisting of long- and short-term goals.

NEED HELP? Review Chapter 1 (pages 8–28).

STEP 1: Develop your treatment plan overview, being careful to consider what you said in Part E of Exercise 3 to prevent any negative bias to your treatment plan.

STEP 2: Develop long-term (major, large, ambitious, comprehensive, broad) goals that *ideally* Kevin would reach by the termination of treatment in order to learn adaptive and/or unlearn maladaptive skills to support his development as a teen and overcome his mirror phobia. If you are having trouble with this step, reread your premise and support topic sentences and transform them into goals that might involve classical conditioning, operant conditioning, and/or observational learning (use the *style* you selected for Exercise 4).

STEP 3: Develop short-term (small, brief, encapsulated, specific, measurable) goals that Kevin and you could expect to see accomplished within a few weeks to chart his progress in learning, instill hope for change, and plan time-effective treatment sessions. If you are having trouble with this step, reread your support paragraphs looking for ideas to transform into goals that (a) might help him learn adaptive or unlearn maladaptive skills using particular modes of learning that are sensitive to his being a teen, (b) enhance factors facilitating or decrease factors inhibiting his ability to learn new skills at this time, (c) utilize his strengths in the learning process whenever possible, and (d) are individualized to his issues as a teen from a neglectful home rather than generic.

Exercise 6

GOAL: To critique behavioral treatment and the case of Kevin.

STYLE: Answer each question in essay format or discuss in a group format.

   A. What are the strengths and weaknesses of this model for helping Kevin (a teenager with a mirror phobia, self-hatred, and problems with aggression)?

   B. What beliefs might Kevin have learned from his family based on the interview, and how might an expansion of your conceptualization to include self-talk, attributions, expectations, and perceptions strengthen your treatment plan?

   C. Based on information from the Domain of Violence, how dangerous do you think Kevin is at this time? In what ways should his propensity toward violent problem solving influence your treatment planning both in the short run and over time?

D. Assume that you were a clinician working at the hospital when 8-year-old Kevin came in to receive treatment for his brain tumor. His doctors referred Kevin to you for support in dealing with his medical condition. What ethical issues would have arisen for you once you learned that Kevin's family never visited or called him? How specifically would you handle the situation?

E. Kevin was quick to take offense at things the clinician said during the interview and has a history of aggressive behavior to things he considers provocative. Reread the interview taking note of your reactions to this behavior. Then, discuss these reactions along with your ideas for how to handle them effectively, within a behavioral framework, to support the development of an effective treatment alliance.

Recommended Resources

American Psychological Association (Producer) & Persons, J. B. (Trainer). (n.d.). *Cognitive behavior therapy* [Motion Picture #4310774]. (Available from the American Psychological Association, 750 First Street, NE, Washington, DC 20002–4242)

Association for Behavioral Analysis International. http://www.abainternational.org/

Ingram, B. L. (2006). Behavioral and learning models. In B. L. Ingram, Ed., *Clinical case formulations: Matching the integrative treatment plan to the client* (pp. 157–190). Hoboken, NJ: John Wiley & Sons, Inc.

Michael, J. L. (2004). *Concepts and principles of behavior analysis* (Rev. ed.). Kalamazoo, MI: Society for the Advancement of Behavior Analysis.

Four

Cognitive Case Conceptualizations and Treatment Plans

Introduction to Cognitive Theory

You received a phone call last week from Marie, a 30-year-old, White widow with two daughters, Amy (age 8) and Nancy (age 5). Marie's husband, Allen, along with two business associates, was killed when their chartered plane crashed during a severe thunderstorm 1 month ago. Allen had been hurrying home to come to the engagement party of Marie's younger sister and had taken the chartered plane because his original flight, on a national airline, was delayed because of the weather. This sudden death ended what Marie described as a happy and satisfying 10-year marriage. She and the girls continue to live in the family home, which is located in a suburb of a large city. Marie is self-referred. She is very concerned about her ability to parent her two daughters in the aftermath of Allen's death. She participated in a mental status interview and psychometric testing last week.

You take the cognitive approach to treatment developed by Aaron Beck (1991; Beck Institute for Cognitive Therapy and Research, 2008). This approach focuses on the role of maladaptive cognitions in psychological distress. From this perspective, it is not the death of her husband and its aftermath that will be the focus of Marie's treatment but rather her cognitive representation of these events. Problems will be a result of self-defeating belief systems (cognitive structures) that increase the power of distorted images and thoughts Marie may have as a result of her husband's death. The goals of treatment will be to assess and modify Marie's cognitive distortions by reappraising her automatic thoughts; teaching her the role of distorted negative thinking in her current difficulties; and recording, challenging, ard modifying her thinking (Beck, 1991; Sudak, 2006).

How has Marie developed her belief systems (cognitive schemata)? Cognitive theory posits that as individuals develop from infancy through old age, they develop and maintain beliefs about themselves and the world. These beliefs develop around important themes or social issues such as success or failure, acceptance or rejection, ard respect or disdain (Beck, 1991). Some of these are core beliefs and have overarching influences on an individual. Others are more specific, intermediate beliefs that consist of working rules and assumptions for more specific situations and events. All of these beliefs become part of the individual's cognitive representations of the world and are reflected in a stream of self-talk or automatic thoughts. This self-talk is the individual's internal communication system. Some individuals are more aware of this internal communication than are others. Through learning, the individual's self-talk comes to include evaluations of the self, others, and the environment as well as recollections of the past and expectations about the future (Beck, 1991).

What impact will this internal communication system have on Marie? Her stream of self-talk will monitor, initiate, and inhibit her behavior. In areas where she shows adaptive behavior (high self-esteem and self-efficacy), this is assumed to result from adaptive beliefs with their concomitant positive stream of self-talk. Conversely, maladaptive behavior (low self-esteem, self-criticism) is assumed to result from maladaptive beliefs with their concomitant negative stream of self-talk. Marie has learned both her adaptive and her maladaptive beliefs.

How does this learning occur? Caretakers and others may explicitly teach these beliefs to children, or children may learn them implicitly through modeling. For example, a child may see a parent drop a glass on the floor. The parent might say, "Oh no, I dropped a glass! Oh well, I can clean it up; it's just a mistake, no big deal." The child might learn from this that everyone makes mistakes and mistakes can be fixed. On the other hand, the parent might say, "Oh no, this is a disaster! I can never do anything right; now the evening is ruined." The child might learn from this that mistakes are awful and cannot be fixed.

From long-term exposure to a positive view of the world, children may develop positively biased cognitive schemata (core and intermediate beliefs) and self-talk in which they interpret their own behavior and that of others with positive expectations, attributions, and evaluations. These individuals have a positive bias to their inferences about the future and their recollections of the past. Mistakes and unpleasant experiences do not in and of themselves lead to the blockage of positive information (Beck, 1991; Sudak, 2006).

In contrast, from long-term exposure to a negative view of the world, children may develop negatively biased cognitive schemata and self-talk, leading to a negative lens for viewing their own and others' behavior. A negative cognitive bias makes people more vulnerable to negative thinking and may prevent them from noticing or being influenced by positive events. Anything that fits the negative worldview is taken in easily. Individuals with a negative bias often interpret anything ambiguous as negative. Beck (1991) postulates the existence of elevated, depressed, anxious, and angry cognitive biases. Cognitive biases can be restricted to specific realms of experience, or they may be comprehensive (Beck, 1991; Sudak, 2006).

Role of the Clinician

How will you help Marie? You will be an educator and a hypothesis generator who takes an active role in directing treatment and helping Marie assess and modify her self-defeating belief systems. First, Marie will be educated about the model so that she understands how her thoughts lead to her feelings and behavior (Beck, 1991; Sudak, 2006). Second, you will help Marie become aware of her self-talk and take on the view that her thoughts are hypotheses that can be tested. This assessment or examination of cognitions involves a partnership between you and Marie. Together you will collect data about, and test the usefulness and validity of, her belief systems using a Socratic dialogue (Beck, 1991; Ingram, 2006). Overall, this process involves you asking Marie questions, pushing her to test out her conclusions, increasing her ability to recognize distortions of thinking, and increasing the imagination and flexibility that she brings to her manner of thinking about her life. Marie will learn to recognize her common errors in thinking in terms of specific here-and-now events in the treatment room and/or in her daily life; this step-by-step refutation of maladaptive thoughts will serve as a means to challenge Marie's underlying maladaptive beliefs (Beck, 1991; Ingram, 2006; Sudak, 2006).

Specifically, you two will investigate (a) the attributions she makes about herself and others, (b) her expectations about the future, (c) her perceptions of what happens including any negative biases she may have, and (d) her perceptions of past events and any biases in her interpretations of these events. Errors in thinking may involve all-or-nothing thinking (dichotomous thinking), arbitrary inference (jumping to conclusions), emotional reasoning (using feelings, not facts, to draw conclusions), fortune telling (believing that the future can be predicted), magnification and minimization (misrepresenting the realistic impact of something), mind reading (believing that you can know what another person is thinking), personalization (assuming something must have something to do with you personally), overgeneralization (overly broad inference), selective abstraction (deleting or ignoring information), and exaggeration or distortion (Beck & Weishaar, 2000; Ingram, 2006).

Marie will investigate her thoughts both within the session and through homework assignments such as keeping a thought log that can make her more aware of how her thinking is connected to her feelings of depression and anxiety. After learning to identify her cognitive errors, Marie will be helped to see the connections between these maladaptive cognitions and her current life stress. She will be helped to understand how constant self-criticism, negative predictions, recollections, and interpretations have all fed on one another to create self-blame, low self-esteem, and low self-efficacy. Then, through in- and out-of-session activities, Marie will be encouraged to notice, catch, monitor, interrupt, and challenge her negative thoughts and then reinforce herself for more adaptive coping responses. She will be helped to identify high-risk situations and consider ways to prepare for, handle, and deal with any failures.

Marie also will be encouraged to engage in activities that promote feelings of competence and pleasure and to make positive self-attributions concerning these activities, such as "I can influence the world" and "I don't have to be a passive victim of life events." These attributions of control are assumed to increase Marie's self-efficacy and enable her to alter the negative attributions she imposes on herself, others, and the environment. As more positive cognitions become part of Marie's automatic stream of consciousness, her mood and overt behavior will be positively influenced (Beck, 1991; Sudak, 2006).

Case Application: Integrating the Domain of Gender

Marie's case will now be examined in detail. There are many domains of complexity that might be relevant to her case. The Domain of Gender has been chosen to examine within a cognitive case conceptualization and treatment plan.

Interview With Marie (M) From a Cognitive Perspective

C: I understand your husband died recently and you have concerns about your children. What are you concerned about specifically?

M: (calmly) My husband and I have always prided ourselves on our parenting. It was very important to both of us that our girls be raised correctly. (pause) Now that I am alone, I feel I am betraying my husband's trust.

C: How do you think you are betraying your husband?

M: (calmly) He was my best friend and perfect husband. We had the same ideas about how to live and raise children; everything was going the way we planned. (with agitation) Now, my 8-year-old, Amy, is having one temper tantrum after another at home, is constantly picking fights with her sister Nancy, and is being rude to her teachers.

C: Your daughter is misbehaving at home and at school. How is this your fault and a betrayal?

M: (regretfully) Amy had a perfect record at school before Allen died. She never missed a day and had the report card of an angel. Now . . . I fight with her every morning just to get her dressed, and she is RUDE to her teacher.

C: You find rudeness unacceptable.

M: (emphatically) Girls do not behave that way. Allen and I never tolerated back talk. He would be so upset by Amy's behavior.

C: What specifically have you tried to do about it?

M: (earnestly) I have always set an example of self-control. I am never rude to anyone, including the children, no matter how badly they have misbehaved.

C: Is it wrong to show anger? (M nods.) Do you think that humans, particularly children, can always control their anger?

M: (sadly) I know that they need to be taught self-control, but the way Amy has been slipping, I just don't know what I am doing wrong that she is . . . (M sobs softly)

C: What thoughts are overwhelming you?

M: (sounding sad and tired) How can I bear it? I am letting Allen down.

C: Would he expect you to set such a high standard for Amy?

M: (back in control) That's the only kind of standard we have in our family. Allen was the best husband and father. He could control the girls' high spirits with just a look or a raise in his voice.

C: Allen did more than set a good example. He also intervened with his eyes and his voice.

M: (emphatically) Yes. He could always control them, so I never needed to.

C: He could set limits on them, but now the limits are gone. (long pause) Should Allen be here?

M: (intently) It's not his fault that he's gone. He was coming to my sister's engagement party; he knew he needed to be there. (long pause, sadly) The weather prevented him from coming.

C: Coming back was the RIGHT thing?

M: (confidently) Yes. Allen would never have intentionally missed the party. It would have been so disrespectful to my family.

C: Can people control the weather?

M: (irritably) We knew the storm wasn't Allen's fault. (pause) But, if you plan well enough, things like this don't happen.

C: You believe bad things don't happen if you plan well.

M: (irritably) The engagement party date was set before Allen's business meeting. He had been consulted about the date out of respect for his work. He felt he had to rush off to this meeting. He knew it was his responsibility to get back. My parents were talking about this, even at the funeral.

C: Did someone tell him that he had to get back for the party?

M: (confusedly) No, it wasn't necessary.

C: The standard was automatic.

M: (confident again) Yes, it was. When the kids act disrespectfully, I can hear Allen's voice in my head saying, "This is not acceptable." There is this little voice—evaluating what is going on and telling me what I should do.

C: What kind of voice?

M: (anxiously) It's just me. Like my conscience. I always hear myself citing the standards . . . keeping me from giving up.

C: What happens if you make a mistake?

M: (sad again) I feel so awful. (pause) I just can't forgive myself.

C: Have you ever felt so bad you thought of harming yourself?

M: (in control again) No. The girls need me. I will not let them down. It's just hard because I keep making mistakes.

C: Does everyone make mistakes?

M: (determinedly) I can't let myself. The girls have only me now; I couldn't forgive myself if I didn't make things right.

C: Can you forgive the girls for their mistakes?

M: (emphatically) Of course. They are just kids. They need to be taught how to behave correctly. (pause) But . . . they have only me now.

C: The standards tell you to be perfect. Does your family expect this perfection too?

M: (stridently) Oh yes. I know my parents are disappointed by the girls' behavior.

C: How do you know?

M: (intently) They have never said anything, but . . . I saw it in their faces for the first time as they watched the girls fight with each other at Allen's funeral. In the past few weeks, they have stopped coming to the house. (pause, M shakes her head) My father says they will be back when I have things under control.

C: You interpret their withdrawal as disapproval of you or the girls?

M: (long pause, desperately) I must be making terrible mistakes as a mother. The girls haven't been well mannered or respectful since Allen died. My parents set a good example for me. My mother is a real lady. She taught me how to keep my temper under control and how to attend to the needs of others. (pause) I am trying to teach the girls . . . (long pause)

C: Your parents hold high standards for you and the girls. You want to reach them. But, are they too high?

M: (emphatically) Standards weren't too high when Allen was alive. We knew we could reach them. He's dead now. I can't let Allen's death ruin my girls' futures.

C: Could their whole futures depend on their behavior now?

M: (uncertainly) I don't know. . . . Behavior can become ingrained. Allen was so proud of my femininity, my manners, my poise. No good men will want to marry my girls if they are rough and undisciplined.

C: You are thinking all the time about your children's welfare. Do you have time to think of anything else?

M: (long pause, calmly) I'm lucky in a way . . . Allen had a lot of life insurance, so I can continue at home with the girls. I don't have to abandon the type of home Allen and I wanted for them. He was always so wonderful.

C: Financially, Allen is still caring for you and the girls; he always cared for you. Now that he's died, are you getting help from anyone else?

M: (calmly) Two of the men from Allen's office have been very kind. They take turns coming over to mow the grass, and they help with home repairs.

C: Were these Allen's jobs?

M: (anxiously) Yes. But . . . (sobbing for a minute, controlled) I may have to tell them to stop coming over because (pause) some of my neighbors are talking.

C: What thoughts are behind your tears?

M: (sadly) They are spreading rumors about me and Allen's friends. (pause) I am lost without Allen. (determinedly) How can people think I would be interested in someone else? (intently) And these men are married!

C: You and Allen's friends know the rumors are untrue. What are you thinking about these rumors that is bothering you so much?

M: (sadly) Clearly, my neighbors have so little respect for me that . . . (sobbing)

C: It's very painful to feel you aren't respected. (M nods) What contacts are you having with your neighbors now?

M: (dismissively) None, really. I don't really know any of them. Our family has moved a lot to help Allen be successful in his work. I never put down roots in any neighborhood. My life was the family.

C: Your neighbors are strangers to you. How could they know anything about you?

M: (pause, uncertainly) I don't know. I should get along with them, and I want them to know I am a respectable woman. I don't want them thinking ill of me. (long pause) I guess I need to tell Allen's friends to stop coming.

C: Do you have any other choices? (long pause) You want help, and Allen's friends are willing to help.

M: (uncertainly) If the neighbors are talking about me, I must be doing something wrong!

C: Must you? (long pause) Could you approach them and let them see who you are?

M: (tearful but no longer crying) Maybe, I could . . . Allen wouldn't want me to cut the grass and things. Those are men's jobs. (pause, controlled) I'm sorry I have acted poorly. You must have no respect for me.

C: You worry about this because your family so highly values self-control. (M nods) Is there anything you feel is under control for you and the girls?

M: (calmly) Well, I took books out from the library about explaining death to children. I know I have helped the girls understand Allen's death better. Right after the accident, the girls had terrible nightmares. Now, these have stopped.

C: In the midst of your own pain, you are still physically caring for your children. You are aware that they are having problems, AND you are trying to help them with these problems. (long pause) Does this mean you are a good mother?

M: (regretfully) No. When you get to know me better, you will see how inadequate I have been since Allen's death. I will be a good mother again when everything is going well for my girls.

C: Your standards are very high. Could anyone reach them?

M: (painfully) You don't think I have to try? (long pause) I feel crazy and out of control without Allen.

C: People in grief feel overwhelmed. It's what happens when a loved one dies.

M: (anxiously) I don't have time to deal with myself. (emphatically) I must take care of these girls!

C: Allen was so important to you. Is grieving realistic?

M: (intently) He would want me to focus exclusively on the girls.

C: You have put yourself under intense pressure. Could you be a good woman and a good mother but not be perfect?

M: (anxiously) If I let go of my standards, I won't know myself. I thought about not wearing makeup yesterday . . . who would care? But, I had to. (desperately) Already, the girls want things from me that I can't give. Allen always used to carry them around the house and play chase games. They miss this fun so much.

C: If the kids need playfulness, can you be playful?

M: (anxiously) I can't take their dad's place. I guess they need me to find them another dad . . . I can't face this now. I am suffocating! (desperately) Will it ever be better?

C: Yes, but it will take some time because Allen was so important. The two of us will explore the standards of behavior for a family in grief.

M: (anxiously) I shouldn't be asking for help. I should be able to control this situation myself.

C: Those are the type of thoughts we will need to explore together.

Cognitive Case Conceptualization of Marie: Diagnosis-Based Style

Whether within her role as a widow, mother, daughter, or friend, Marie is feeling depressed and anxious and is suffering from feelings of low self-esteem and personal efficacy. Marie has experienced a negative cognitive shift, in which she has trouble perceiving anything positive about herself, her children, or her immediate social environment. This negative shift, and its accompanying symptoms, began after her husband was killed suddenly in a plane accident. Marie has no prior history of depression; however, she does have a history of core perfectionist and rigid belief systems, along with strong intermediary beliefs about the proper role of men and women that are serving to complicate her ability to grieve effectively for her husband. Although she shows significant symptomatology at this time, her continued positive attention to her children's developmental, academic, and social needs reflects an individual with significant intellectual and functional competencies. Her total constellation of behaviors is most accurately reflected in a diagnosis on Axis I of V62.82 Bereavement. Marie exhibits signs of obsessional and perfectionist thinking. Her past high level of functioning, however, suggests that these reflect her personal style based on core beliefs rather than a personality disorder. Thus, she has no diagnosis on Axis II. There is also no diagnosis on Axis III, as Marie has no current medical conditions influencing her functioning. In terms of Axis IV, Marie currently has inadequate social support as she has no friendships of her own and her parents have recently withdrawn their emotional support. On Axis V, her current level of adaptive functioning is estimated at 65, and her highest level of adaptive functioning in the past year is estimated at 90. Because of her high level of distress, her strong motivation for treatment, and her prior history of adaptive functioning, treatment prognosis is considered good to excellent.

How does Marie view herself as a widow? She believes that she and her husband had a strong and satisfying relationship that lasted for 10 years. Sharing core and intermediary beliefs on gender role stereotypes and ideal family functioning, they were each other's strong support system. Due to their frequent moves in support of Allen's career, they maintained an isolated family unit. As a result, Marie has lost her husband and only intimate friend. Her ability to grieve has been inhibited by her rigidly held gender role beliefs. These intermediary beliefs contain assumptions such as "women cannot be angry," "women cannot lose control," and "women must always help others." These gender role stereotypes are superimposed on perfectionist core belief systems that dictate to Marie that "only the highest standards are acceptable," "if you plan properly, things do not go wrong," and "you are either perfect or inadequate." These maladaptive belief systems are reflected in a stream of self-talk that criticizes Marie for experiencing her very normal reactions of grief and exhorts her to perfection even in the immediate aftermath of loss. At a time when she really needs the support of others, her negative lens leads her to view all the "others" in her environment as disapproving. Even in the face of positive support from the clinician, she reinterprets his support as misguided: "When you get to know me better, you will see how inadequate I have been since Allen's death." Using overgeneralizations and distortions, she looks back at her husband as a perfect spouse and evaluates herself now as betraying his trust through her inadequacies; she did have positive thoughts about herself as a woman and wife before her bereavement.

How does Marie view herself as a parent? Based on her belief systems, Marie strives to be a perfect mother and despite her loss has continued to provide well for most of her children's needs. She attends well to their physical needs, she communicates regularly with their teachers, and she has helped them understand the reality of their father's death. Her perfectionist and gender-typed beliefs, however, are inhibiting her from recognizing her abilities as a mother and maintaining a sense of competency in her role. Furthermore, these beliefs lead to negative assumptions about her children's recent acting-out behaviors; she views their misbehavior as unacceptable rather than as understandable stress reactions to the death of their father. Marie exaggerates the seriousness of their difficulties even to the point of making catastrophic predictions about their futures. She sees their only hope for life success as tied to their ability to always be little ladies even in the direct aftermath of their father's death. She views her role in their lives strictly in terms of setting standards, being a perfect role model, and taking care of their physical needs. The role of a father is that of financial supporter and perfect playmate. Marie sees remarriage as her only option to providing for her children's need for this perfect playmate. In addition to her own critical voice, Marie hears the voice of Allen and sees the looks of her parents as a critical chorus disapproving of her every parenting move. Despite feeling overwhelmed by their current behavioral outbursts, she does perceive her daughters to have achieved well academically and socially prior to Allen's death.

How does Marie view herself as a daughter? She and Allen remained actively involved with her family after their marriage. She recognizes that she took her core beliefs, and her beliefs about how to be a perfect woman, from her mother, who she describes as "a real lady." Her parents continue to reinforce her belief systems involving perfectionism and rigid gender role stereotypes. Even after Allen's death, her parents do not consider him rushing home during a storm as inappropriate. They say things such as "He knew it was his responsibility to be back on time; he was doing what he was supposed to do." Perhaps there was some softly voiced criticism of Allen at the funeral from extended family members such as "If he had planned better, this wouldn't have happened." Marie may be sharing this criticism implicitly when she says, "The engagement party date was set before Allen's business meeting . . . He had been consulted about the date . . . He felt he had to rush off . . . He knew it was his responsibility to get back." Marie does not believe that women should be angry, but deep down, she may be angry at Allen for going to the business meeting. She may also feel guilty that he got killed flying home for a party in her sister's honor. Allen and Marie both knew that her family would accept no excuses for his absence from the party. Marie's extended family is not providing Marie with any emotional support for her own grief reactions or for her parenting dilemmas. Her parents plan to stay withdrawn from Marie and the children until Marie has "gained control" of the situation. Marie does not complain about this withdrawal. She interprets it as their justified reaction to her "failings" as a woman and a mother.

How does Marie view herself as a female friend and neighbor? Her past roles were as perfect wife and mother. She had no other role for herself and no friends of her own because she always put Allen and the children first. She has tried to maintain her past perfectionist standards by dressing and acting like a perfect lady at all times despite her state of bereavement. She has not directly solicited help from her neighbors because of her beliefs that "everything will turn out right if you plan enough, and it's shameful to be out of control of your children." This may have led her neighbors to assume that she does not need help or in fact is not really grief stricken. It may also be part of the reason why her neighbors gossip about the role Allen's friends are currently playing in her life. Their gossip unintentionally serves to reinforce Marie's assumption that she is betraying Allen's trust and that her parenting "mistakes" mean she is defective and unacceptable. Marie has the social skills to develop positive relationships with her neighbors, as well as to develop personal friendships, if she develops the belief that it is acceptable for her to have these relationships.

In many ways, Marie's family is functioning well in the aftermath of Allen's death. Everyone is getting enough to eat, everyone is living in the family home, the children are attending their neighborhood school, and after only 1 month, they have progressed through the denial stage of grief. Unfortunately, maladaptive belief systems are inhibiting Marie from proceeding further in the grief process, leaving her feeling depressed, anxious, and incompetent. These beliefs are also preventing her from recognizing that her children's acting-out behaviors are legitimate grief reactions and that a relaxation of her "high standards" is appropriate at this time. The behavior of Marie's parents, in reinforcing her perfectionistic core beliefs, may serve to impede Marie's ability to function more flexibly at this time. However, Marie's stress level has become so intense that she has violated one of her own standards and is actively seeking help from a clinician. She is also questioning whether all her assumptions of what it means to be a perfect lady, such as wearing a lot of makeup each day, are really necessary at this time of loss. This may represent a window of opportunity in which she can be helped to reevaluate the efficacy of her current belief systems in guiding her behavior and that of her children.

Cognitive Treatment Plan: Diagnosis-Based Style

Treatment Plan Overview. Marie is verbal, intelligent, in distress, and motivated for change; thus, she is a good candidate for treatment, and her prognosis for improvement is good to excellent. The treatment plan follows the *assessment format*.

SUBJECTIVE DATA: Marie comes in expressing concerns about her children. She views their behavior to have seriously deteriorated following the recent death of their father from a plane accident. She finds herself to be inadequate and a failure as a woman and a mother. She is guilt ridden that she is failing her own and her husband's standards as a parent. She considers her own functioning as irrelevant at this time; only her children are important.

OBJECTIVE DATA: Standardized intellectual testing using the Wechsler Adult Intelligence Scale-Revised (WAIS-R) revealed that Marie has an average level of intelligence. Personality testing utilizing the Minnesota

Multiphasic Personality Inventory-2 (MMPI-2) revealed signs of rigid, perfectionist thinking; traditional sex role stereotypes; mild cognitive confusion; significant personal turmoil; and distress. Her profile is most consistent with a diagnosis of bereavement.

ASSESSMENT: Marie is depressed, anxious, and suffering from feelings of low self-esteem and personal efficacy. Due to a negative cognitive shift, she has trouble perceiving anything positive about herself, her children, or her immediate social environment. Marie is a highly functioning and competent woman and parent who is involved in a pathological grieving process. Normal grieving is inhibited by her core beliefs involving perfectionism and her intermediary beliefs involving rigid gender roles. Although she is showing significant symptomatology at this time, her continued positive attention to her children's developmental, academic, and social needs reflects an individual with significant intellectual and functional competencies.

Her working diagnosis at this time is:

Axis I	V62.82 Bereavement
Axis II	V71.09 No diagnosis
Axis III	None
Axis IV	Inadequate social support
	Good social skills
	Financial stability
	Average intelligence
Axis V	GAF 65 (admission)
	GAF 90 (highest level past year)

PLAN:

Treatment Plan Overview: Marie's adaptive and maladaptive belief systems will be explored within her roles as a widow, a mother, an adult daughter, a friend, and a neighbor.

LONG-TERM GOAL 1: Marie will become aware of her belief systems about herself as a newly widowed woman and how these are helping her or creating stress for her.

Short-Term Goals

1. Marie will become aware of her self-talk around the issue that a good woman is never angry and how it is or is not helping her cope realistically with the sudden death of her husband.

2. Marie will become aware of her self-talk around the issue that a good woman never loses control and how it is or is not helping her cope realistically with the sudden death of her husband.

3. Marie will become aware of her self-talk around the issue of whether a good woman must always focus on helping others and how it is or is not helping her cope realistically with the sudden death of her husband.

4. Marie will hypothesis test about whether these thoughts are realistic through reading books on bereavement, talking with the clinician, and initiating discussions with other people who are grieving.

5. Marie will replace any perfectionist and unrealistic thoughts with more adaptive ones based on her greater knowledge of bereavement issues in her discussions about herself with others and within her own head when she considers her own "performance" as a recent widow.

6. Other goals will be developed as appropriate.

LONG-TERM GOAL 2: Marie will become aware of her belief systems around herself as a mother and how these are helping her or creating stress for her.

Short-Term Goals

1. Marie will become aware of her self-talk around the behavior of her daughters and whether it represents a realistic appraisal of the behavior of recently bereaved children.

2. Marie will become aware of her self-talk around her disciplinary strategies with her daughters and whether they represent realistic interventions for young girls in grief.

3. Marie will hypothesis test around her self-talk through reading about grief and young children, talk with the clinician, and observations of other parents with their young children.

4. Marie will replace any perfectionistic or unrealistic self-talk with constructive self-talk based on her new level of understanding of child development and grief in her interactions with her daughters.

5. Other goals will be developed as appropriate.

LONG-TERM GOAL 3: Marie will become aware of her belief systems around herself as an adult daughter and how these are helping her or creating stress for her.

Short-Term Goals

1. Marie will become aware of her self-talk that she learned as a daughter and that her parents continue to emphasize (if you plan, things always turn out "right").

2. Marie will become aware of her self-talk that she learned as a daughter and that her parents continue to emphasize (it is an adult's responsibility to do things "right").

3. Marie will become aware of her self-talk around Allen that she learned as a daughter and that her parents continue to emphasize (it was his responsibility to get back for a family party, etc.).

4. Marie will hypothesis test about whether this self-talk is adaptive or not based on reading about the differences between rational and unrealistic thinking and the differential impact these types of thinking have on moods such as anger, depression, and anxiety; discussing these issues with the clinician; and keeping a thought diary to monitor her own emotions in relation to her thinking in these absolutist terms.

5. Marie will replace any negative self-talk with more adaptive self-talk that will support more positive emotions and adaptive, flexible behavior free of perfectionism in her interactions with her parents.

6. Other goals will be developed as appropriate.

LONG-TERM GOAL 4: Marie will become aware of her belief systems around herself as a female friend and neighbor and how these are helping her or creating stress for her.

Short-Term Goals

1. Marie will become aware of her self-talk around her role as a female friend and neighbor and how it requires her to always look perfectly groomed, always be in emotional control, and always be in complete control as a parent.

2. Marie will hypothesis test around her ideas that she cannot show the world that she is grieving and in distress and cannot ask for help for anything or

else she isn't a lady and deserving of respect through reading about the importance of social support, discussing the issues with the clinician, and watching other adults interacting with their peers.

3. Marie will replace any maladaptive talk with adaptive talk that will enable her to request help when needed with her home, her children, and her feelings of loneliness following the death of her husband and best friend.

4. Marie will consider what adaptive talk would help her in discussing with her neighbors the current false rumors that have begun circulating about her since her husband's death.

5. Other goals will be developed as appropriate.

Practice Case for Student Conceptualization: Integrating the Domain of Sexual Orientation

It is time to do a cognitive analysis of Eric. There are many domains of complexity that might provide insights into his behavior. Within this analysis, you are asked to try to integrate the Domain of Sexual Orientation into your case conceptualization.

Information Received From Phone Intake

Eric is a 16-year-old White male living in a poor and deteriorating section of a large Midwestern city. He is presently a junior in high school. He is an average student with no record of school adjustment problems. His parents were divorced 7 years ago, but they remain in a conflictual relationship. Over the past 7 years, Eric has switched households five times. In addition to living with his parents, sometimes he has gone to live with his maternal aunt and uncle. These moves have also involved his switching back and forth among three school systems. Eric was referred to a clinician, who provides treatment at the high school, by his history teacher, Mr. Jenkins. Mr. Jenkins considered Eric to be depressed, and he was also worried about whether Eric's home environment was safe.

During a brief mental status exam, there were moderate signs of distress but no indications of suicidal or homicidal ideation or severe psychopathology. Eric showed some anxiety during the discussion of the limits of confidentiality. However, he said he would agree to treatment in order to please Mr. Jenkins.

Interview With Eric (E) From a Cognitive Perspective

C: Mr. Jenkins told me a little about you. Could you tell me what's on your mind?

E: (angrily) Well, I feel like a bouncing ball all the time. Sometimes my mom seems to want me, sometimes my dad, and sometimes neither does and I end up at my aunt and uncle's house. My dad always has to control everything. He always tries to jerk me around. (pause) I've never been sure if there was anything about me he liked. It was pathetic how much I tried to please him when I was little. (pause) But I've given up on that now. When I am at his house, I just keep out of his way. (reflectively) My dad and mom seem to hate each other. My mom has let her new drinking buddy move into our home. One thing I'm sure about is that he hates me.

C: What makes you think that?

E: (reflectively) If I even say hello to Mom, he screams his lungs out. She has to give him 100% of her time. (shaking his head, intently) HE is the intruder, not ME.

C: When your mom pays attention to you, he gets angry?

E: (caustically) That's an understatement. If I say hello to Mom when I come in from school, she'll ignore me if he's home. Even the sound of my voice alone often starts him screaming.

C: How exactly does your mom react to this?

E: (furiously) She tells me to shut up. She says if I drive him away we'll starve.

C: What do you think will happen when she threatens you with this?

E: (resignedly) She'll kick me out for a while, and it's back to my aunt and uncle again.

C: What will happen there?

E: (desolately) They let me stay. They feed me. (pause) Once when I needed a new coat, they bought it for me. They never really talk to me . . . but they don't talk to each other either. At school, it's the same deal. I have no one.

C: What stops you from making friends at school?

E: (sadly) I have changed schools so many times I've never had a chance to make any real friends. (long pause) I feel alone, different. I don't fit in anywhere.

C: You can't think of any times when you thought you fit in.

E: (anxiously) I have to figure out who I am beside the fact that my parents can't waste their time on me. (explosively) This can't go on!

C: Are you pressuring yourself for insight? (pause) You feel alone in this struggle. Have you noticed any other teens struggling with this?

E: (dejectedly) No one has gone through what I have.

C: You say this to yourself, and it increases your distress.

E: (pause, reflectively) Maybe. Other people seem to have close friends. I want that, but whenever I start to make a friend, I think, what if it is just more pain?

C: Your family relationships are painful. Does this mean all relationships must be that way?

E: (intently) Well, my folks can't do anything but hurt each other. Their new relationships don't seem so great either. (with resignation) Good relationships seem impossible.

C: If I tell you good relationships are possible, what goes through your mind?

E: (confidently) I'll get hurt, I'll be rejected, and I won't be able to take any more pain.

C: If someone rejects you, you think everyone will?

E: (matter-of-factly) Everyone rejects me. Only Mr. Jenkins cares.

C: I understand you spend a lot of time with him.

E: (explosively) WHAT'S WRONG WITH THAT?

C: You sound angry. What are you thinking?

E: (long pause, intently) Yesterday, some guys harassed me in the locker room. They called me a queer with a crush on Mr. Jenkins. One of them had been mouthing off in class to Mr. Jenkins, so I sort of shoved him in the hall after class. Then he got a bunch of his friends to shove me around by the lockers.

C: Are you OK?

E: (surprised) Yeah. They just wanted to make me feel small. Once they felt they had done it real well, they left me alone.

C: They shoved you out of revenge. But why did they call you a queer?

E: (explosively) I HAVE NEVER THOUGHT ABOUT IT. (long pause, calmly) I don't know. (dejectedly) Maybe I am.

C: You have slumped down in the chair. What's on your mind?

E: (sarcastically) Well, it's not like it's a good thing to be queer.

C: What do you think is good or bad about being gay?

E: (shaking his head, tensely) I can't talk about this with you or anyone else.

C: It might be hard for you to talk about. (pause) Our sexuality is an important part of who we are. (long pause) I don't know if you're gay or not. (long pause) Could it be OK if you are?

E: (firmly) I'm only willing to talk about this if I am gay. (pause) How will I know?

C: When you think about Mr. Jenkins right now, what specific thoughts and feelings do you have?

E: (quietly) I think I would rather be with him than anyone else. If he says hello to me, I feel great. If he is sick, I feel low. I think about him all the time, what he would think of everything I do. Does this mean I'm gay?

C: Mr. Jenkins is important to you. Is there a difference between feeling very emotionally close and the desire for something more?

E: (uncertainly) What do you mean?

C: Well, when teens go through puberty, most of them begin to have special thoughts, wishes, or fantasies about a particular person or type of person that are different from how they think about most people.

E: (dejectedly) I think I'm a dud like those guys said.

C: Are you a dud or something else? (pause) Are you shaving yet? (E shakes head no) Could you have a lot more growing to do? (long pause) Is it possible that it isn't time yet for you to have these feelings?

E: (sarcastically) The guys who beat me up made a big deal about my size.

C: Is it a big deal to you? (long pause)

E: (frankly) I didn't really care till I got into that fight. I could have used some extra inches then. (long pause) What does this all mean about Mr. Jenkins and me?

C: I don't know if you have special feelings about Mr. Jenkins or not. You don't seem to know either. If I give you some stuff to read and you give yourself time to grow up, might it all become clear to you in time? (E shakes his head no) Questioning is a normal part of learning who you are.

E: (furiously) I can't take my whole life to figure this thing out. (long pause, calmly) I've wondered a lot if I should tell Mr. Jenkins about this. This is the one important thing I haven't shared. He knows something is up.

C: What are you imagining he will do if you tell him?

E: (desperately) I hear him screaming abuse in my mind, just like the guys in the locker room; then I see myself disintegrating, alone, no one caring about me.

C: Those consequences are catastrophic. Could anything else be possible?

E: (dejectedly) I can't imagine anything else.

C: I don't know what he would do. He could freak out, or he might understand and talk to you about it. What risks are involved in telling or not telling?

E: (sadly) Sometimes I think to myself that he won't want me, but he will pity me instead and still let me hang around him.

C: What else might happen?

E: (intently) Nothing. He's very into right and wrong. I know that from our talks about my parents. He will be my teacher and nothing else. I guess I must be a real jerk to consider anything else.

C: You say very harsh things to yourself. Do you think any other students may have had personal thoughts about their teachers?

E: (hopefully) Yeah, I guess. (long pause, agitatedly) My dad would just hate me if I was gay.

C: What makes you expect this?

E: (anxiously) He never has had much interest in me. I've heard him say a lot of ugly stuff about fags . . . if he thought I was one, it might just push him into hate.

C: Have you met any gay or lesbian individuals?

E: (uncertainly) I think I did once. I was walking down the street with my dad, when some guy brushed up against him. I thought it was an accident, but Dad said the guy was a faggot and beat the crap out of him. (long pause) I think Dad just takes me sometimes to drive my mother nuts.

C: What was that guy like, the one your dad called a faggot?

E: (confusedly) He looked like anyone else, but my dad says he can always tell. (pause) He hasn't seemed concerned about me yet. If he did, he might beat the crap out of me like he did that guy on the street.

C: Some dads do that. But, some parents and friends learn to understand. Could anyone in your family try to understand? (long pause) Would they all be extreme and beat you up or kick you out?

E: (intently) My parents do everything to the extreme. They married young. They drank a lot, fought a lot. My dad finally walked out after so much fighting and jealousy. (pause) I don't have that crap with Mr. Jenkins; with him it's calm. On my own it's a nightmare. (long pause, yelling) IF I DON'T WHIP MYSELF INTO SHAPE, RIGHT NOW, I'LL BUST!

C: Are things bad enough that you are thinking about hurting yourself or running away?

E: (calmly) No. I'm OK.

C: Are you safe at home?

E: (calmly) Home is an angry place, but no one hits me or anything.

C: What about school?

E: (calmly) No one but those guys have ever threatened me. The principal overheard them the other day and threatened them with something. They avoid me now.

C: OK. If you come back next week, we need to focus on your thoughts about yourself and others and how this self-talk might be influencing you. I'd like you to keep a record of your thoughts about yourself and being gay.

E: (anxiously) If I do the assignment, will it tell me if I'm gay?

C: It's normal to need time to question and explore. You may need to allow yourself to be like everyone else and take time to work it out.

Exercises for Developing a Case Conceptualization of Eric

Exercise 1 (4-page maximum)

GOAL: To verify that you have a clear understanding of cognitive theory.

STYLE: An integrative essay addressing Parts A–C.

NEED HELP? Review this chapter (pages 122–125).

A. Develop a concise overview of the assumptions of cognitive theory (the theory's hypotheses about key dimensions in understanding the role of belief systems in adaptive and maladaptive living; think broadly, abstractly).

B. Develop a thorough description of how each of these assumptions is used to understand a client's thought processes, emotions, and behavior (for each assumption provide specific examples).

C. Describe the role of the clinician in initiating cognitive change (consultant, doctor, educator, helper; treatment approach; technique examples).

Exercise 2 (4-page maximum)

GOAL: To aid application of cognitive theory to Eric.

STYLE: A separate sentence outline for each section, A–D.

NEED HELP?   Review this chapter (pages 122–125).

A. Create a list of Eric's weaknesses (concerns, issues, problems, symptoms, skill deficits, treatment barriers) and indicate which Eric wants help with.

B. Create a list of Eric's strengths (strong points, positive features, successes, skills, factors facilitating change) and indicate which Eric is aware of having.

C. How is what Eric thinks related to these weaknesses and strengths considering his (a) belief systems, (b) self-talk, (c) attributions about himself and others, (d) perceptions of current and past events and any biases in these perceptions, and (e) expectations about the future. If you have not already done so, consider how his thinking influences his affect, behavior, and motivations within his strengths and weaknesses.

D. What is Eric's overall worldview, what forces in the environment are reinforcing or contradicting this worldview, and overall, how adaptive is his thinking at this time?

Exercise 3 (4-page maximum)

GOAL: To develop an understanding of the potential role of sexual orientation in Eric's life.

STYLE: A separate sentence outline for each section, A–F.

NEED HELP?   Review Chapter 2 (pages 73–78).

A. Assess where Eric is in the process of identifying his sexual orientation, in terms of desires, fantasies, attitudes, emotions, and behavior related to sexuality and whether his identification is stable, ambivalent, questioning, or shifting at this time.

B. Assess the past and present environments that are influencing Eric's comfort with his sexual identification including opportunities or barriers within the school environment, family relationships, social relationships, and level of access to information and resources.

C. Assess the potential benefits there might be if Eric comes out at this time as a sexual person and which aspects of Eric's world might benefit the most from coming out considering

      his personal identity, family relationships, peer relation-
ships, educational relationships, and safety within the
neighborhood he lives in.

D. Assess the potential costs there might be if Eric comes out at
this time as a sexual person and which aspects of Eric's
world might be most at risk to the "coming out" process
considering his personal identity, family relationships, peer
relationships, educational relationships, and safety in his
neighborhood.

E. Considering your assessment of potential costs and benefits
from Parts C–D, how strong are the real-world constraints
on Eric fully exploring his sexuality at this time?

F. Assess whether Eric needs to find a common ground
between his sexual identity and other aspects of his identity
such as his identity as a student or family member and consider how to connect him with resources and decrease barriers to this process.

G. Assess whether any aspects of your identity or your treatment approach might lead to negative bias, marginalization,
or invalidation of Eric's sexual identity or minimize the
potential negative impact of societal homophobia on Eric's
well-being and consider what can be done to increase the likelihood of a positive outcome (be thoughtful and detailed).

Exercise 4 (6-page maximum)

GOAL: To help you integrate your knowledge of cognitive
theory and issues relevant to sexual orientation into an
in-depth conceptualization of Eric (who he is and why he
does what he does).

STYLE: An integrated essay consisting of a premise, supportive
details, and conclusions following a carefully planned
organizational style.

NEED HELP? Review Chapter 1 (pages 7–28) and Chapter 2 (pages
73–78).

             STEP 1: Consider what style you could use for organizing your
cognitive understanding of Eric that (a) would support you in
providing a comprehensive and clear understanding of his

beliefs, self-talk, attributions, perceptions, and expectations and (b) would support language that he might find persuasive in his current state of desperation.

STEP 2: Develop your concise premise (overview, preliminary or explanatory statements, proposition, thesis statement, theory-driven introduction, hypotheses, summary, concluding causal statements) that explains Eric's overall level of functioning as an individual who is struggling to understand his sexuality amidst family chaos. If you're having trouble with Step 2, remember it should be an integration of the key ideas of Exercises 2 and 3 that (a) provides a basis for Eric's long-term goals, (b) is grounded in cognitive theory and is sensitive to sexual orientation issues, and (c) highlights the strengths he brings to cognitive treatment whenever possible.

STEP 3: Develop your supporting material (detailed case analysis of strengths and weaknesses, supplying data to support an introductory premise) from a cognitive perspective that integrates an in-depth understanding of Eric, a homophobic teen. If you're having trouble with Step 3, consider the information you'll need to include in order to (a) support the development of short-term goals, (b) be grounded in cognitive theory and sensitive to sexual orientation issues, and (c) integrate an understanding of Eric's strengths in analyzing his beliefs and self-talk.

STEP 4: Develop your conclusions and broad treatment recommendations including (a) Eric's overall level of functioning, (b) anything facilitating or serving as a barrier to his developing more constructive beliefs at this time, and (c) his basic needs as he evaluates his thinking, being careful to consider what you said in Part G of Exercise 3 (be concise and general).

Exercise 5 (3-page maximum)

GOAL: To develop a theory-driven action plan for Eric that considers his strengths and is sensitive to his sexual orientation issues.

STYLE: A sentence outline consisting of long- and short-term goals.

NEED HELP? Review Chapter 1 (pages 8–28).

STEP 1: Develop your treatment plan overview, being careful to consider what you said in Part G of Exercise 3 to try and prevent any negative bias to your treatment plan.

STEP 2: Develop long-term (major, large, ambitious, comprehensive, broad) goals that *ideally* Eric would reach by the termination of treatment and that would lead to an adaptive worldview and a healthy integration of his sexuality into his identity. If you are having trouble with Step 2, reread your premise and support topic sentences for ideas, paying careful attention to how they could be transformed into goals that are realistic to Eric's needs and situation (use the *style* of Exercise 4).

STEP 3: Develop short-term (small, brief, encapsulated, specific, measurable, subsidiary) goals that Eric and you could expect to see accomplished within a few weeks to chart Eric's progress in learning to analyze, challenge, and replace his maladaptive thoughts, particularly around sexuality; instill hope for change; and plan time-effective treatment sessions. If you are having trouble with Step 3, reread your support paragraphs, looking for ideas to transform into goals that (a) might help Eric hypothesis test about his specific beliefs or replace maladaptive thoughts with adaptive ones, (b) might enhance factors facilitating or decrease factors inhibiting his ability to explore his sexuality at this time, (c) might utilize his strengths in analyzing his life whenever possible, and (d) are individualized to him as a neglected teen rather than generic.

Exercise 6

GOAL: To critique cognitive treatment and the case of Eric.

STYLE: Answer Questions A–E in essay format or discuss them in a group format.

    A. What are the strengths and weaknesses of this model for helping Eric (a teen with sexual orientation issues)?

    B. Consider how taking a cognitive-behavioral perspective, where you help him integrate an understanding of the role of his thoughts with an understanding of his learning history, would change the treatment plan. What modes of learning does Eric seem to use most? What role models have influenced his thoughts and behaviors? Which approach do you consider most valuable to Eric at this time, and why?

    C. Assume that Eric's comments about his mother's boyfriend and his father are understatements and that there are realistic threats to his safety at this time. Considering what you know from the Domain of Violence, what issues must you assess, and what specifically will you do, to encourage the change process without jeopardizing Eric's safety?

D. Considering Eric's family situation and the research on sexual orientation, discuss Eric's current risk for suicide. Are there particular issues you need to assess in more depth to develop an accurate assessment of this? What could happen if his family becomes aware that his treatment with you focuses on issues related to his sexuality? Might this increase or decrease his risk for suicide?

E. What did you learn about your own attitudes toward sexuality and helping teenagers with their sexuality as you were working through the case of Eric?

Recommended Resources

American Institute for Cognitive Therapy. (2003). *What is cognitive therapy?* Retrieved April 8, 2009, from http://www.cognitivetherapynyc.com/default.asp?sid=768

American Psychological Association (Producer) & Beck, J. S. (Trainer). (n.d.). *Cognitive therapy* [Motion picture, #4310736]. (Available from the American Psychological Association, 750 First Street, NE, Washington, DC 20002–4242)

Beck Institute for Cognitive Therapy and Research. (2008). Retrieved April 8, 2009, from http://www.beckinstitute.org/Library/InfoManage/Guide.asp?Folder ID=200&SessionID={1C10428F-9375–4F78–89AF-E9B106C7DD19}

Ingram, B. L. (2006). *Clinical case formulations: Matching the integrative treatment plan to the client* (pp. 191–228). Hoboken, NJ: John Wiley & Sons, Inc.

Sudak, D. M. (2006). *Psychotherapy in clinical practice: Cognitive behavioral therapy for clinicians.* Philadelphia: Lippincott Williams & Wilkins.

Five

Feminist Case Conceptualizations and Treatment Plans

Introduction to Feminist Theory

John is a 56-year-old White male who wants an immediate appointment to discuss a marital problem. He is the chief executive officer (CEO) of an international corporation that has its corporate headquarters across the street from your office in a large, northeastern city. Your office location was his sole reason for choosing you as his clinician. He has been married to 53-year-old Margaret for the last 30 years. He came home from a business trip last week to find that she had moved out of the house. He has only been able to locate her via cell phone, and she has refused to come home. Starting a few days ago, she stopped answering his calls. They have two daughters, Juliet (age 25) and Kimberly (age 22), who recently moved to California. They are starting their own company using trust fund money recently inherited when Margaret's father died.

As a proponent of Empowerment Feminist Therapy (EFT), you recognize the power of the environment, in terms of social and political forces, to shape John's values, expectations, and behaviors within his marriage to Margaret. Your first step will be to help John deepen his understanding of his complex personal and social identities and the roles power, privilege, and oppression play in them. Through consciousness raising, John will recognize that rather than developing his own unique marriage with Margaret, he has been adapting to the status quo and following many unconscious "shoulds" within a socially designed marriage. Socializing forces have led John and Margaret to take on rigid gender roles within their marriage that deny them the right to express themselves as individuals. John's current mindset is that Margaret's behavior is pathological and stems from internal causes such as a psychotic breakdown or midlife crisis. You will help him recognize how differential power, within society and within their marriage, is what is actually behind Margaret's current behavior. She has been actively discriminated against, oppressed, and denied opportunities for expressing herself as a unique individual and setting her own unique life goals. While John will not be blamed for Margaret's distress, as he, like her, has been shaped by external pressures, he will come to recognize that to have a healthy marriage, he must work to develop an egalitarian relationship with Margaret in which her values as a woman are respected (Worell & Remer, 2003).

Who is John? While he may view himself primarily as a successful businessman, in fact, according to the first principle of EFT, he has multiple social and personal identities that are interdependent and that, taken together, serve to define him (Worell & Remer, 2003). Each of his identities may be more or less salient to John depending on the time period and the social context. You will help John become consciously aware of this complex matrix of personal and social identities that together govern his thoughts, feelings, behaviors, and values within different aspects of his life. How these identities may support his strengths, as well as contribute to his current difficulties, will be considered in depth. Each carries with it a potential "seat of advantage" within the dominant society where John experiences privilege or a potential "seat of oppression" where John might have experiences that deny him power or freedom of choice (Worell & Remer, 2003, p. 58). Power is intrinsic to all relationships. The person with more power in a relationship experiences more privilege. For example, as the CEO of a company, John has the most power. This means he has the ability to decide when a meeting should be held, what the agenda should be, and who at the meeting will be assigned what tasks to do. He could make fair or unjust decisions. Other people at the meeting are in a one-down position relative to him and, depending on what John does, may be treated with respect and fairness or may experience oppression.

A gendered, social order promotes the myth that men and women are fundamentally different from each other and that individuals within each gender are highly similar to each other; thus gender homogenization is made to seem natural and healthy, and anyone who departs from rigid gender roles is pathologized. Sexist society has determined that males have more privilege than females within the institutions of society, including the institution of marriage. Thus, women are oppressed within marriage in a parallel manner to how they are oppressed within public institutions. For example, society has given John, as a husband, more power than Margaret, as a wife. This illustrates the second principle of EFT, "the personal is political"; the same oppression that exists in society also exists in personal relationships (Worell & Remer, 2003, p. 6). In treatment, John's consciousness will be raised so that he can recognize how traditional sex role stereotypes homogenize people by gender. Men are socialized into the role of breadwinner, and women are socialized into the role of caretaker of home and children. Even within her role as caretaker of the home, Margaret still has to defer to John on important family decisions. Men are allowed to pursue their own personal goals, as long as they earn money, and they are free to use direct power in their relationships. For example, John can directly tell Margaret what to do, such as prepare a party for his business colleagues. Margaret has been placed in a subordinate role and is expected to support John's goals. As subordinates, women may have only indirect methods of gaining power, such as through manipulating, rather than asking, men to do what they want (Worell & Remer, 2003). Women are expected to become attuned to the moods of their husbands and adapt their behavior accordingly. They pick what to fight about, and when, in an effort to keep their marriage secure (Goodrich, 2008). Thus, if Margaret is sick and doesn't want to prepare for a party, she might suggest that the weather is predicted to be better next week and mention that she knows how much John likes to grill outside at parties. She doesn't directly express her needs. She couches her needs within a framework John might find motivating. John and Margaret are likely to view their behavior as guided by personal choice. However, through consciousness raising they could learn to recognize the influence of gender role socialization and institutionalized sexism on their functioning and consider the value of living a more androgynous lifestyle.

What is needed for a healthy marriage? According to the third principle of EFT, egalitarian relationships foster healthy thoughts, emotions, and behaviors. While John's genuine strengths will be supported and prized, all of his oppressive thoughts, feelings, and actions will be explored for their impact on others. Treatment would seek to transform the hierarchical, power-imbalanced relationship between John and Margaret into an egalitarian one in which both partners could thrive as individuals. John will have to take responsibility for his oppressive behavior within and outside the marriage; however, social pressures will work against this change from the status quo. John will need to be aware of these pressures and take responsibility for resisting them within his personal identities, as well as, ideally, within his social identities. He will be encouraged to use the knowledge he gains in treatment to become an agent of positive social change in his personal, social, and work relationships.

Society has encouraged John and Margaret to take on gendered perspectives. In addition, it has socialized them to believe that male values are superior to female. John will be encouraged to throw off this bias and treat Margaret's perspective as equal to his own. The mindset that "women's perspectives are valued in addition to men's" represents the final principle of EFT (Worell & Remer, 2003, p. 73). From a male point of view, meaning is constructed out of life through wielding power in the workplace. It is important to be a leader and take initiative in setting the agenda and solving problems. To be successful at taking on this role, men are taught to value independence and emotional detachment; it is assumed that emotional detachment is needed for logical decision making. From a female point of view, meaning is constructed through nurturing others and building emotional attachments. Society encourages women to develop an expressive orientation to the world where warmth, nurturance, kindness, and a concern for the welfare of others are paramount over competition in the workplace. Yet, society devalues women who are successful at taking on this role, treating their achievements as if they were commonplace (American Psychological Association, 2006; Worell & Remer, 2003). The devaluation of women may occur overtly or subtly. In society, John's opinion might be taken over Margaret's at a parent-teacher conference. In the home, John may override Margaret's economic choices whenever she disagrees with him, citing his greater business savvy. Or, John might just grimace when Margaret makes a suggestion about finances. Even subtle slights have been found, when they are repetitive, to undermine the self-esteem and emotional well-being of women (Goodrich, 2008). To have a just society, the achievements of men and women must be given equal respect. To improve their marriage, John will need to listen to Margaret and treat her perspective as valuable; Margaret will need to do the same for John.

Treatment will empower John to view himself as a human being who can freely choose what behaviors and attitudes are most relevant to him within each specific situation in which he finds himself; he will no longer be a gendered male who must fit neatly into a prescribed identity.

Role of the Clinician

How will you help John? You will actively use a variety of techniques that challenge John to consider a fuller range of choices in how to act, think, and feel as an individual rather than as a gendered self. The first step will be to work toward an egalitarian relationship with him. While a truly egalitarian relationship is more of an ideal than a reality, as John is here for help and you are here to help him, there are two major strategies you can use to establish a collaborative relationship. The first strategy is to discuss, with John, the values embedded in EFT. It is important to demystify the treatment process so that he is an educated consumer. John should be educated about the theory and the techniques that are available to help him. After an initial session, John will be given the opportunity to provide you with feedback about the session and whether he feels that you and EFT can help him.

You will also make selective self-disclosures when you feel these will help him understand his experiences more fully. You will make self-involving statements with John that show him your emotional responses to what he is saying and doing. Empathy, nurturance, and mutual respect will be modeled, as will a nonblaming attitude. You will actively explore John's strengths and encourage him to value his selfhood at the same time as you will discourage any of his oppressive thoughts, feelings, and behaviors. Finally, John will be treated as the expert on his experiences.

In addition to building a collaborative relationship, you will help John identify each of his personal and social identities. Within each, you will help him identify how much, and what type, of privilege he experiences and how much, and in what ways, he is oppressed in any of them. He will then identify which of his many identities are most salient to him at this time and how they may be influenced by sex role socialization and environmental pressures. He will be educated as to how interdependent his identities are and how together they give him a sense of who he is.

What will you do next? Feminist clinicians can choose from the myriad of treatment techniques to use with John as long as they aren't inconsistent with the principles of EFT. Commonly used techniques include reframing and relabeling, cultural analysis, bibliotherapy, assertiveness training, consciousness raising, gender role analysis, and power analysis; the last two techniques are unique to feminist treatment.

If you use the technique of reframing, you're shifting John's definition of his problem. This will usually involve changing an intrapersonal definition of the problem to one in which interpersonal, social, or political pressures are suggested as causative. You might help John see how Margaret's problems are not caused by something internal, such as being menopausal. Rather, they are caused by her lifelong experiences of being homogenized and devalued as an individual.

In relabeling, you take something that the client has viewed with a negative lens and relabel it using a positive lens or vice versa. You might relabel John's "marital crisis" as a "life opportunity." This might get John to examine his situation from a different perspective and may open up the possibility of him trying new solutions.

In a cultural analysis, you will help John see how his White culture has provided him with a context for understanding his presenting concerns. The definition his cultural group gives for understanding marital problems will be explored along with any cultural myths that may exist relevant to these problems. This will include an analysis of how the very language or labels typically used by White culture to describe his marital problems will suggest intrapersonal causality and personal blame, such as that Margaret is suffering from "the empty nest syndrome." He will be educated about the incidence rate of his problems within White culture. Through understanding the full power of the cultural context in which his difficulties are embedded, he will come to see how the pressures from his White culture played an important role in "causing" his marital problems.

In bibliotherapy, John will be encouraged to read articles and books that are relevant to helping him understand his marital problems and the cultural context in which they are embedded. He will engage in a dialogue with you about what he is learning. This will help him become more aware of experiences he is having that are a result of privilege or oppression.

In assertiveness training, John will learn how to stand up for his own rights without trampling the rights of other people. This might be a particularly valuable treatment option for John. In the past, he has always expressed his needs and wishes through the exertion of power; this has led to the oppression of others. Consciousness raising is a significant part of assertiveness training and can be done individually or in groups. The intent is to help John become aware of how gender role socialization has encouraged men to use domination and control to get what they want without regard for the needs and wishes of others; thus John is following the path in his marriage that men have been socialized to take.

Men and women may differ in their thoughts, feelings, and actions, but these differences are caused by socialization pressures, not biology. In gender role analysis, John will be helped to see how men and women have been socialized differently and how this is the direct cause of their differences. How gendered expectations for males may have helped or hindered his development will be discussed. This will include helping him identify both direct and indirect messages and pressures he has experienced to fulfill specific gender role tasks and to experience things in a gender-prescribed manner. He will be taught skills for breaking free of these gendered pressures so he can think, feel, and behave in ways that support his uniqueness as an individual.

Finally, in a power analysis, John will be made aware of the types of power that exist and the differential power that exists between groups. For example, society has been structured to give men more power than women, Whites more power than people of color, wealthy people more power than the poor, physically able people more power than people with disabilities, and so forth. Power can be exerted either directly or indirectly. Being male and having access to personal resources such as accumulated wealth, possessions, and high-quality health care make John highly privileged and thus give him access to a great deal of power. People who are privileged are free to use direct power strategies. Less privileged people must rely on more indirect strategies to get what they need. John will be encouraged to explore both the direct and the indirect ways he has expressed power over other people. Rather than controlling others, John will be encouraged to develop egalitarian relationships and use constructive power, which is the power to create personal or external change.

The treatment process will be considered effective when John has become empowered to recognize external causes of stress and respond effectively to them, have an increased resilience in the face of stress, thrive within his social and personal spheres, and work to end oppressive practices against others. Feminist treatment attempts to foster a more just society. Thus, the deepest form of change would occur if John worked to end sexism on a social level.

Case Application: Integrating the Domain of Race and Ethnicity

John's case will now be examined in further detail. While there are many domains of human complexity that could provide insights into his behavior, the Domain of Race and Ethnicity has been selected to integrate within a feminist case conceptualization and treatment plan.

Interview With John (J) From a Feminist Perspective

C: I understand that your wife has suddenly left you, and this is what you want help with.

J: (tensely) Yes. I'm probably wasting time, but I'm out of ideas for fixing things.

C: You sound angry.

J: (angrily) I'm feeling trapped. My wife has me in a vice. She won't return my calls. My daughters deny they know what's going on. I'm stuck with being here.

C: You're angry and stuck without a good option. Choices are important. If at any time you are dissatisfied with what is going on with me, I want you to bring it up. If you decide not to see me again, I will help you locate someone else if you want me to.

J: (calmly) Fair enough. You need to understand that I must get this problem under control by the end of next week when I'm leaving the country to complete crucial business.

C: Time keeps coming up. You really value it and don't want to waste any of it.

J: (surprisedly) Doesn't everyone?

C: It seems normal to you. Part of the business culture is to have a huge respect for time and to feel pressure never to waste it. You say the business deal is crucial. That sounds like there is a great deal of work pressure on you right now.

J: (impatiently) Of course I'm under pressure. I'm the CEO. Closing deals like this is my job.

C: I can hear how powerful and successful you are at closing business deals. But, on the phone, you said you're confused about why your wife left. (long pause) Do you expect that you can resolve the problem in 2 weeks?

J: (angrily, changing subject) Margaret left me suddenly, (emphatically) and she won't answer my calls. I need more data to figure this thing out.

C: The suddenness of it is shocking. (long pause) You want more information, but she won't talk to you. (pause) Has she ever done this before?

J: (frustratedly, changing subject again) I've given Margaret everything. She has a beautiful home, a closet full of gorgeous clothes, memberships in exclusive clubs.

C: John, you may not realize it, but twice now, I've asked you a question and you've changed the subject. What do you think this means?

J: (emphatically) I gave you information that was more relevant.

C: You are a leader at work. You set the agenda of what is important and what isn't. (J nods) But, this isn't your office, and we aren't engaged in a business deal. Might I know anything about what is relevant to discuss?

J: (emphatically) I need you to understand that this deal is not just a deal. It's "THE DEAL." Margaret and I have been working for this since we graduated from college.

C: It's been the goal of your life, and you're assuming it was Margaret's too. Did you ever discuss this with her?

J: (irritably) We didn't have a meeting about it, if that's what you're asking. This is our marriage; she knew what she was signing on for.

C: You're sounding like a CEO, not a husband. That's a very important part of your identity. But, I think we need to explore your husband role more. Society pushes all of us to accept stereotypical and gender-typed behavior. As a man, you were under a lot of pressure to put your work first and leave the home front to Margaret. Do you think she wanted that?

J: (reflectively) I met Margaret at college; she had a clear head. She was analytical, ambitious, and busy planning her own future in the business world. Of course, once we married, she got pregnant and needed to stay home. It took her time, but she came to excel at it.

C: You and Margaret both had business aspirations. But, you also shared expectations that getting married meant her ambitions needed to change but yours didn't. This is typical. We fulfill society's expectations, not necessarily our own.

J: (hostilely) Are you trying to tell me Margaret didn't want to put our family life first?

C: Society encourages men to be ambitious and make a success of making money using their unique talents and abilities. Women are homogenized as if they are all the same and should all want to channel their energies exclusively into family life. Some find this satisfying; others do not. You suggested that, at least at first, Margaret might not have been happy with making this shift in her ambitions.

J: Both my mother and hers helped her adjust. She has been great at it for the last 30 years. Now she's just cutting herself off—right when I'm at the peak of my success. (scornfully) My golf foursome thinks she's just gone menopausal. Could that be it?

C: She might've started going through menopause. Stop and think about what you just said from Margaret's point of view. She's taken the very serious step of moving out. Yet, your golf buddies are trivializing it as if it's unimportant and irrational.

J: (insistently) Well, women do go through menopause and get too emotional. I need to help her get back on a rational track, but she won't return my phone calls.

C: Society puts a lot of pressure on men to be analytical and logical. But, it really isn't logical for human beings to discount feelings. Feelings are very powerful and have a big influence on people. I'd like to help you seriously consider Margaret's point of view about the health of your marriage.

J: (angrily) My marriage is fine!

C: If you really thought that, you wouldn't be here. (J looks down) It's OK to be angry and confused. You're on uncharted ground. Is it possible that Margaret left when you were out of the country and avoids your calls in order to avoid giving you the opportunity to make her serious decision seem stupid and unimportant?

J: (hostilely) It's ironic. She's avoiding my calls after years of complaining I didn't call enough.

C: You were aware that she was dissatisfied.

J: (dismissively) I knew she was lonely sometimes, but she needed to adjust to it. I was on the fast track, and she benefited from it as much as I did.

C: You're very ambitious and successful. Society has rewarded you with status and money. Your expectations for life as an adult have been met. You were the CEO, both at work and at home. It sounds like Margaret was like one of your subordinates, needing to adjust her expectations and goals to fit in with yours

J: (insistently) She needed to be a wife and mother if that's what you're talking about. (pause) Maybe Margaret has that empty nest syndrome?

C: Blaming Margaret's behavior on some cause that's internal to her would feel good to you right now. (pause) She may have found taking care of the home and the girls satisfying when your daughters were children. She might be sad or anxious now that her "nest" is empty. On the other hand, societal pressures for her to only be a wife and mom, rather than that ambitious student you met, may have decreased since your daughters became adults. She may be reconnecting with her own individual ambitions.

J: (frustratedly) What is this social pressure you keep bringing up?

C: You both grew up in a White, upper-class culture that emphasized the importance of money and status. You and Margaret were raised to share similar expectations for how wives and husbands should behave. When Margaret was struggling with this, society, in the forms of her mother and yours, pressured her to make herself fit into the role of the wife of a successful man.

J: (angrily but quietly) I don't like your suggestion that I've been forcing anything on her. Sure, her original plans were to start a business, but I allowed her total control of the house and the girls.

C: These socialization messages are ingrained so deeply that you are just confused and angry to consider that Margaret might have wanted something else than what she got. From your position, as the leader of your family, everything was going smoothly according to your plan. You are angry that your wife is rejecting the plan.

J: (furiously) You bet I'm angry. You can't even begin to imagine the time I've put in, the ideas I've had to generate, and the crises I've had to resolve in order to make my company as strong as it is. Margaret knew I was going to be out of the country to orchestrate a new deal, and while my back was turned, she pulled this power play on me.

C: After all of your hard work, ingenuity, and success, you have come to expect that everyone, including Margaret, will treat you with deference, and you're feeling infuriated, right now, by what you feel is her disrespectful behavior.

J: (angrily) I have a right to respect!

C: Was Margaret leaving when you were gone a mark of disrespect, or was it a sign that she did in fact know how powerful you are? Maybe, she only had enough power of her own to leave if you were absent. .

J: (hostilely) She should have faced me with this. What she did was very cowardly. I always faced my bosses whenever I was moving on to another job.

C: Whenever we begin to talk of you and Margaret as husband and wife, your business role of CEO keeps coming up. This identity is so salient to you it pervades every aspect of your life.

J: (argumentatively) Are you telling me it's wrong to be a leader?

C: I'm trying to tell you that there are a lot of social and political forces bearing in on each of us that we aren't consciously aware of but that strongly influence us. They are pressuring you to put work first and take control in relationships. I want you to be consciously aware of all these influences. Then, you have the freedom to make your own unique choices apart from the stereotype of male success.

J: (furiously) I can make any choices I want!

C: You do have a lot of privilege. You are a powerful businessman. (J looks calmer) As wealthy, White Protestants, you and Margaret can live in any neighborhood you choose. You have money for buying beautiful possessions and can afford quality health care and so on. One thing you don't seem to have is time. (long pause) Work is pressuring you to leave the country in 2 weeks. If losing Margaret is a crisis for you, does work have the right to pressure you to take only 2 weeks to try to resolve such a serious situation? You've always given so much to work. Shouldn't it be possible to delay this trip so that you can focus on your marriage?

J: (furiously) If I delay the trip, the deal is off.

C: The CEO part of you says take the trip. What about Margaret's husband? Do people at work ever have the choice to give a family crisis top priority?

J: (long pause, reflectively) Most of the men I know are divorced, sometimes from marriages 2 and 3.

C: How would you feel if divorce papers were waiting for you after the trip?

J: (quietly) I would be angry at Margaret for forcing it on me.

C: You look more sad than angry as you say that.

J: (furiously) Don't try to push that emotional crap on me that it's good for men to cry.

C: You certainly seem angry now. Society pressures men to ignore their feelings of depression or anxiety. Only anger is considered manly, so sometimes men express anger instead. That's not logical or natural. Humans, both male and female, have a variety of emotions. They're real, and they have a potent impact on human relationships.

J: (intently) I don't want a divorce, but you can't tell me to blow off this deal.

C: I don't tell people what to do. We are collaborating. You're bringing your strengths to the table; I am bringing mine. You have highly developed strategy skills. (pause) But, I'm wondering if you were taught that if you related to people on an emotional level, it would impede your success as a man.

J: My father trained me well if that's what you mean.

C: What did your father tell you being a man meant?

J: He showed me more than told me. He was very busy. I wanted to see him more than I did, so I tended to listen in on a lot of his phone conversations when he was at home. He didn't stop me as long as I didn't interrupt. I come from a long line of successful businessmen; it's instinctual, inborn.

C: It feels natural. Like you automatically knew it, but you were taught. He taught just by letting you listen in on his phone conversations. But, what did it feel like, as a son, having him at home but having him thinking about work and not the family?

J: (confusedly) I don't know. What kind of question is that? Dad did what he had to do. I knew what I needed to do. My part was to get the most out of my education so I would be ready for success. I worked really hard at school to show him I could do it. He bought me a car when I was valedictorian of my high school class—his note said this was a family tradition. (pause) But, I wished he had shown up at graduation. (pause) His absence really infuriated my mother.

C: How did you know?

J: (dismissively) She embarrassed the family by drinking too much at my graduation party.

C: She was in a lot of pain, and she drank too much to dampen it. What do you think she should have done?

J: (matter-of-factly) Just accept it. Dad was always going to put work first; it was necessary. He would have made it up to her with a present—usually jewelry. She needed to be happy with that.

C: He showed that he cared by buying her beautiful things. You learned to do this for Margaret. You were both trained by society to think that women should be satisfied with what men give them and not ask for anything else.

J: (angrily) You think I'm not being a good husband?

C: I think you are doing everything that you thought a good husband was supposed to do. But, I don't think you recognize how much power and control you were exerting over Margaret. Did you ever ask her if she wanted to continue with her plans to work after graduation? (He shakes his head no) Did you ask if what she wanted from you was lots of money?

J: (angrily) Of course she wanted money. She came from a very wealthy family. She could never have been happy with a dinky little house in the suburbs.

C: Margaret's family background was similar to yours. She had a lot of privilege in terms of money and housing. What she didn't have was the power and control to set her own life goals.

J: (intently) Sacrifices are part of life. I can't remember a week when I didn't have to skip a game of golf or miss out on a party to close a deal.

C: You missed out on things that you would have preferred to do. You were trying to be an excellent provider, and you did provide everything money can buy. (pause) What's your relationship like with your daughters?

J: (intently) I've given them everything they've ever asked for. I sent them to private schools and paid for all their special clubs and activities. I did plan to be around more for them than my dad was for me, but their recitals and events always conflicted with important work.

C: Do you have any intuition about what they might say about their mother moving out?

J: (angrily) Intuition is crap. I need facts and logical reasons for Margaret disappearing. They refuse to answer my questions. I'm their father. I deserve their respect.

C: You expect this, and you feel you aren't getting it. I agree with you that logic is a valuable tool for understanding things, but it only gives you some of the information you might need. Intuition is a way of bringing your emotional experience in to help you with this situation. Could you think about your girls for a moment and see if you have any gut feelings about what they would say about your marriage?

J: (long pause) To be honest, my gut feeling is I don't really know what they would say.

C: Your voice sounds a little sad as you say that. (pause) It is very sad that you didn't achieve your goal of knowing them better than your dad knew you.

J: (long pause, reflectively) I do have some regrets; I can admit that. I'm proud of them. They're very independent. They started a new life far away, not asking for anything from me although the money they inherited when Margaret's dad died 3 months ago sealed the deal.

C: You aren't as proud because they received some money from their grandfather?

J: (emphatically) It would have been a bigger achievement if they had made their own money before inheriting it from the family. That's just my point.

C: Why did they move so far away?

J: (matter-of-factly) I've got no idea. A lot of this happened last month when I was out of state. I don't have many facts to go on. Like Margaret, they just took off.

C: Why don't you take a moment to consider Margaret's feelings and why she might have left while you were away.

J: (long pause, looking down) I guess if Margaret had been home and told me she was going to walk out . . . (long pause) I probably would've told her to forget it because she couldn't make it without me.

C: Would you have listened to her point of view before telling her what to do?

J: (intently) Probably not. I'm feeling very stupid. I should have seen this thing coming.

C: You aren't the least bit stupid. You are an expert at a lot of things but not at recognizing the emotional needs of other people. This is because society didn't take the time to teach you those skills. In fact, your father, and your whole social background, has actively discouraged you from learning them. You could learn them quickly if you wanted to. Would you be willing to try?

J: (sincerely) I don't know. I really want to hear your opinion of why Margaret left.

C: I haven't spoken to Margaret, so I can only take an educated guess. The moment we are born and people see that we are male or female, they treat us as if this defines . . .

J: (interrupting) It does define us.

C: Did you realize you interrupted me? You have done this several times before. This is how you use your power to control the agenda. It makes me wonder if you consider my ideas of any value to you.

J: (pause, sincerely) I do want to know your opinion.

C: Sex defines what we physically look like. However, scientific research has made it clear that men and women are not "opposite sexes." It is society that imposes different expectations and standards for how men and women should behave, and this isn't logical. It restricts what both men and women are allowed to think, feel, and do if they are going to be "good" men and women. Margaret may be trying to figure out what her identity really is rather than living an identity she thinks she should be. If you want to come back, we would work on how you have developed strengths, following the "shoulds" of manhood, and also explore how these "shoulds" may have contributed to your problems with Margaret.

J: (calmly) I need more time to think about this. I don't know if I buy into your ideas.

C: You've made a lot of important decisions by weighing the facts. Let me give you some things to read that will give you more facts about what we've been talking about today. I think you should take as much time as you need to decide, rather than following a schedule dictated by work; decisions about your marriage are vital and deserve careful thought. I will wait to hear from you one way or the other about whether you want to talk with me again.

J: (quietly but emphatically) I won't give up being strong!

C: The goal would be to give you more choices and more strengths.

Feminist Case Conceptualization of John: Assumption-Based Style

John's most prominent identity is that of a CEO; however, his other identities of being White, wealthy, and male are also having a potent impact on him at this time. These identities consume most of his time. In contrast, he has allowed his identities as a husband and father to fall by the wayside. There are no egalitarian relationships in John's life. He wields the same power in his relationships with his wife and daughters that he wields at work with his employees, and he is unaware of this parallel or the injustices that derive from it. His reaction to his wife setting the agenda for his marriage is to demean her thoughts and emotions; only his perspective as a husband is valid. From the perspective of White culture, he is fulfilling his role as a male to perfection—he is powerful, wealthy, analytical, and in control of his emotions. John's strengths include the ability to learn quickly and analyze the pros and cons of a decision. In addition, he has the financial resources to gain greater work flexibility and gain more of that commodity "time" that his White culture has taught him to consider so precious. These will serve him well if he is willing to form an egalitarian treatment relationship that allows him the freedom to explore how powerful socialization messages, rather than "inborn abilities," are playing a role in both his business successes and his personal failures.

John's identity as a CEO is his most salient identity, but how his identity as a White person eased his path to this position goes unrecognized. He considers his success a result of his internal qualities of independence, ambitiousness, and aggressiveness. White culture encouraged him to develop these qualities, but it was the environmental resources of inherited wealth and an excellent education that gave him an entry into the world of financial success. His father directly modeled absolute dedication to work and reinforced the White cultural message that a man's success is measured by the amount of money he earns. Currently, John's business identity thoroughly dominates his personal identities as a husband and a father. He uses business metaphors to try to understand his current family crisis. He has been treating his family members as subordinates, ignoring their wishes and values as if these were irrelevant. He isn't interested in giving up some of his authority in the family so that his wife and daughters will feel more respected. In addition, John hasn't even considered using his professional status and power to change the timing of his upcoming business deal. "Time" has become his dictatorial and oppressive boss, and he has become the loyal subordinate who automatically makes any sacrifice demanded of him. John may have difficulty recognizing that by keeping his personal and social identities so closely aligned, he may lose his family roles as husband and father. Man as head of the family and economic provider is a cultural icon for White Protestants. Thus, John may find it very difficult to recognize how oppressively he has treated Margaret and his daughters and that a different type of family life is possible. However, he has learned to work very hard and persist when trying to solve complex problems within the business world; he could learn to do this within his personal world.

John's identity as a wealthy man is entwined and interdependent with his identity as a member of the White culture. The "Whiteness" exists outside his conscious awareness, but he is very aware of his inherited wealth and considers it a natural part of himself. John started his work career already buoyed up by economic privilege. He passed this privilege on to his daughters by giving them a private school education and membership in exclusive clubs and activities—those that are dominated by Whites. He considers these privileges a result of his hard work and dedication to success, and thus he has the "right" to be treated deferentially. He is unaware that society has given White people and wealthy people unearned privilege that has been systematically denied to people of color and the poor. John's feeling of entitlement was passed down to him, just as his Whiteness and inherited wealth were. He, in his turn, has passed it down to his daughters. The ability they had to start their own business in their 20s is a concrete example of how inherited wealth and white skin have brought John's family a lot of power. They can select high-status employment and relocate to the community of their choice; no neighborhoods or business opportunities will be closed to them. John may be resistant to the idea of developing egalitarian relationships as society has encouraged him to consider himself superior to many other people. He may struggle with the idea that empowering others, through treating their thoughts and feelings with respect, is an issue of social justice. John may also struggle with developing respect for a female perspective on what is important since emotional intimacy doesn't equate with dollars and cents.

John's view of himself as a man entails taking on rigid gender role stereotypes that in many ways had their origins in his White culture. This culture emphasized independence, achievement, and emotional control over nurturance and emotional connection as well as workforce achievements over family achievements. John began learning his gender role through watching his father and mother. They had a hierarchical relationship with his father clearly having the most power. His dad chose when and how he would relate to his family. His mother's only recourse was to dampen her disappointments with alcohol. White culture carries with it the myth of a just society. Thus, if his mother was powerless, she must have deserved it. John regretted his father's frequent absences but came to believe that his father was doing what he had to do—that it was natural for a father to always put work first. His mother was to supply the "impeccable background" of a beautiful home and high-achieving children. Unlike Latino culture where the mothering role carries a great deal of respect, within the White culture his mother's work was unpaid and therefore unimportant. John learned that autonomy (a male value) was more important than emotional connection (a female value). John learned to view his dad's behavior as strong and worth emulating and to treat his mother with condescension. Finally, John came to believe that less powerful family members, children and wives, should appreciate what they are given and adjust to their powerlessness in the family. Thus, while he recognized his mother's unhappiness, John doesn't understand that his father's devaluation of her role as a woman, wife, and mother was the cause of her turning to alcohol, not a weak character. John is not aware that his parents' marriage, and his own with Margaret, faces challenges caused by an oppressive society that tries to enforce gendered behavior patterns. While John is currently relating to family members as a stereotypical male, husband, and father, he recognizes that he has lost something he valued by doing so.

John's view of himself as a husband maintains the same rigid marital pattern that he observed between his parents; this was a common pattern amongst the White and wealthy community he grew up in, and it had a powerful impact on John's expectations. While he was initially attracted to a personally ambitious Margaret, he considered it natural and inevitable that she would take on the homemaker role once they were married. As a wife, Margaret was given access to any resources that money could buy except power within her relationship with John or the freedom to choose her own life goals. To be a successful husband, John was socialized to believe he must supply a lot of money and possessions; he assumed Margaret preferred this to time with him. This led him to work very long hours and bring work home. Margaret was often psychologically, if not physically, alone. Margaret succumbed for many years to taking on the role prescribed by her gender, under pressure from John, her own mother, and his.

Now, he is both puzzled and confused by his sudden loss of power in their marital relationship. John had been unwilling to seek out help for these marital problems as they were building up over years; this is in keeping with his White cultural beliefs in extreme independence and self-sufficiency. However, Margaret's act of desertion was too dramatic to be ignored. Why she left is unknown; however, the money Margaret inherited from her father gave her access to money that John couldn't control. She may have finally felt capable of exerting power to control her own destiny. Margaret's identity as an independent woman may have become more salient, and she may be pursuing goals relevant to her past wishes to enter the business world. If she believed John would respect and value her viewpoint, she might not have left abruptly without attempting to negotiate a more satisfying and perhaps egalitarian relationship with him. While John doesn't want to give up his greater authority within the family, he doesn't want a divorce; this may serve as an opening to his developing a less oppressive relationship with Margaret.

What about John's identity as a father? John is only vaguely aware that he didn't make good on the promise he made to himself—to be around more for his daughters than his father was for him. He couldn't find the type of balance between his personal and work identities that would have allowed him to know his daughters better, and he does regret this; it is unlikely that there was anything in his White business community or White, affluent neighborhood to guide him in achieving such a balance. His daughters did learn many of the life lessons he values; they pursued higher education, and they are currently valuing business success over family life. Their choice to leave the East Coast and build their company out in California may be an indirect exertion of power. They may need physical distance between themselves and their dad to maintain a sense of control over their own lives. They may be following John's example and allowing their work identities to dominate their lives. If so, they may be identifying with the male perspective and placing more value on financial success than on developing emotionally intimate relationships. The social pressures, within their White community, may have led them to believe this was a choice they "had" to make. John is torn between pride in their achievements and confusion as to why they're making choices independent of his influence; he may not have experienced this type of internal struggle if these were his sons rather than his daughters. In a reciprocal fashion, rigid gender roles may be limiting the quality of the relationship between John and his daughters. John's vague dissatisfaction with his fathering may serve as an opening for him to reconsider his devaluation of the female perspective.

John might find a new role, that of a client in treatment, difficult to embrace as in many ways this role is counter to the values that White, male, Protestant society has taught him. However, through the course of his first appointment he did not walk out when he wasn't allowed to be in charge of the session. He didn't refuse to come back when it became clear he would have to take responsibility for his own role in his marital difficulties, as well as consider the role societal pressures may have played in it. John has noticed that many of his successful White peers have had more than one marriage fail; he doesn't want to follow this pattern. In addition, he is a highly skilled learner who enjoys being challenged by complex problems. Thus, while he is currently still on the fence about changing, should he commit to treatment, it won't take long for him to recognize that a clash between the male and female perspective is at the root of his current marital crisis. The time may be right for John to take on a new challenge, that of being a more androgynous male.

John, as a family man who is a CEO, is struggling to decide if his goals of salvaging his marriage and understanding his daughters are important enough to overcome his desire to close another business deal. This decision is causing him significant emotional distress because his White cultural background and status, as a successful CEO, bring with them powerful environmental pressures to maintain the status quo. He has been brought up to be "a man" and regard expressing emotions and sharing power as weaknesses; yet, these are the very skills that might help him build bridges to Margaret and his daughters. However, his highly developed problem-solving skills, learned on the business front, may motivate him to want to have this same edge on the home front, thus opening up some willingness to consider learning new skills. John hasn't developed the skills needed to be attuned and responsive to the needs of others because society has not helped him develop these skills. This may be why his marital problems are currently hitting him like a ton of bricks. John is at an important choice point within his social identities; he needs to decide if developing more emotionally connected relationships with Margaret and his daughters is "worth his time."

Feminist Treatment Plan: Assumption-Based Style

Treatment Plan Overview. John's White cultural background has reinforced his oppressive use of power within all his relationships; thus, becoming aware of this will come first. Then, the identities that are most salient to him right now, those of being male, a CEO, and from a wealthy background, will be addressed simultaneously. The plan will follow the *basic format.*

LONG-TERM GOAL 1: John will examine how his social identity as a White person was shaped by socialization forces and consider the ways it has brought him privilege, as well as prevented him from engaging in thoughts, feelings, and actions that would have helped him develop mutually satisfying relationships with White and non-White individuals.

Short-Term Goals

1. John will take notes on his role as a White individual both as a member of the community where he resides and on his international trips.
   a. He will read materials on "White" as a race and consider the validity of this within his note taking.
   b. He will discuss his notes, within the treatment session, and consider the pros and cons of being consciously aware of his Whiteness rather than having it influence his thoughts and actions on an automatic level.

2. John will explore his thoughts, feelings, and actions as he relates to non-White individuals and whether these differ when he is relating with White individuals.
   a. In treatment sessions, he will discuss his recent interactions with White and non-White people.
   b. He will explore how White culture has pressured and continues to pressure him to relate to people differently based on skin color.

3. John will discuss the justice of his unearned privilege based on being White and how he may or may not have used this privilege to intentionally or unintentionally oppress non-White individuals or businesses and consider making them more egalitarian.

LONG-TERM GOAL 2: John will examine how his social identity as a male was shaped by rigid gender role socialization and how his gender has brought him privilege, as well as limited his choices in developing a mutually satisfying relationship with Margaret.

Short-Term Goals

1. John will read literature on gender role stereotypes and then analyze his behavior, for a week, as he relates to men and women and come to tentative conclusions about the validity of gender stereotypes for his own values, attitudes, emotions, and behavior.

2. John will consider his childhood and analyze what socialization pressures from his family, his community, and the media might have shaped his current gender role and gendered expectations about marriage and family life.

3. John will discuss, in sessions, the way his being male has given him a privileged or dominant relationship to women and in what ways taking on this role has limited his freedom of choice in relating to his wife, Margaret, and his daughters.

4. John will read articles about relationship-building skills and use his analytic skills to determine which skills might be useful as he attempts to develop an egalitarian relationship with Margaret and his daughters.

LONG-TERM GOAL 3: John will examine how his social identity as a CEO was shaped by socialization forces and the ways this has brought him privilege and financial success while at the same time reducing his success as a husband and father.

Short-Term Goals

1. John will observe interactions between the president, vice presidents, and department heads of his company over the course of a week, and he will take notes on their communication styles and the direct and indirect uses of power he witnesses.

2. John will compare his behavior toward subordinates at work with his past behavior toward Margaret and his daughters.

3. John will use role-plays to practice different relationship skills and then decide which skills he would like to try in reconnecting with Margaret and those he would like to try in reconnecting with his daughters.

LONG-TERM GOAL 4: John will examine how his primary social identity as a wealthy individual was shaped by socialization forces and the ways this has brought him privilege as well as prevented him from engaging in egalitarian and mutually satisfying relationships with Margaret and his daughters.

Short-Term Goals

1. John will read articles about the history of wealth accumulation in the United States and create a new family biography based on this to discuss within treatment sessions.

2. John will create a history of his own accomplishments on a timeline and consider the role of inherited wealth in these accomplishments.

3. John will create a strengths-and-weaknesses chart and then evaluate the role that unearned privilege versus earned privilege played in each strength and weakness.

4. John will consider what values, attitudes, emotions, and behaviors support him in experiencing success within his work and family identities without oppressing others.

Practice Case for Student Conceptualization: Integrating the Domain of Socioeconomic Status

It is time to use Empowerment Feminist Therapy to do an analysis of Sharon. Within this analysis, you are asked to integrate the Domain of Socioeconomic Status into your case conceptualization and treatment plan.

Information Received From Brief Intake

Sharon is a 34-year-old White female living in a small city set within a large rural county. She has currently been married for 1 year. This is her second marriage. Her first marriage lasted for 10 years and ended in divorce due to her husband's long-term alcohol abuse. She has two children with her first husband, Adrian, age 10, and Susie, age 8. Sharon and her children lived alone for a year before she began dating Edward, her second husband. They married after 6 months of dating. Edward is the regional manager of a large bank, and Sharon is the manager of one of these banks. She was referred by her internist due to losing weight steadily over the past year and exhibiting signs of anxiety and depression.

During a brief mental status exam, Sharon expressed significant anger over her physician's referral for treatment; however, out of respect for him, she agreed to come. Sharon showed no signs of homicidal or suicidal ideation or serious pathology. She repeatedly insisted she was happily married and excited by her work at the bank.

Interview With Sharon (S) From a Feminist Perspective

C: Would you like to start by talking about your work at the bank?

S: (earnestly) I love my work at the bank. I had been a stay-at-home mom. I love my kids, but it feels very exhilarating to have responsibilities that test my limits.

C: You love it because you are intellectually challenged. (pause) Can you tell me more?

S: (smiling) I started as a teller, and I was petrified my first week on the job. But, I was amazed how easily I took to the whole banking process. I began studying on my own, and the manager noticed my work and promoted me for the first time. (excitedly) It really felt thrilling to have my work acknowledged.

C: I can see the pleasure in your face when you talk about this. It feels good to me too when people recognize my efforts.

S: (smiling) It was just the start of an exciting ride. The bank helped pay for me to go to college part-time. I loved the university setting and taking courses. Once I got my degree, I was promoted again first to assistant manager and now to manager.

C: Your hard work and top skills were appreciated . . . (S starts frowning) What's wrong?

S: (dismissively) It's not a big deal. Most people did recognize my skills, but I was just thinking about some rumors that started circulating since I was promoted last year.

C: Can you tell me about them?

S: (angrily) I have been accused of sleeping my way to the top. It's because Edward and I were married around the time of my last promotion. I met Edward at church. I only found out once we started dating that he was the regional manager. He had been promoted a few weeks before from a bank 2 hours away; we had never met!

C: Edward had nothing to do with your promotion. You deserved it and deserve to feel good about it. Unfortunately, there is still a lot of sexism in our country that tends to invalidate the achievements of women.

S: I think it was just spiteful people at my office. I don't believe feminist nonsense.

C: You know what happened in your office, and of course, I don't. However, government statistics show men earn more, at every job classification, than women. It's possible that understanding what's happening to women in general could enhance your understanding of what's happening to you now.

S: (irritably) I don't mean to contradict you, but Edward and I feel very strongly that we live in a country of equal opportunity. He isn't going to want me coming in here if you are going to be indoctrinating me with propaganda.

C: You can contradict me whenever you want to. I would never want to indoctrinate you into anything. I do have a treatment philosophy that influences everything I do. I believe that men and women should be treated equally and accorded the same respect for their efforts.

S: (sincerely) Well, I agree with that. I just don't want to be told what to think.

C: I can understand that. Since you enjoyed your time at the university so much, I wonder if you'd like to take out some of the books that I have on this subject. You could read the federal statistics and come to your own conclusions.

S: (sincerely) I think I would enjoy that. But, what if I don't agree with you?

C: You can tell me what you don't agree with, and we can discuss it. If you find that my treatment philosophy is wrong for you, I have a list of the other clinicians in our community that you can use to find someone you would feel comfortable with.

S: (intently) You say I can disagree. I need to know you mean it. I want you to tell me what you're thinking since I said your beliefs were feminist nonsense.

C: I don't agree that it's nonsense, but we don't have to agree on everything. I am very impressed with how you have educated yourself, learned banking, and raised two children at the same time. You don't need me or anyone else to tell you what to think.

S: (matter-of-factly) Good. For a start, my life is just great right now. Work is going great; the rumors are just irritating; there is no point in talking about them further.

C: What does seem worth discussing?

S: (looking anxious) I'm worried about my kids. They are having a hard time adjusting to my new marriage. Even when I was married to their father, it was really just them and me—their dad took a hands-off approach to child rearing. Edward is very different. He has rules, and Adrian and Susie are having trouble adjusting.

C: Did Edward discuss these rules with you?

S: (intently) No. He started from Day 1. I really appreciate his efforts; however, he is older than I am and lived a long time without children. He doesn't realize that I know a lot more than he does about children. He expects too much.

C: Have you discussed this with him?

S: (earnestly) What I enjoy so much about our relationship is that we can share our interest in finance. Even at home, we tend to talk about banking business. I periodically raise the issue of the children, but it seems we get quickly back to business. He really appreciates having a partner who shares his work interests.

C: Even as a couple at home, it is your work identities that are most important.

S: (confusedly) I don't understand what you mean.

C: Everyone has many identities that define who they are. For example, you are a bank manager, a newlywed, a mother. Each of these identities is interdependent with the others. It sounds like even when you are in your wife role, your banking skills come to play. Each identity carries with it a certain level of power or oppression in relationships with other people. At work, you are the manager. All the other people at the bank are your subordinates. So, you have more power than they do to decide how the bank should be conducted.

S: (defensively) Well, I worked hard to be in a position of authority.

C: You did work hard, and you deserved your position. I'm trying to point out that your position brings with it power and control to make things happen at the bank. On the other hand, Edward, as the regional manager, has still more power than you.

S: (sincerely) Yes, of course that's true.

C: If you talk about work, even when you're at home, he is still in a position of greater power. Does Edward ever feel more like your boss than your husband? (S looks confused) You said whenever you bring up the children, he changes the topic back to work. Bosses set the topic with subordinates.

S: (reflectively) Thinking about it, yes, he does control the topic of conversation most of the time at home. He also decides what we do at home, but it's because he is introducing us to new things.

C: What does he decide for you?

S: (defensively) Nothing big—just things that will help me fit in with his friends. He wanted me to take up tennis because we belong to a country club. He's been champion of the men's singles tournament for a long time.

C: Edward really enjoys competition.

S: (emphatically) He does, and he was a little disappointed to find out that we didn't play tennis and golf—we are all in lessons now. Edward grew up in a wealthy home. He still doesn't really understand what it was like for me when I was growing up. I worked at any dead-end job I could get. In my first marriage, we lived paycheck to paycheck. Expensive sports were not an option.

C: Edward grew up with wealth. He takes for granted many of the privileges that are new to you, like playing sports that require expensive equipment. I'm wondering if he also had the privilege of a faster career path than you.

S: (calmly) That's an understatement. His father was in banking too. Edward had to start on his own, but he had the benefit of his dad's advice. This job has been a big step up for me and my family; I'm so thankful. I took the first steps myself, but Edward is a huge help. (excitedly) He feels we will be an unstoppable team!

C: You've really experienced a change in personal power.

S: (pause, uncertainly) Yes, it's all been great except Adrian really isn't enjoying golf lessons, but Edward says he needs the golf to be successful in business.

C: Edward is trying to help Adrian with a future goal, being successful in business. But, Adrian is still young. Should he have a choice in what he does in his free time?

S: (defensively) Edward is really dedicated to Adrian. He wants to make a success out of him. I really appreciate that. After all, Adrian isn't really his son.

C: Does your family spend time just relaxing?

S: (softly) Edward feels that it is just wasting time to do what Adrian calls "hanging out." (pause) I realize Edward can be domineering, but that's only one side of him. He's been very generous to us. The day we got home from our wedding, he had surprised the kids by changing two rooms in his house to be their bedrooms. He made a study corner with a personal computer in both their rooms. We were all stunned.

C: I've noticed that you use "we" rather than just giving me your own reaction.

S: (intently) I meant the children and me. Edward picked our wedding day for the delivery so everything would be a big surprise when we got back to the house.

C: He is very generous with possessions. (pause) But, would you like to be consulted about these decisions rather than being surprised by them?

S: (intently) He's not intentionally leaving me out. He is a very action-oriented person and makes quick decisions. He's not the type to consult with other people.

C: Does this ever make you feel that your opinions aren't valued?

S: (anxiously) He values my opinion, but his experience is wider.

C: In our society, the husband and father often has the most power in making decisions.

S: (irritably) I don't think I'm letting him do it because he's the man. I really admire his intellect and his decision-making abilities. I think he just underestimates my experiences as a mother.

C: How serious a problem do you think this is?

S: (defensively) I don't think it's serious. Adrian and Susie are getting so much out of having him as a father. But, Susie has been crying a lot, and I don't like that. It also makes Edward edgy; he feels she should have more self-control. I keep trying to remind the kids of all Edward has given us. They do love the clothes and the house. We lived in a very small apartment before. The children had to share a room; we didn't have money for extras like going to the movies.

C: You gained a lot of resources since your marriage. Why was Susie crying?

S: (angrily) She's getting bullied in ballet class because they say her clothes are stupid. Everybody else has been together in classes since kindergarten, and she's the newcomer. I've told her things will get better with time and her clothes are beautiful.

C: Women and girls are under a lot of social pressure to look certain ways. It can squelch their individuality.

S: (emphatically) I agree. That's what's happening to Susie. I wish I had more time to help her. One regret I have about my life changing is my time is so limited with the kids. When I was a stay-at-home mom, I could put them first and give them a lot of my time. But, they didn't have nice clothes and toys. Now it's the reverse; I'm always in a rush, but I can get them pretty much anything money can buy.

C: As a mom you wish you could give more time to your children. At this point, there's constant tension between your identity as a wife and that of a mother.

S: (sadly) It does feel like that. I feel pulled between them. Edward doesn't understand. I just want to be with my kids. Whenever I've planned a weekend just to be quietly at home with them, I find that Edward has signed them up for something. My role is just to drive them somewhere and drop them off.

C: I can see the pain in your face. Does Edward know how you feel?

S: (sadly) He tends to minimize my concerns—without a plan, he feels time is wasted. My mother thinks I'm nuts to ever disagree with Edward.

C: She doesn't validate your concerns. (pause) You have a right to have them. You love your kids, and it makes sense that you want time with them.

S: (irritably) Mom actually told me I'm crazy to worry. She just reminds me how bad things used to be and how Edward really has been the savior of the family. He's helped her refinance her home so that she's a lot more comfortable financially now.

C: When it comes to money, Edward really comes through for everyone. When you are struggling to stay out of debt, more money does really seem to be the savior of the situation. However, has the money you have now made the children happier?

S: (sadly) The kids are happy right after they have been given something. But, they don't seem to like the new private school they're enrolled in. Those other kids are brats, and I really don't want my children to be like them. (anxiously) I'm worried about the kids, but Edward thinks they just need time to adjust.

C: Change is hard. People often need time to adjust, but you don't want to be adjusting to something that isn't healthy for you.

S: (long pause) Adrian is having the most trouble with Edward. He works hard in school, but sometimes he just wants to lie around and not do anything. I wish Edward could understand this. Last week, Edward really lost it when Adrian's baseball bat accidentally broke a vase in the living room.

C: What do you mean, "lost it"?

S: (sadly) Edward hit him on the butt a few times. I definitely wouldn't call it abuse, but I don't hit my kids. Adrian yelled into Edward's face that he was a child abuser, and then Edward grounded him for a month; this is too long. Adrian was disrespectful, but kids lose their cool sometimes. (anxiously) I wish Edward could understand this.

C: Has Edward ever left bruises or other marks on one of the kids after he disciplined them?

S: (intently) No, he does spank both of them; however, he's never left any marks. Edward's sharpest weapon is his tongue. He says demeaning things if he's displeased with them. He is trying to motivate them to try harder. He believes that his father helped him by setting hard standards and making him live up to them. He believes Adrian is really intelligent but too emotional. I guess I have encouraged my kids to talk to me about their feelings. Edward thinks Adrian's a wimp and needs to toughen up.

C: Do you want this?

S: (calmly) I think Adrian's fine, but it wouldn't hurt him to try to learn from Edward.

C: Edward is very powerful both at work and in the home. What about you? It doesn't seem as if your role as the mother is being given as much respect as you deserve.

S: (nervously) He's given me so much.

C: He's given you material possessions and training opportunities at work. Have you given him anything?

S: (intently) Yes. I've been a good wife to him, supported his interests, cared for him. But, (long pause) I don't know really what I could want that I don't have.

C: It's up to you to define a good marriage for yourself. But, I believe that both partners' opinions should have equal say and equal respect. Edward has the right to be treated with respect for his knowledge of banking, but your knowledge of parenting also deserves respect.

S: (uncertainly) I'm new to feeling like I deserve respect.

C: Edward has been a good partner in many respects. But, like many powerful men, he isn't stopping to consider if you have valuable knowledge he doesn't—about how to raise children. How are you handling the stress of Edward not understanding the kids?

S: (anxiously) I guess I need to tell you that I've lost a lot of weight recently. I just don't feel like eating. I know that's crazy. (sadly) Edward likes it. (emphatically) He says I'm going to be the most beautiful woman at the country club.

C: What did your doctor say about your weight?

S: (uncertainly) He says I'm too thin. But, I'm not hungry, and I'm getting a lot of compliments.

C: There is a lot of social pressure on women to be thin. It comes from TV, movies, and advertisements. It sells a lot of diet products, but it's not healthy for women.

S: (sadly) I'm really not trying to diet. But, Susie has begun to copy me and eat less. I don't want that for her!

C: There are a lot of positives from building this new family of yours. I know it made you angry when your doctor said it, but I have to be honest with you, and say that you do seem anxious and depressed. I think it may be coming from the terrible pressure you are under to be a good wife and a good mother in this new family.

S: (anxiously) I don't want to lose Edward.

C: If you choose to come back, we need to think about the ways you can balance your identities as a wife and mother without losing your appetite.

S: (long pause, calmly) I guess I do need to come back.

Exercises for Developing a Case Conceptualization of Sharon

Exercise 1 (4-page maximum)

GOAL: To verify that you have a clear understanding of Empowerment Feminist Therapy.

STYLE: An integrative essay addressing Parts A–C.

NEED HELP?   Review this chapter (pages 151–157).

A. Develop a concise overview of the assumptions of feminist theory (the theory's hypotheses about key dimensions in understanding the impact of social forces on individual males and females; think broadly, abstractly).

B. Develop a thorough description of how each of these assumptions is used to understand how privileged or oppressed a client is (for each assumption provide specific examples).

C. Describe the role of the clinician in supporting the empowerment of the client (consultant, doctor, educator, helper; treatment approach; technique examples).

Exercise 2 (4-page maximum)

GOAL: To aid application of feminist theory to Sharon.

STYLE: A separate sentence outline for each section, A–D.

NEED HELP?   Review this chapter (pages 151–157).

A. For each of Sharon's identities as a mother, wife, daughter, and bank manager, discuss where appropriate:

1. The role, if any, of past gender role stereotypes in the development of this identity.

2. The role, if any, of current pressures from family and/or society in maintaining gender stereotypes within this identity.

3. How much privilege or oppression Sharon experiences within each identity.

4. How much or how little of a woman's perspective is valued within this identity.

5. How egalitarian Sharon's relationships are with others when she functions in this identity.

6. What, if any, significant changes have occurred in the identity since Sharon's first marriage.

7. What Sharon's current weaknesses (concerns, issues, problems, symptoms, skill deficits, treatment barriers) are at this time within this identity.

8. What Sharon's current strengths (strong points, positive features, successes, skills, factors facilitating change) are at this time within this identity.

B. Discuss how interdependent her identities are with each other at this time, which identity or identities are most salient to her, how empowered Sharon currently is, and how androgynous her current lifestyle is.

C. In what ways are her current environmental and social contexts facilitating or inhibiting her growth as an individual at this time, how aware is she of how societal expectations for her to be a gendered female are influencing her life, and what role do these social pressures play in her weight loss, anxiety, and depression?

D. How well is Sharon functioning overall, how might her strengths be utilized to support her greater empowerment and her development of egalitarian relationships with other adults, and what specifically might EFT have to offer her at this time?

Exercise 3 (4-page maximum)

GOAL: To develop an understanding of the potential role of socioeconomic status in Sharon's life.

STYLE: A separate sentence outline for each section, A–E.

NEED HELP?   Review Chapter 2 (pages 79–84).

Answer the following questions in detail, providing specific examples to support your points about Sharon and her family:

A. How has Sharon's high socioeconomic status (SES) influenced her current access to resources within her new marriage (attention she can get and give other family members; help she can give and get from other family members; her access to resources such as food, water, privacy, safe housing, and recreation), and how has this been a change from the past?

B. How does SES influence Sharon's current access to resources outside of the family (educational, vocational, medical, legal, and social/political), and in what ways has this been a change from the past?

C. Considering A and B above, assess the impact of Sharon and her husband's economic and social class on their self-esteem and personal welfare; their family welfare; their ability to make independent decisions at home, at school, and/or within the work setting; and their ability to influence their own life circumstances versus their lives being under the control of others within the work, social, or political spheres. Has this been a change from the past, and has this differed between the spouses?

D. Considering A–C above, is SES serving more to constrain or support Sharon's life at this time, how is SES related to her strengths and/or weaknesses at this time, and how does her current SES inhibit or facilitate her ability to make changes in her life at this time?

E. Assess the role that your economic and social class might have in your expectations and perceptions of Sharon and her family, as well as how classist values might be implicitly embedded within your treatment orientation, and consider what might be done to increase the likelihood of a positive outcome.

Exercise 4 (6-page maximum)

GOAL: To help you integrate your knowledge of Empowerment Feminist Theory and the role of socioeconomic status into an in-depth conceptualization of Sharon (who she is and why she does what she does).

STYLE: An integrated essay consisting of a premise, supportive details, and conclusions following a carefully planned organizational style.

NEED HELP?   Review Chapter 1 (pages 7–28) and Chapter 2 (pages 79–84).

STEP 1: Consider what style you could use for organizing your feminist understanding of Sharon that (a) would support you in providing a comprehensive and clear understanding of her identities and her power in the world and (b) would support language she might find persuasive in spite of her ambivalence toward EFT.

STEP 2: Develop your concise premise (overview, preliminary or explanatory statements, proposition, thesis statement, theory-driven introduction, hypotheses, summary, concluding causal statements) that explains Sharon's strengths and weaknesses as a newly upper-class woman who is concerned about how her children and their new stepfather are relating to each other. If you're having trouble with Step 2, remember it should be an integration of the key ideas of Exercises 2 and 3 that (a) provides a basis for Sharon's long-term goals, (b) is grounded in feminist theory and sensitive to issues of social class, and (c) highlights the strengths she may bring to feminist treatment.

STEP 3: Develop your supporting material (detailed case analysis of strengths and weaknesses, supplying data to support an introductory premise) from a feminist perspective that integrates within each paragraph an in-depth understanding of Sharon, a woman whose struggle to find a balance between her personal and work identities has resulted in anxiety, depression, and weight loss. If you're having trouble with Step 3, consider the information you'll need to include in order to (a) support the development of short-term goals, (b) be grounded in the principles of EFT especially as they relate to SES, and (c) integrate an understanding of Sharon's strengths in evaluating the role of social forces in her life whenever possible.

STEP 4: Develop your feminist conclusions and broad treatment recommendations including (a) Sharon's overall level of functioning, (b) anything facilitating or serving as a barrier to her empowerment at this time, and (c) her basic needs as she tries to develop egalitarian relationships that allow her to develop her own unique abilities (be concise and general).

Exercise 5 (3-page maximum)

GOAL: To develop an individualized, theory-driven action plan for Sharon that considers her strengths and is sensitive to issues of socioeconomic status.

STYLE: A sentence outline consisting of long- and short-term goals.

NEED HELP?   Review Chapter 1 (pages 8–28).

> *STEP 1:* Develop your treatment plan overview, being careful to consider what you said in Part E of Exercise 3 to try and prevent any negative bias to your treatment plan.

> *STEP 2:* Develop long-term (major, large, ambitious, comprehensive, broad) goals that *ideally* Sharon would reach by the termination of treatment that would lead to her empowerment. If you are having trouble with Step 2, reread your premise and support topic sentences and transform them into goals that would meet her needs as a mother, wife, and bank manager (use the *style* of Exercise 4).

> *STEP 3:* Develop short-term (small, brief, encapsulated, specific, measurable) goals that Sharon and the clinician could expect to see accomplished within a few weeks to chart Sharon's progress toward understanding the impact of social forces in her life, instill hope for change, and plan time-effective treatment sessions. If you are having trouble with Step 3, reread your support paragraphs looking for ideas to transform into goals that (a) might facilitate change that is relevant to a principle of EFT and issues of SES, (b) might enhance anything facilitating or decrease anything serving as a barrier to her empowerment at this time, (c) utilize her strengths whenever possible in understanding the role of societal pressures in her life, and (d) are individualized to her needs as a newly married mother of two rather than generic.

Exercise 6

GOAL: To critique Empowerment Feminist Therapy and the case, of Sharon.

STYLE: Answer Questions A–E in essay format or discuss them in a group format.

> A. What are the strengths and weaknesses of this model for helping Sharon (a newly married mother of two who went from the lower to the upper class)?

> B. Discuss the power of using cognitive theory with this case, looking for any signs in the interview of thinking errors such as absolutist standards, right/wrong thinking, and so forth. Then, compare and contrast the power of using a cognitive versus a feminist

approach to this case. Conclude with a discussion of which theory you consider most powerful for helping Sharon at this time, and explain why.

C. Apply the Domain of Gender to Sharon and Edward. Then, discuss whether you think gender or SES is having the greatest impact on Sharon's spousal relationship at this time. Also, discuss how the dynamics in her spousal relationship might change if Edward was the owner of a small landscaping business and she was still the manager of the bank.

D. What ethical issues arise in working with Sharon considering her overt rejection of the idea that gender role stereotypes are relevant to her and her marriage? A principle of EFT is that Sharon has the right to find her own unique identity. What specifically will you do if, after a few weeks, she tells you that her choice is to allow Edward to remain in control of family decisions and she wants your help in discussing this with her children?

E. What did you learn about your own gender role assumptions as you tried to implement this model for Sharon? How did you react to Sharon's comments that involved her relationship to Edward and his relationship to her children? How might this support or inhibit your ability to develop a positive working relationship with her?

Recommended Resources

American Psychological Association (Producer) & Brown, L. S. (Trainer). (n.d.). *Feminist therapy: Part of the Systems of Psychotherapy Video Series* [Motion picture, #4310828]. (Available from the American Psychological Association, 750 First Street, NE, Washington, DC 20002–4242)

Chappell, M. (2008, May 5). *Who we are.* Retrieved June 5, 2009, from http:// www.feminist-therapy-institute.org/index.htm

Worell, J., & Remer, P. (2003). *Feminist perspectives in therapy: Empowering diverse women.* New York: John Wiley & Sons, Inc.

Six

Emotion-Focused Case Conceptualizations and Treatment Plans

Introduction to Emotion-Focused Treatment

Ellen calls and leaves a message on your answering machine. She is a 32-year-old White female who has recently divorced Frank, her husband of 10 years. She is currently living in the city with her two sons, ages 8 and 10. Ellen divorced Frank, after a chronically unhappy marriage, when she recognized that she was a lesbian. She says that Frank has not yet accepted the divorce or her sexual orientation. Ellen wants help in resolving her relationship with Frank and in developing a constructive relationship with another lesbian adult. Her parting words are "Don't call me back if you think my lesbianism is the problem. I want it clear from the start that it's part of the solution to my problems."

You provide a form of Emotion-Focused Treatment with roots in the traditions of Client-Centered Therapy, Existential Therapy, and Gestalt Therapy (Perls, Hefferline, & Goodman, 1951; Rogers, 1951) as well as the research in cognitive science and neuroscience on emotions (Greenberg & Goldman, 2007). You believe that people have an innate, emotion-based system that helps them derive meaning from their experiences and motivates them to grow and develop. Ellen comes to you in a state of distress and doesn't want you pointing her in the wrong direction. She doesn't need to worry about that. You would never tell her that her lesbianism is a problem or is not a problem. She is the expert on her experiences, and only she will be able to decide if something is adaptive or maladaptive for her. She also has a natural capacity to grow and change in an adaptive way, if she can trust herself to fully process her experiences. Your role will be to facilitate this process (Greenberg & Goldman, 2007; Rogers, 1951). The following more detailed analysis of Emotion-Focused Treatment is drawn from Elliot and Greenberg (1995).

Ellen is constantly creating meaning from her experiences so that she can understand herself, others, and her situation. Healthy functioning results when she processes her internal and external experiences thoroughly so that the meaning derived from them can guide her flexibly and adaptively. As she does this processing, she needs to keep her emotional arousal at a level that is optimal for her. There are times when she will need to access her emotions, heighten them, and tolerate them so that she can recognize the importance of the situation (the meaning of it) and take appropriate action. At other times, the meaning creation process will be blocked unless she can reduce her state of arousal by containing or distancing herself from these emotions so she'll be able to think adaptively about the situation and act appropriately. Emotional regulation is critical to Ellen's adaptive functioning and consists of knowing when to be more in touch with her emotions so that they can guide her and when she needs to keep her emotions under control so that she can process her experiences using reason. If Ellen's present functioning is maladaptive, it is the result of blocked emotional processing.

Ellen has recently begun trusting her internal experiences. This has led her to redefine herself as a lesbian rather than a heterosexual. She is now struggling with the meaning this shift in sexual orientation has for other aspects of her life. Ellen did not change her view of herself in the world overnight. Rather, this has always been in a state of construction as she integrated new and old experiences. Old experiences, in the form of emotion schemes, serve as a filter for new experiences. Emotion schemes develop during childhood and then operate automatically and unconsciously to guide behavior in an anticipatory and pattern-determined fashion. This innate, emotion-based system provides a holistic sense of how things are going for Ellen on a moment-to-moment basis.

An emotion scheme could be developed around a primary or secondary emotion. Primary emotions occur in direct reaction to something that has happened. If Ellen is angry at her father, this anger is a primary emotion. However, if immediately upon experiencing the anger Ellen experiences fear that her father will hit her if she expresses anger, then fear becomes a secondary emotion that serves to cover up the primary emotion of anger. To gain constructive meaning from these experiences, Ellen will need to work through the fear until the primary emotion surfaces and then fully process her anger. Negative emotions always serve as cues to areas of experience that need further processing for meaning.

Emotion schemes are not simple feelings. Although feelings play a key role in their development, emotion schemes represent high-level organizing structures in which feelings, bodily sensations, cognitions (beliefs, perceptions, expectations), and motivational tendencies or action tendencies are brought together to help Ellen understand who she is, how she relates to others, and what is important to her. While these emotion schemes automatically influence her behavior, Ellen's processing of new experiences, or further processing of older experiences, can serve to modify or transform her already created emotion schemes as well as serve to create new ones.

Ellen's strengths come from healthy emotion schemes and adaptive emotions while her difficulties are the result of either maladaptive emotion schemes or adaptive emotions to problematic experiences. Healthy schemes will help guide Ellen to get her needs met in a life-enhancing manner. They will each contain feelings, bodily sensations, cognitions, and motivations or action tendencies. Incomplete, unhealthy, and/or contradictory schemes will not guide Ellen adaptively but will still be an attempt to get her legitimate needs met.

What might a healthy emotion scheme be? Ellen always did well in school. This may be due to a healthy scheme that guides her in learning academic material effectively. This might contain feelings of confidence, expectations that she can learn new things, and perceptions that she has been successful in learning in the past. This might be coupled with motivational tendencies to pay attention in class and study. This scheme would be adaptive in helping Ellen learn within an academic environment and would bode well for her being able to learn new things within the treatment environment.

What is an adaptive emotion? It is an emotion that guides Ellen adaptively in her present circumstances. If someone insults Ellen at work, she might feel angry. If in response to this anger she responds with assertive behavior to defend herself, then the anger is functioning as an adaptive emotion that leads her to take adaptive action. Similarly, if she is in a situation with a romantic partner and being treated with kindness and love, Ellen might feel love in return. If she responds by expressing love and affection to the partner, then this love would be acting as an adaptive emotion.

Ellen has some emotional processing problems, so all of her experiences are not organized into healthy and fully complete emotion schemes. What goes wrong if Ellen has an incomplete scheme? Ellen could have a desire or motivational tendency to form an emotionally intimate relationship with another adult. However, this scheme could exist solely as inchoate longings for emotional connection (an unclear felt sense). This scheme is incomplete and therefore not helpful in guiding Ellen in how she should act to get this need met. In treatment, you would help Ellen become more aware of her longing for emotional connection. She could discuss it and put into words what the longing means to her (symbolize it). Through focusing her attention on her bodily sensations, she may come to label these sensations as reflecting a feeling of sadness that she doesn't know how to develop emotional intimacy even though she's very motivated to experience it. By processing this longing more deeply, Ellen may recognize that she doesn't know how to share her feelings with another person. From this further emotional processing, her unclear felt sense has been transformed into a complete and adaptive scheme in which she has feelings of hope, cognitions that she has learned effectively in the past and can continue to do so, and a motivation to try hard and practice new social skills so that she can develop emotional intimacy with another person.

What about a complete but maladaptive emotion scheme? Due to her father's abusive behavior, Ellen may have developed a scheme for interacting with men that includes cognitions that all women need to be submissive in order to be safe. Her motivational tendencies may be to engage in submissive behavior including the bodily responses of looking down, speaking quietly, and always agreeing with men. She might feel unfulfilled but safe. While this scheme might have been functional in decreasing her father's abusive behavior, it is rigidly guiding her behavior with both violent and nonviolent men. Thus, it couldn't guide her to have an emotionally satisfying relationship with Frank.

How might two conflicting schemes influence Ellen? She might have two emotion schemes that guide her in incongruent ways; this may cause a self-evaluative split in which Ellen is torn between two competing aspects of her experience. For example, she could have an emotion scheme guiding her sexual behavior. This developed through her childhood as she watched her parents, and other visible sexual partners, interact. Ellen also heard a lot of homophobic comments as she was growing up, so the scheme guiding her sexual behavior might include cognitions that appropriate sexual behavior occurs only between a man and a woman and that lesbian and gay sexual behavior is always unacceptable. In contrast to this scheme that developed in childhood, as an adult Ellen has a newly developed scheme that supports her in a lesbian personal identity. At this time, this scheme might consist of feelings of hope and contentment; sensations of excitement; and cognitions that she understands herself better, that she wasn't a loser as a marital partner, and that being a lesbian is part of the solution to her problems. This scheme might contain motivational tendencies for reaching out to date other lesbians. However, her "sexual behavior" scheme that tells her how to behave in sexual relationships is incongruent with her "personal identity" scheme that motivates her to date lesbians. This leaves Ellen in a state of confusion and internal conflict, unable to date unless she is drunk so that alcohol can dampen her contradictory cognitions and action tendencies.

Finally, Ellen could experience problems due to an adaptive emotion that developed in response to problematic experiences during childhood; this would lead to a feeling of vulnerability and overarousal whenever she was aware of this emotion. Since Ellen underwent the trauma of physical abuse as a child, fear may have become an adaptive emotion. Whenever her dad raised his voice, her fear may have motivated her to be submissive, and this may have moderated her father's rage—thus it was adaptive. Now, this formerly adaptive emotion may be limiting her ability to express anger herself or work through problems with others who are angry. Treatment could help her fully explore this emotion and decrease its potency for her so that she could understand its role in her relationships. Ellen could then decide if her submissive actions are functional for her in dealing with angry people and if it is safe for her to be angry with other people.

She may have predominately healthy emotion schemes and adaptive emotions guiding her in processing meaning from her experiences and have only minimal or circumscribed emotional processing problems. On the other hand, she may have developed a problematic global processing style that interferes with appropriate emotional regulation much of the time. This problematic processing style could reflect being emotionally overregulated (person is cut off from emotions), being emotionally underregulated (person is a sea of emotions), relying too heavily on experiential processing (person overuses emotional or bodily awareness), or relying too heavily on conceptual processing (person overuses reasoning strategies).

If Ellen has a problematic processing style, it is associated with intensely painful emotions (core pains) or overwhelming thoughts (core issues). These emanate from one of four causes: difficulty in putting her experiences into words so that she can conceptually process them; intrapersonal dynamics such as struggles with self-esteem or self-definition; interpersonal dynamics such as struggles in forming attachments that balance her needs for intimacy with her needs for autonomy; and existential dynamics where she struggles with the meaning of death, loss, life, and so forth. Ellen could have more than one core pain or issue. Each of these will be a component of a dysfunctional or underarticulated emotion scheme or an adaptive emotion to a problematic experience.

As long as Ellen is not fully processing her experiences, her freedom of choice and action is limited. Treatment will focus on helping her (a) become more fully aware of her experiences, (b) process them more fully for meaning, and (c) decide if any aspect of an emotion scheme is not functional for her. If she decides this, then she will modify it, transform it, or create something new that was missing. As a result of this functional processing of her emotions, Ellen will have a new view of herself in the world, a new view of others, and a greater understanding and acceptance of herself.

Role of the Clinician

How will you help Ellen? Overall, you will follow two overarching principles. The first is to foster a collaborative, prizing, and genuine treatment relationship. To do so, you will focus on developing empathetic attunement to Ellen's frame of reference, you will develop a prizing relationship with her, and you will involve her in a process of mutual goal setting and participation in treatment tasks. The second principle is that, while you will be nondirective as to the content of the treatment session, as Ellen is an expert on what she needs to discuss, you will facilitate her self-exploration through providing opportunities for her to engage in specific treatment tasks. The tasks will facilitate her fully processing painful emotional states and thematic material and incorporate these new experiences into her constructions of herself and her situation. Your challenge is to create a balance between therapeutic attunement to Ellen's self-exploration, which is critical to helping her learn to trust her internal experience, and the introduction of specific tasks, which aid Ellen in constructing meaning from her experiences.

How will you decide what tasks will help Ellen in the moment? You will listen attentively and track her emotions in the moment. You will look for markers that indicate an emotional processing problem (unresolved cognitive-affective problems) and then suggest a task that could help with this in-the-moment block to fully experiencing her internal and external world. You can also examine the quality of Ellen's voice as she relates her experiences as this can provide clues to what she needs from you. Four different vocal qualities have been identified. If she speaks with a focused voice, it indicates she is ready to put into words some new aspect of experience. An emotional voice indicates that she is tuned into her feelings. If she is speaking with a limited voice, it indicates she is concerned about what would happen if she got in touch with her emotions. In this situation, Ellen needs to develop trust and a greater sense of safety within the treatment relationship before she can explore her experiences more fully. Finally, if Ellen has an external voice, she is describing her experiences in a rehearsed or rote manner with her attention on the reaction this description will evoke in you rather than on developing an internal understanding of their meaning. In this case, you will help her turn inward and reenact each experience in a vivid way so that it can be processed within the immediacy of the moment. Will Ellen proceed with a task you suggest? Her autonomy and self-directed exploration are critical, and thus she will only take on a task if she feels she is ready to do so.

Ellen is always in the process of incorporating new experiences into her sense of self and her world; as she does this she is re-creating herself and what she needs in the moment. As a result, no plan of action carries directly over from one session to another. She will determine the pace and direction of each session. However, you expect that if she has a core pain or core issue, it will reoccur across sessions. Each time you see Ellen, you will wait to see what emerges from her and follow her lead as you build a collaborative, egalitarian treatment relationship. You will never impose meanings on her experiences as this could impede the treatment process and prevent her from reorganizing her experience in the manner that is most helpful to her.

Markers of experiences that should be explored cou come from Ellen's global processing style of overregulating her emoti. Thus, at the first sign, or marker, that she is minimizing her ex ence of emotions, you could suggest a task that would facilitate her fully experiencing them instead. A marker could also be something s that occurs within the immediacy of the moment, such as an as of nonverbal behavior. For example, Ellen might look down of discussing something (nonverbal expression). You would draw attention to her bodily sensations around this behavior and help her f symbolize it (put it into words) and then consider what it might mean.

Six different types of emotional processing problems (process diagnoses) will be discussed. For each type, there is a related treatment task that could help Ellen explore and/or transform it for adaptive meaning. The first type is called a problematic reaction in which Ellen recognizes that there is a discrepancy between her expected reaction and her actual reaction; she finds the experience puzzling or troubling in some way. The task that is helpful in this case is Systematic Evocative Unfolding. Ellen will be helped to vividly reexperience and explore this problematic reaction while you respond empathically. You will slow down the processing of the puzzling experience so you can help Ellen more deeply examine every small piece of it. She will come to recognize the perceptual trigger (what happened immediately before the reaction), the immediate thoughts she has around it (further symbolization of the experience), her feelings in response to it (how the experience feels), and her motivations (what she wants to feel and think about it). As a result, Ellen will be able to draw more adaptive meaning from the problematic experience.

People have a multiplicity of selves, not a single executive self. Ellen is in a constant state of constructing a unified sense of herself. If she has a second type of processing problem, a self-evaluative split, two aspects of herself are working against each other rather than being fully integrated within her sense of herself. For example, one aspect of her identity could be critical or coercive to another. One may criticize her as incapable of a relationship since her marriage failed. The other may insist that it was sexual confusion, not an inability to relate, that led to the failure. These two aspects need to be integrated adaptively into Ellen's self-concept. The treatment technique of a two-chair dialogue is helpful in this situation. Ellen will personify each aspect of herself (the critic of her role as a wife vs. her newly developed identity as a lesbian). You will coach her in having one aspect talk to the other until the messages of both voices are

d. This will aid her in integrating both voices. She may have fully proce. _ denied some aspect of her experience because it was traumatic previou table to her. Ellen will be helped to show compassion toward or un d accept this aspect of her experience as a valid part of herself.

her related vein, a third type of problem is a self-interruptive split. It's _ble that Ellen went for years with one aspect of herself (the part _ng to be the good wife) interrupting or minimizing her ability to _xpress or fully experience her emotion of dissatisfaction in the marriage. In this case, a two-chair enactment task might be helpful. Ellen will slowly process this split by bringing the interrupting good wife (who is overregulating her emotion of dissatisfaction) under her deliberate control. Ellen will then be able to fully express her dissatisfaction and process it for constructive meaning.

A fourth type of problem is called a sense of vulnerability. This represents painful emotions relevant to some aspect of her experience that Ellen may have kept secret from everyone in the past. Perhaps Ellen always believed that she deserved the abusive treatment she got from her father as she wondered if she was inherently bad or worthless. Whenever this sense of vulnerability begins to surface, she may shy away from experiencing it, fearing that to take in this experience will mean she is bad and worthless. In this case, the task of empathic affirmation is needed. You will demonstrate to Ellen that you understand and value her for who she is—a divorced, lesbian mother of two who was abused as a child and so forth; you value her whole self. This acceptance will help Ellen develop a greater sense of hope and strength so that she can accept all aspects of herself.

A fifth processing problem is an absent or unclear felt sense. This is relevant to Ellen if she has a confusing or an absent physiological reaction around some aspect of her experience. Experiential focusing is a task that is particularly helpful in this situation. Assume Ellen always feels numb when she turns off the lights prior to going to bed, but she has no idea why. You help Ellen turn inward and pay close attention to this numbness while giving herself permission to process it more. She is helped to intensify her feeling of numbness so that she can give it a label that helps her visualize this sensation. She says the numbness is like being an ice cube, frozen and suspended until it melts and she is lost. Keeping this ice cube metaphor in mind, Ellen can now symbolize (put into words or further symbols) that as an ice cube she didn't have to feel pain as her father beat her. Afterward she melted away because her mother treated her as if the experience didn't occur. Ellen can construct new meaning from this intense focusing on this unclear felt sense. While her past cannot be changed, the meaning of the beatings can. She can stop believing she is just water melting away. She can now believe that her father was abusive and that her mother was in denial of this. Her sense of self now contains recognition that as an adult she can protect herself from abuse. She may now turn off the lights at night, remaining fully aware, as the adult Ellen is safe in bed.

The last type of processing marker is called unfinished business. Perhaps Ellen's mother died when she was 5, and Ellen has unresolved feelings of abandonment or anger over this event. A dialogue using an empty chair (where her mother is imagined to be sitting) can be a valuable task in this situation. First Ellen talks from her own perspective while looking at the empty chair. Then, Ellen moves to sit in the "mother's chair" and continues the dialogue from her mother's perspective. Ellen keeps changing chairs, and points of view, until she has fully fleshed out all aspects of the unfinished business. She can now come to an adaptive conclusion where she has resolved her feelings toward her mother's death.

All process diagnoses (recognition of markers) are tentative and may or may not be confirmed by further emotional processing. All six treatment tasks serve to bring unconscious and automatic emotion schemes into Ellen's awareness, where they can be explored in depth. If Ellen finds a scheme that can guide her constructively but that she has minimized in the past, she can pay more attention to it to increase its potency in guiding her. If she discovers that one of her guiding schemes is destructive, she can reorganize it, transform it, or create a different scheme that is more helpful to her.

What will Ellen have gained at the end of treatment? She will have full access to her emotions and be able to use them to guide her actions. If she is feeling overwhelmed with her emotions, she will have learned skills to reduce her arousal using strategies such as self-soothing, seeking support from others, and distracting. In contrast, if she is cut off from her emotions, she will have learned skills such as how to attend to her bodily sensations and take an inner focus so that she can become aware of her emotional states. Overall, she will be able to trust her own experience, make use of a greater range of emotional information, and develop an ability to reflect on her own way of thinking and feeling about her experiences. She will learn that she can be herself in a relationship with someone else because she is a worthwhile person and can guide her own destiny.

Case Application: Integrating the Domain of Sexual Orientation

Ellen's case will now be examined in detail. There are many domains of complexity that might be relevant to her case. The Domain of Sexual Orientation has been chosen to be examined within an emotion-focused case conceptualization and treatment plan.

Interview With Ellen (E) From an Emotion-Focused Perspective

C: Welcome. Where would you like to start?

E: (sadly) I am lonely. I met my husband in high school. He was my first and only serious relationship. He started everything. Now that I am alone, I just don't know where to begin to start things up myself.

C: You're seeking a way out of the loneliness (pause) but (pause) how?

E: (embarrassedly) I have been trying going to bars. I end up drinking way too much. I have only started one "date." I was so drunk I don't remember the woman's name. (pause and then disgustedly) I felt sick afterwards. I had slept in my clothes, and I couldn't REMEMBER what I had done.

C: It was disorienting because you couldn't remember what happened. (pause) This isn't what you are looking for.

E: (firmly) No, it's not. This wasn't the first time I had a blackout. Before I got my life together, I spent a lot of time drunk. I am not going to get drunk again! I am through with that trap.

C: How often do you drink now?

E: That was the first time in the past year. I really don't like alcohol. I never have.

C: But you have abused alcohol in the past?

E: (sadly) Yes. I was hiding from myself. (pause and then firmly) Now that I know who I am I don't need to do that anymore.

C: You sound confident. (Pause) I am still wondering what it meant that you got drunk recently.

E: (irritably) It didn't mean anything, and it won't happen again. When I woke up, I realized how serious my dating fears were. (firmly) That is why I am here. I am facing these fears, not using alcohol to cover them up.

C: I irritated you when I asked about the drinking. It seemed like you felt insulted.

E: (calmly) Yes, I did feel insulted. I don't like you suggesting I might get drunk.

C: It is very important that I understand you and not jump to the wrong conclusions. (pause) You are turning to treatment, not alcohol. (pause) Is there anything besides treatment helping you avoid the alcohol trap?

E: (thoughtfully) My boys need an attentive mother. They have never done well in school. (pause, painfully) I have been so caught up with my own struggles that I neglected them like my parents ignored me. They both were held back last year, and (pause, choked up) I never helped. The teachers never suggested anything either. (long pause, determinedly) I let myself be drunk and uncaring—that's over.

C: Your concern for your boys has increased your determination not to drink. (E nods) You are willing to struggle to understand yourself and be a good parent.

E: (smiling) Yes, I am determined to discover who I am, but (softly) there is so much I don't know about being a good mother. I feed and clothe them, but that's about it. If they misbehave, I just . . . scream at them. (sobbing)

C: (long pause) I can feel so much pain in this room.

E: (tearfully) I don't want my boys to hate me. I've already been such a bad mother. (slumped down in chair) How will they react if they know I'm a lesbian?

C: So much pain. (pause) So much worry. (pause) Your body looks overwhelmed.

E: (long pause, calmly) Overwhelmed is the old me. The new me will learn to be a good mom. (pause) But, I can't hide who I am. I need to be accepted for who I am.

C: You have such a strong and determined look on your face now.

E: (smiling) I do feel determined. Frank and I should have divorced years ago. (pause) I have left him before but gone back because I became so lonely. He only needs the sad, submissive me—even though she drank. (desperately) I need more.

C: You knew things weren't right, and you tried to find your way. You have a growing awareness of what you need, but you're still unsure.

E: (calmly) During my last hospitalization, I suddenly realized I was just trying to escape from myself. I don't know what made me see it; one moment I was confused, and then it clicked—I realized I was a lesbian. I didn't feel lost anymore . . . But, I hate loneliness, and Frank still wants me.

C: In the past, you tried to end your loneliness with Frank, but something always felt very wrong. Now you know why it didn't work.

E: (energetically) Knowing I'm a lesbian didn't solve all my problems, but it did make it easy to quit drinking. Sober, I know I don't want to keep using Frank.

C: In your face I can see the freedom you feel after accepting something that is so important about yourself. It has energized and freed you to explore your life.

E: (smiling) Yes, I do feel free sometimes, but I also feel so angry whenever Frank suggests that being a lesbian is my problem. (tensely and loudly) Frank said you would cure me of this lesbian thing and then I would come back home!

C: This new sense of who you are feels so right that it makes you tense to have it scoffed at by Frank. (pause) I wonder how you are feeling as you speak so loudly.

E: (confusedly) I don't know. (pause) I just don't know.

C: Can you allow yourself to focus on what your body is saying?

E: (long pause) I'm angry. (pause) I have to let go of it or people will move away from me, and I am lonely enough.

C: (pause) I won't move away if you want to experience your anger more.

E: (long pause, then furiously) I am just boiling inside a lot of the time. My family has never really accepted me for myself. I was a punching bag for my dad. My mom ignored me most of the time.

C: You felt neglected. You used the word *boiling*. That sounds so hot, so intense, yet you looked contained, as if no steam is rising from your boiling insides.

E: (panicky) I can't let the steam out; I might explode.

C: There is so much anger inside you. Will it destroy you to experience it more?

E: (tensely) I can control it, push it down.

C: You can control it. It is yours to control. Yet it is an important part of you.

E: I don't want it to be important.

C: If it wasn't important, you wouldn't be afraid to let it out.

E: (timidly) I do not feel afraid now. (pause, looking furious) I feel angry.

C: You look angry. (pause) Yet, you aren't exploding. What does that mean?

E: (pause) I guess I won't explode. I don't want to explode and destroy anything with my anger. I want acceptance from my parents and Frank.

C: (long pause) You deserve acceptance.

E: (plaintively) I need it to be OK with everyone that I'm a lesbian. If I could feel safe about retaining custody of my boys . . . (long pause, E looks off in space)

C: Why are you looking away? (long pause) Are you afraid you will lose custody?

E: (softly) I don't know. Frank has never threatened me with it. When he finally realizes I'm not coming back, he might become spiteful—he can be that way.

C: (whispering) Your voice has gotten softer and softer.

E: (painfully) I heard nothing but insults about lesbians as I grew up. I guess this is part of why I hid from myself for so long. If it came to a court fight, my parents would work against me. (pause) What would the judge do if Frank said he had to get the kids because I was a bad influence? (questioningly) What if I just denied the truth in court, (pause) just said I made it up to punish Frank?

C: You sound ambivalent.

E: (firmly) I don't want to lie. I've done that for too long. I want my kids to know who I am and understand it's alright. One of them might be gay. I wouldn't want either of my sons to suffer like I have. I want them to like themselves.

C: Self-acceptance is important.

E: (painfully) I'll be in chaos if I lie again. I might drink again. (pause, confidently) No. I won't do that. Things are going to be different. I'm starting with my name.

C: I felt despair turn to something else when you mentioned your name.

E: (smiling) I have created a new name for myself. I hated my dad. He was an alcoholic and abusive. My marriage to Frank was really a lie, so his name isn't mine either. I am going to have my own name to mark my new beginnings.

C: I can really feel your power as you talk about this.

E: (smiling) I do feel more important somehow when I consider what name to pick.

C: You're smiling. You look relaxed.

E: (sincerely) I know what I want even though I'm not sure how to start, (pause) but I'm not going into a coma this time to avoid feeling lonely.

C: Lonely feels bad, but being in a coma was worse—you lost yourself. There is so much excitement ahead as you come out of the coma and truly experience life.

E: (long pause, anxiously) I'm going to need help.

C: I'm here. (pause, E smiles) You smiled and sank lower in that chair.

E: It's a relief to realize that Frank was wrong. You aren't going to make me change.

C: You were afraid that I wouldn't accept you or accept your goals for yourself. (E nods) Let me be sure I've understood everything. You feel good about yourself as a lesbian. You feel more personal control, and you're symbolizing it by picking a new name. (E nods) What's confusing is how to integrate this new understanding of yourself into your role as a mother, an ex-wife, a daughter, and a partner in a lesbian relationship. Alcohol is no longer a part of your life—you don't need to hide because you can trust yourself now. You know that, somehow, you can grow and be the woman and mother you want to be.

E: (smiling) Yes. (pause) I know I can. Thank you for listening!

Emotion-Focused Case Conceptualization of Ellen: Interpersonally Based Style

In the past, Ellen's views of herself and how to develop interpersonal relationships were based on the assumption that she was heterosexual. In this regard, Ellen saw herself as a loser who had been a failure as a wife and a mother. In processing these experiences, she used a global style of avoiding her emotions; her alcohol abuse served to support this style. However, it left her with deep-seated fears of loneliness and unresolved anger. Recently, these negative perceptions and feelings in relation to herself have undergone a substantial change. Her awareness of her internal experiences has deepened, and this has led her to the recognition that she is a lesbian. Through this greater self-knowledge, she has reevaluated the meaning of her past "failures." She has realized that a denial of internal experience around her sexuality was a root cause of her difficulties. Although her self-awareness has grown, she continues to overregulate her emotions. She needs help fully processing the meaning her lesbianism has for her within her relationships with an intimate partner, her children, and her extended family. Ellen's strengths lie in her increased awareness of the value of attending to her internal experiences, her recognition and acceptance of her sexual feelings for other women, and her trusting her internal felt sense of "wrongness" when she was drunk that led her to stop drinking.

Ellen learned recently that she wants to relate to another woman in an intimate relationship. She had entered a hospital for treatment of alcohol abuse. Something of which she's not consciously aware triggered a deeper understanding of a previously unclear felt sense around her sexuality. This increased understanding helped her construct an understanding of why she had "failed" to establish a satisfying intimate relationship with her husband. She has tried to reach out to form new relationships based on her greater sexual awareness. She found, however, that she could reach out only when abusing alcohol because she was afraid and conflicted about how to behave. In reflecting on her experience after an alcohol-precipitated date, she recognized that it "felt wrong." Processing this problematic reaction point on her own, Ellen recognized that her behavior was not congruent with her motivation to respect herself within her relationships with others. She recognized that she is unsure of how to guide herself to develop a healthy intimate relationship. While still feeling confused about what actions to take, a strength Ellen brings to this challenge is her increased awareness that, in the past, she entered into relationships out of a sense of loneliness and vulnerability and gave in to the wishes of others to gain their acceptance. Her deep craving to remain true to herself and relate authentically to others, when more completely processed, will help her discover the behaviors she needs to actualize this motivation. A final strength is Ellen's new awareness that alcohol inhibited her ability to process her internal and external experiences, which has strengthened her resolve to keep a clear head so that her meaning construction will be adaptive.

Ellen has come to recognize that she was an uninvolved and passive mother. She came to these conclusions after focusing her awareness more intensely on her parenting behavior and her children's welfare. She recognized that, while her boys have been experiencing problems in school for a long time, she never helped them with their schoolwork and did not request any meetings with their teachers to try to assess what help her children needed. Ellen also has some awareness that she was neglected as a child by her mother and only screamed at or beaten by her father. She hasn't processed these experiences beyond a vague sense that she doesn't want to parent like they did, but she has not constructed meaning that would help her parent her own children in a positive way. Ellen may have a self-evaluative split in which "a critical voice" demeans her past mothering behavior while a "passive voice" plaintively expresses confusion over how to do things differently. Ellen needs to fully integrate and accept both aspects of herself as a mother. This will facilitate her search for parenting behaviors that will enhance her boys' welfare. She is also unsure if, or how, her lesbianism should influence her parenting and when, and how, she should explain her sexuality to them. Her strengths, as she seeks to develop a positive mothering role, lie in her recognition that for her boys to develop a positive sense of themselves as males they need to respect their own internal experiences; she does not want them to undergo the same struggles in understanding their sexuality that she has undergone in understanding hers. In addition, she may have begun to develop an emotion scheme around effective parenting as signified by her inchoate hopes that she has the potential to develop into a good mother. Her concern for her boys has also increased her resolve to avoid alcohol as it served as a barrier to her taking constructive actions.

Ellen has reflected on her adult relationships with her ex-husband and parents and recognized that they provide her with no emotional support. After constant avoidance, she has finally allowed herself to become aware of just how great a fear of loneliness and vulnerability she has in her relationships with them and how these feelings have negatively affected her relationships. While her relationship with Frank was unsatisfying, as he was underaware of her needs as an individual and didn't show concern over her self-destructive use of alcohol, she could only briefly separate from him before her fear of loneliness would send her back. Similarly, Ellen has remained motivated to emotionally connect with her parents, despite their inability, or lack of interest, in meeting her physical and emotional needs in the past. Currently, Ellen recognizes that Frank and her parents may not share her motivations, particularly if she maintains a lesbian identity. Frank wants her back as a wife, but she fears he may turn on her and "be spiteful" if she clearly rebuffs his desire for reconciliation and openly maintains a lesbian identity; this may represent a realistic fear as some judges have made homophobic custody decisions. In addition, she fears that her parents, due to homophobia, might go from passively ignoring her needs to actively uniting with Frank against her in a custody dispute. Despite these fears, she is aware that she cannot return to a time when she denies her own needs as a human being. Her strengths lie in her desire to transform her dysfunctional relationships with family members into constructive ones, her awareness that to deny aspects of her identity is to return to personal self-destruction, and her commitment to a course of personal choice and strength.

Ellen has recently developed a stronger relationship with herself as a result of trusting her internal experience and discovering the truth about her sexuality. Prior to this, Ellen used alcohol to keep herself unaware, or only partially aware, of many of her internal experiences; this prevented her from developing a positive identity and engaging in constructive relationships with others. Her fears of rejection and loneliness were the motivations behind her using alcohol as a barrier to fully processing her experiences. Her mental numbness has now ended. Despite continuing to be fearful, her increased sense of agency and her desire for self-determination are propelling her toward adaptive growth. She has been empowered by exploring her feelings and trusting her intuitions about herself. She is symbolizing this change by selecting a new last name to identify herself with. Thinking about this name fills her with feelings of confidence and excitement. Fully articulating this fledgling emotion scheme may help further power positive self-growth. A barrier to her continued growth at this time is her realistic fears about losing custody of her sons as an "out" lesbian mother. However, she is open to personal collaboration with someone who is willing to listen and treat her self-knowledge with respect. She is highly motivated to continue on her path of self-discovery through processing her experiences for constructive and life-enhancing meaning.

Emotion-Focused Treatment Plan: Interpersonally Based Style

Treatment Plan Overview. Ellen's long-term goals are interpersonal in nature. They may be refined or refocused as treatment progresses and she comes to a deeper understanding of her feelings and needs. Ellen will determine which interpersonal relationship is a focus of the treatment session at any given time. The clinician will need to monitor Ellen's alcohol usage due to her past history of abuse. The treatment plan follows the *basic format.*

LONG-TERM GOAL 1: Ellen will fully explore how to relate to other adults in a same-sex, intimate relationship.

Short-Term Goals

1. Ellen will fully process the problematic reaction she had when she was drunk and on her first lesbian date.
   a. She will intensify the feeling of "wrongness" and put into words as she remembers this experience how it served to increase her motivation to respect herself when relating to a lesbian partner.

   b. Ellen will intensify her feeling of fear in initiating same-sex relationships and put into words the relationships among this fear, her abuse of alcohol on her date, and her "wrongness" feeling.

2. Ellen will become aware of her feelings of loneliness and experience how quickly they intensify in terms of their accompanying bodily sensations.

   a. Ellen will articulate the cognitions accompanying these sensations.

   b. Ellen will consider how the intensity of these emotions may have stopped her from trying to form new relationships.

3. Ellen will fully process her feelings of "wrongness," fear, and loneliness to develop constructive meaning that will guide her to take actions that might bring a feeling of "rightness" when on a date.

LONG-TERM GOAL 2: Ellen will explore how to relate to her children as a lesbian parent.

Short-Tem Goals

1. Ellen will fully explore her conflicting cognitions of self-criticism and passivity through personifying them and taking turns speaking with the voice of each one until they are fully understood.

   a. Ellen will become aware of her body as she takes on the role of each voice and identify the emotion, motivation, and action tendencies that go along with these physical sensations.

   b. Ellen will draw new meaning from this processing that allows her to accept the constructive aspects of both voices into her parenting.

2. Ellen will fully explore her inchoate hopes and feelings of determination around parenting.

   a. Ellen will put these feelings into words that describe her beliefs about being an effective parent.

   b. Ellen will focus attention on her desire to be an active parent and consider what type of actions might bring this desire to fruition.

3. Ellen will explore the confusing thoughts she has about coming out to her sons including her fear that her boys will hate her for being a lesbian.

   a. Ellen will put into words her concern that her boys may internalize homophobic ideas and hate themselves if they are gay if she remains closeted until they are adults.

   b. Ellen will fully explore the outcomes that might result from coming out and the meaning these outcomes would have for her and decide on a course of action.

LONG-TERM GOAL 3: Ellen will explore the contradictory feelings guiding her in relating to her ex-husband and extended family members as a lesbian family member.

Short-Term Goals

1. Ellen will explore the boiling-over-with-anger feeling that she experiences in her relationships with her ex-husband and extended family through focusing on her bodily sensations as her anger builds.

   a. Ellen will put into words the motivation that comes from this experience and if it is tied to others wanting her to be submissive and not true to herself.

   b. Ellen will fully process her more deeply understood anger and determine if directly communicating her needs to family members would serve her well at this time.

2. Ellen will explore her vulnerable feelings of pain and isolation that she feels when relating to her ex-husband and extended family through experiencing these feelings vividly.

   a. Ellen will put into words the motivation that comes from this experience.

   b. Ellen will construct meaning from this vividly re-created experience and decide whether it would be adaptive to try and change her role in relating to her ex-husband and extended family at this time.

3. Ellen will become aware of how her feelings of pain and isolation are motivating her to behave very differently than are her feelings of anger in trying to relate to her ex-husband and parents.

   a. Ellen will focus her attention first on her motivation to approach them (to avoid the pain of isolation) and then on her motivation to avoid them (to increase her sense of personal control and self-affirmation).

   b. Ellen will further process these discrepant tendencies until she can develop meaning that will guide her adaptively at this time of self-discovery when she has realistic concerns about losing custody of her sons.

LONG-TERM GOAL 4: Ellen will explore her feelings of confidence and excitement evoked by her new name and how this influences her relationship to herself as a lesbian.

Short-Term Goals

1. Ellen will reexperience her feelings of confidence and excitement associated with her new name.

   a. Ellen will use words to describe what this new name means to her including her motivations and behaviors in regard to it.

   b. Ellen will consider whether alcohol will be a part of this newly named person's life.

   c. Ellen will consider whether heterosexual behavior will ever be a part of this newly named person's life.

2. Ellen will reexperience her feelings of freedom and self-acceptance that occurred when she recognized her new sexual motivation, allowing herself the psychological space to stay fully aware of these emotions.

   a. Ellen will use words to describe the meaning these feelings have for her.

   b. Ellen will consider what behaviors will be most valuable to her in maintaining these positive emotions.

   c. Ellen will discuss her new narrative of herself, how she wants to interact with others, and how she will maintain a healthy lifestyle.

Practice Case for Student Conceptualization: Integrating the Domain of Violence

It is time to do an emotion-focused analysis of Nicole. There are many domains of complexity that might provide insights into her behavior. For this case, you are asked to integrate the Domain of Violence into your case conceptualization and treatment plan.

Information Received From Brief Intake

Nicole is an 18-year-old White female living in a rural town. She is presently a senior in high school. She has an excellent academic record and will be attending college next year. She comes from a nuclear family in which she has three older brothers who are still living at home. Her father is the proprietor of a car mechanic's shop, and his sons work for him. Nicole says that her father and brothers have made a lifestyle out of beating women, including herself and her mother. She now has the opportunity to leave home and move in with her boyfriend Tim; however, she is afraid to go. She wants help making the decision about whether she should leave or stay. Nicole referred herself for treatment after completing a high school psychology course. Her parents are not aware that she has sought treatment, and Nicole wants this information kept private.

During a brief mental status exam, there were no clinical signs of homicidal or suicidal ideation or severe psychopathology. However,

Nicole showed some anxiety when the limits of confidentiality were raised. This anxiety subsided when she was reassured that, at 18, she is no longer under the purview of Child Protective Services. She preferred to receive help from the first clinician who had an opening.

Interview With Nicole (N) From an Emotion-Focused Perspective

C: Hello, Nicole. How can I help?

N: (earnestly) My boyfriend is pressuring me to move in with him when we graduate this spring. (confusedly) I don't know what to tell him. (pause) We've been hanging out together since our freshman year. He's really my best and only friend but . . .

C: (pause) But . . .

N: (uncertainly) I do care, but he wants more, and I don't know if I can give it.

C: He wants more than friendship, and you aren't sure if you do.

N: (certain) I do want him physically. This edgy feeling just overwhelms me whenever I think of having sex with him. Just kissing is hard enough.

C: Do you know what this edginess means?

N: (anxiously) I don't know, and whenever I have tried to talk to Tim about it, he gets angry and avoids me for a while. (pause) Then we just forget about it.

C: It's confusing. You don't really understand it and haven't been able to work it through. Would you like to try to experience it more now?

N: (long pause, then panicky) It's like my skin is crawling. I feel doomed. (whispering) I am not going to keep doing this.

C: (pause) When you experienced it more, it went beyond edgy into something threatening that you had to get away from.

N: (anxiously) This is just great. I come here to get help for this, and I can't stand talking about it. (pause) I am such a loser.

C: The feeling is overwhelming now, but does this mean it always will be?

N: (sadly) Do you think this is a waste of time?

C: You want to work it out, but at this particular moment it feels too hard.

N: (tentatively) Maybe if we talk about something else first, I can handle it later.

C: What feels right to discuss?

N: (long pause, anxiously) I want you to tell me everything is going to work out.

C: It would feel reassuring if I could promise that.

N: (sadly) You won't promise anything, huh?

C: I will promise to listen, to attend to what you say, and to put all my energy into understanding you.

N: (pause, hopefully) Would you really do that for me?

C: You are important. (N smiles) You smiled. It would feel good to experience someone as finding you important.

N: (cautiously) I can't really take it in somehow. I know I'm important to Tim, but I don't feel it. (pause, anxiously) I don't want to lose him.

C: He is important to you. You don't want to lose feeling valued.

N: No . . . I don't . . . but this moving-in thing . . .

C: You don't want to lose Tim, but you feel uneasy about moving in with him.

N: (confusedly) It's weird because I have always hated living at home, and here is my chance to get away.

C: (long pause) You're wondering what's stopping you from escaping from it.

N: I'm a punching bag at home, and so is my mom. I can't remember a time when one of us didn't have bruises healing up somewhere.

C: I'm worried that you're in danger.

N: (emphatically) No. I am OK. I have been living with this all my life. I know how to escape from the house when I need to.

C: This dangerous situation is commonplace to you. (pause) How bad is it?

N: (matter-of-factly) I used to be hurt really bad when I was younger. I didn't know how to recognize the signs of impending disaster. A few times I ended up with a broken arm or leg. Since I've been a teenager, I haven't gotten more than a few bruises. I can tell when things are heating up and can back out the door and get to Tim's house fast. I've done it many times.

C: How do you back out the door?

N: (matter-of-factly) After the first blow, I can always escape. I may pretend to back down and act like I'm going to do what they want, or I get them fighting with each other; that's EASY to do. Then, I take off out the bathroom window or through the front door, whichever is closer.

C: Once you're out of the house, how do you get to Tim's?

N: He's just a few blocks away. His parents have him living in their basement. I can go in the basement door, and they don't even know I'm there.

C: What if Tim's gone?

N: I have a key. (sincerely) Really, this is commonplace for me. I have never needed it, but I know where the battered women's shelter is if I ever do.

C: You have thought about this a lot. You have an escape plan (pause) but . . .

N: (interrupting) Honestly, I know I have to get out at some point. I want to, (pause) but what will happen when I do?

C: There is danger at home, (pause) but you know how to escape. In a new situation, there is the unknown.

N: Exactly. (long pause, anxiously) Maybe it will be worse somewhere else.

C: A frightening thought.

N: (hurriedly) I'm scared. I want to feel safe.

C: You sound anxious. You want to feel safe. Have you ever been safe?

N: (calmly) At school I am. There isn't any hitting at school.

C: School has been a safe place. Anyplace else?

N: (ambivalently) Tim has never hit me. He gets MAD but . . . (pause)

C: But?

N: (hurriedly) I haven't LIVED with him.

C: Tim has gotten mad, and nothing scary has happened so far. You wonder if this would change if you lived in the same house.

N: (anxiously) When people live together, things get very intense.

C: Living together increases intensity, and maybe scary things happen.

N: (pause) It's risky. I don't think I can stand this. (pause) Let's talk of something else.

C: Your fear is filling the room.

N: (desperately) Help me (pause) please.

C: You're trembling. All the fear inside is pouring out.

N: (yelling) I AM GOING TO EXPLODE!

C: (whispering) So much fear. Fear you have had all your life. If it all comes out . . .

N: (anxiously) I don't like this. It feels TERRIBLE.

C: Even though the fear is washing over you, it is safe here to be aware of it.

N: (with forced calm) I need to escape from this before I do something bad. (pause, panicky) I need to stop this NOW!

C: (whispering) Escape if you need to.

N: (desperately) SCHOOL. It will be OK if we talk about school more.

C: (long pause) School . . .

N: (taking deep breaths) School is calm. If you do your work, the teachers smile at you. The worst thing that happens is the teachers jerk you around a little.

C: Calm, smiles, maybe some jerking around.

N: (relaxedly) The jerking stuff is nothing. The teachers make the decisions. They can be bossy. I can go with it. They tell you what to do, but they don't hurt you. A lot of them have encouraged me; that has felt good.

C: Teachers have more power than you, but some have believed in you.

N: (amazedly) They like me. I don't know if I would've ever realized I was smart enough for college if so many of them hadn't told me so.

C: They helped you see yourself as an intelligent person. How does it feel?

N: (reflectively) Nice, I guess. It's the only place I feel at ease with myself.

C: How do you feel here? (long pause, N looks thoughtful) I can see that you're thinking deeply about something. Can you tell me about it?

N: (calmly) I do feel safe here too. It's strange in a way because I just met you and I don't believe in jumping to conclusions.

C: What do you mean?

N: (calmly) There's a lot of uncontrolled anger in the world. I have to be very careful to protect myself.

C: Anger is out there in the world, and it feels dangerous to you.

N: (anxiously) I don't want more hurt. I might escape from it by moving in with Tim. Tim says he wants to share a safe place with me.

C: He needs a safe place; you need a safe place.

N: (seriously) No one is threatening Tim. He's just ignored by his family—kind of an outcast. I'm really his family. I like it, but . . . (N is looking overwhelmed)

C: You look lost. (N nods) You need physical safety; he needs emotional safety. You each get some of that with each other. (pause) But you fear that if Tim gets too close, he might stop being a safe person for you.

N: (anxiously) He would go ballistic if he heard me say that. He has been my best friend through a lot of scary stuff at home.

C: He has been your best friend. But this fear of anger is always with you.

N: (nodding her head) Yeah . . . I can't . . . (long pause) I don't . . . (long pause)

C: You are really struggling to put your feelings into words.

N: (longingly) I need to understand this more. I don't want to fear my best friend. Sometimes I think it is so weird that I could ever be scared of Tim. He knows how much pain I have been in sometimes over my family, and I know he cares for me.

C: But, the fear is still there. It's real. It surrounds you.

N: (sadly) It's never completely gone. (pause) I always hold back.

C: How does it feel in your body when you hold back?

N: (puzzled) I don't know. Tim gets engrossed in me all the time. I see the love in his eyes. I do love him. (looking away) There is always a part of me looking on from afar, kind of examining what is going on at a safe distance.

C: He doesn't fear you, so he can let himself go fully into the relationship. You hold back a part of yourself so you can feel safe.

N: (nodding) Sometimes I have to rush off to the bathroom for a breather. In the mirror I see this look on my own face. (pause) I don't know what it means, but I have seen this look on my mother's face.

C: You don't understand it, but you recognize it. Would your mother understand?

N: (dismissively) I don't know. We don't talk much. What's the point? (pause) She has never helped me. She never will.

C: You share a look with your mother, but you don't share your thoughts. (long pause) Why doesn't she help you?

N: (angrily) I used to cry out for her help when I was little until I figured out she was a total puppet for my dad. The only thing she ever did was keep my hiding place in the kitchen a secret when my dad was hunting for me.

C: She never actively helped you, but did she show she cared by letting you escape?

N: (unconvinced) I don't know if she was showing that she cared. I think she was just showing how passive she was—never doing anything unless she was told to do it. (long pause, angrily) I used to ask myself why my teachers cared more about me than my own mother. (pause, with resignation) I'm used to it now.

C: The attention from your teachers felt good, but it also made you angry because you weren't getting this attention from your mother. What do you think was going on?

N: (long pause, thoughtfully) My dad could never tolerate my mom paying the smallest amount of attention to me; he demands constant attention on himself. When my brothers and I were little, we were all getting slammed by him constantly. Now that they can hold their own against him, he treats them as buddies. He laughs if one of them punches my mom for not doing something fast enough for them. They try to treat me as their slave, but I escape a lot.

C: First your dad and now your brothers use force to keep your mother their slave. You are trying to escape from this.

N: (slumping down in the chair) I feel exhausted. I have really had it for the day.

C: You have experienced a lot of difficult things today. You are ready for a rest. Still, I'm worried about you being safe at home.

N: (tiredly) It's kind of you to care but unnecessary. My dad and brothers work late during the week; I only cross their paths on the weekend. If things look ugly, I can take off. If I get caught by surprise, after the first blow, I can always escape.

C: Even one bruise is too much. You deserve safety. If you were 17, I would be calling Child Protective Services in to protect you from this abuse.

N: (skeptically) Child Protective Services was called in a few times when I was younger. My dad always outsmarted them. Don't worry; I'm going to be OK.

C: I respect your right to decide. I just strongly believe in your right to be safe.

N: (reflectively) I can tell that you mean it. (pause) I'll think about it.

Exercises for Developing a Case Conceptualization of Nicole

Exercise 1 (4-page maximum)

GOAL: To verify that you have a clear understanding of Emotion-Focused Treatment.

STYLE: An integrative essay addressing Parts A–C.

NEED HELP?   Review this Chapter (pages 190–199).

A. Develop a concise overview of the assumptions of Emotion-Focused Treatment (the theory's hypotheses about key dimensions in understanding the role of emotions in adaptive and maladaptive functioning; think broadly, abstractly).

B. Develop a thorough description of how each of these assumptions is used to understand the client and the client's ability to process emotions to develop an integrated understanding of herself, others, and her situation (for each assumption provide specific examples).

C. Describe the role of the clinician in helping the client fully process her experiences (consultant, doctor, educator, helper; treatment approach; technique examples).

Exercise 2 (4-page maximum)

GOAL: To aid application of Emotion-Focused Treatment to Nicole.

STYLE: A separate sentence outline for each section, A–G.

NEED HELP?   Review this Chapter (pages 190–199).

A. What does Nicole view as her weaknesses (concerns, issues, problems, symptoms, skill deficits, treatment barriers, areas in which her growth is blocked) at this time?

For each of these consider the following:

1. What marker of an emotional processing problem, adaptive emotion to a problematic experience, or aspect of a maladaptive emotion scheme might each weakness represent?

2. Looking across all the information above, what maladaptive emotion schemes might be operating in Nicole's life?

   a. Several weaknesses could be part of the same emotion scheme.

   b. Maladaptive schemes can be incomplete, complete but guiding the client in maladaptive ways, or providing conflicting guidance in relation to other schemes.

B. Looking across the markers of emotional processing problems and their underlying emotion schemes, does Nicole have a global processing style (emotionally overregulated, emotionally underregulated, engaged in mostly conceptual processing, engaged in mostly experiential processing)?

   1. Based on your responses to A and B, what core pain(s) or core issue(s) is (are) associated with this global processing style?

   2. Does the core pain(s) or issue(s) relate to an inability to symbolize internal experience, intrapersonal problems, interpersonal problems, or existential concerns?

C. Discuss the type of voice (focused, emotional, limited, external) Nicole uses over the course of the interview, giving specific examples to support your choice. Then, discuss the implications of this for her ability to profit from Emotion-Focused Treatment, in general, and the types of techniques she may profit from most at this time.

D. For each marker you indicated in Part A, discuss the type of emotional processing task it suggests Nicole might profit from at this time. Does the voice you indicated she has in Part C have any influence in facilitating or inhibiting how much Nicole would profit from each task at this time?

E. What does Nicole view as her strengths (strong points, positive features, successes, skills, factors facilitating change, areas in which her growth is not blocked) at this time?

For each of these consider the following:

   1. What signs of healthy emotional processing, aspect of an adaptive emotion scheme, or adaptive emotion might each strength reflect or have developed from?

   2. Looking at all the information above, what healthy or incomplete but partially healthy emotion schemes seem

to be operating in Nicole's life (several strengths could be part of the same scheme)?

3. How might her strengths reflect a positive tendency toward self-growth, and how could these strengths be given more attention so that they could help Nicole with her current difficulties?

F. Considering the information from A–E, what types of meaning is Nicole currently creating from her experiences about herself, others, and her situation, and how does this relate to her overall level of functioning?

G. What barriers or windows of opportunity currently exist to Nicole's fully processing her experiences and drawing adaptive meaning from them at this time?

Exercise 3 (3-page maximum)

GOAL: To develop an understanding of the potential role of violence in Nicole's life.

STYLE: A separate sentence outline for each section, A–D.

NEED HELP? Review Chapter 2 (pages 84–91).

A. Assess the risk factors for Nicole engaging in/being a victim of violence and the protective factors for discouraging violence that are currently in place considering:

1. The *internal* factors within Nicole such as her ability to control impulses, set limits on her own behavior, regulate emotions, engage in reflective problem solving, and understand the emotions and behaviors of others.

2. The *long-term* social network and environment during Nicole's childhood and whether they supported or constrained violence such as the existence of (a) traumatic, ambivalent, or nonexistent emotional bonds; (b) positive emotional bonds; (c) family violence; (d) level of family toleration for violence as a problem-solving strategy; (e) positive or negative school experiences or neighborhood experiences; and (f) religious background.

3. The *current* environmental supports or constraints on violence such as Nicole's (a) family relationships, (b) peer relationships, (c) educational attainment, (d) current neighborhood, and (e) current religious beliefs.

4. Any *immediate* eliciting or triggering factors that might serve to justify and/or make a violent or prosocial response more likely such as (a) presence or absence of a weapon, (b) level of alcohol or drug use, (c) level of frustration/anger, and (d) encouragement or discouragement of violence from others.

5. Nicole's worldview, including a consideration of how generalized or circumscribed a role violence plays in it, and whether Nicole is currently generating/promoting violence or generating/promoting prosocial behavior.

B. Assess Nicole's safety and that of others within her environment at this time and if, and how, safety could be enhanced in both the immediate and the longer term including careful consideration of the *characteristics* of the perpetrators of violence.

C. Assess the overall psychological and physical impact of violence on Nicole and others, whether there are more forces supporting violence or supporting nonviolence, and the prognosis for Nicole living a life free of violence at this time.

D. Assess whether your past experiences with violence, your stereotypes of Nicole's violent lifestyle, or biases embedded in your treatment approach might lead to negative bias, marginalization of her point of view, or an increase in danger to her and others and consider what you might do to modify your approach to increase the likelihood of a positive outcome (be thoughtful and detailed).

Exercise 4 (6-page maximum)

GOAL: To help you integrate your knowledge of Emotion-Focused Treatment and violence issues into an in-depth conceptualization of Nicole (who she is, why she does what she does).

STYLE: An integrated essay consisting of a premise, supportive details, and conclusions following a carefully planned organizational style.

NEED HELP? Review Chapter 1 (pages 7–28) and Chapter 2 (pages 84–91).

STEP 1: Consider what style you should use in organizing your emotion-focused understanding of Nicole that (a) would support you in providing a comprehensive and clear understanding of how she processes emotion and (b) would support language she might find persuasive in her current state of confusion.

STEP 2: Develop your concise premise (overview, preliminary or explanatory statements, proposition, thesis statement, theory-driven introduction, hypotheses, summary, concluding causal statements) that explains Nicole's difficulty deciding where to live. If you are having trouble with Step 2, remember it should be an integration of the key ideas of Exercises 2 and 3 that (a) provides a basis for her long-term goals, (b) is grounded in Emotion-Focused Treatment and is sensitive to issues of violence, and (c) highlights the strengths Nicole brings to Emotion-Focused Treatment.

STEP 3: Develop your supporting material (detailed case analysis of strengths and weaknesses, supplying data to support an introductory premise) from an emotion-focused perspective that integrates within each paragraph a deep understanding of Nicole as a victim of violence. If you need help with Step 3, consider the information you'll need to include in order to (a) support the development of short-term goals, (b) be grounded in Emotion-Focused Treatment that is sensitive to violence issues, and (c) integrate an understanding of how her strengths could be used in processing her emotions for further meaning whenever possible.

STEP 4: Develop your conclusions and broad treatment recommendations including (a) Nicole's overall level of functioning, (b) anything facilitating or serving as a barrier to her fully processing her experiences at this time, and (c) her basic emotional processing needs at this time in order to enhance her natural tendency for positive growth, being careful to consider what you said in Part D of Exercise 3 (be concise and general).

Exercise 5 (3-page maximum)

GOAL: To develop an individualized, theory-driven action plan for Nicole that considers her strengths and is sensitive to violence issues.

STYLE: A sentence outline consisting of long- and short-term goals.

NEED HELP?   Review Chapter 1 (pages 8–28).

STEP 1: Develop your treatment plan overview, being careful to consider what you said in Part D of Exercise 3 to try and prevent any negative bias to your treatment plan.

STEP 2: Develop long-term (major, large, ambitious, comprehensive, broad) goals that *ideally* Nicole would reach by the termination of treatment that would lead her to be free to grow adaptively from her new experiences and live in a nonviolent environment. If you are having trouble with Step 2, reread your premise and support topic sentences looking for ideas to transform into goals that would support emotional processing of internal and external experience (use the *style* of Exercise 4).

STEP 3: Develop short-term (small, brief, encapsulated, specific, measurable) goals that Nicole and you could expect to see accomplished within a few weeks to chart her progress in processing her experiences, instill hope for change, and plan time-effective treatment sessions. If you are having trouble with Step 3, reread your support paragraphs looking for ideas to transform into goals that (a) might help her fully process her experiences of violence and nonviolence, (b) might enhance factors facilitating or decrease barriers to her developing new meaning from her experiences, (c) utilize her strengths in processing her experiences whenever possible, and (d) are individualized to her needs as a victim of abuse rather than generic.

Exercise 6

GOAL: To critique Emotion-Focused Treatment and the case of Nicole.

STYLE: Answer Questions A–E in essay form or discuss them in a group format.

A. What are the strengths and weaknesses of this model for helping Nicole (a teen with a history of violence)?

B. Discuss the pros and cons of taking a feminist approach with Nicole instead of an emotion-focused approach (include consideration of its compatibility with Nicole's view of her difficulties, her potential motivation to work on a treatment plan within its framework, and its responsiveness to issues of violence).

C. Using the Domain of Age, describe how Nicole's childhood exposure to violence influenced her cognitive and psychosocial functioning. Include an analysis of how it influenced her strengths and her weaknesses as an emerging adult.

D. What ethical issues are raised by using a treatment approach with Nicole that gives her the power to decide if she does or does not discuss her physical safety during the course of a session? Can you try to ensure Nicole's safety while continuing to treat her as an expert on her own experience and an equal partner in the treatment relationship?

E. The clinician in Emotion-Focused Treatment uses a process-directive but content-nondirective approach. Discuss your own personal style as a clinician and consider how compatible this is with this type of treatment approach. Does your style fit best overall with the more directive forms of treatment such as behavioral and cognitive or the more nondirective ones such as emotion-focused and constructivist?

Recommended Resources

American Psychological Association (Producer) & Greenberg, L. S. (Trainer). (n.d.). *Process-experiential therapy: Part of the Systems of Psychotherapy Video Series* [Motion picture, #4310290]. (Available from the American Psychological Association, 750 First Street, NE, Washington, DC 20002–4242)

Applied Psychology Institute. (2009). *Welcome to EFT!* Retrieved June 5, 2009, from http://www.emotionfocusedtherapy.org

Elliot, R., Watson, J. C., Goldman, R. N., & Greenberg, L. S. (2004). *Learning emotion-focused therapy.* Washington, DC: American Psychological Association.

Greenberg, L., & Goldman, R. (2007). Case-formulation in emotion-focused therapy. In T. D. Eells (Ed.), *Handbook of psychotherapy case formulation* (2nd ed., pp. 379–411). New York: Guilford Press.

Johnson, S. (2007). *International Centre for Excellence in Emotion Focused Therapy (ICEEF).* Retrieved June 12, 2009, from http://www.eft.ca/home.htm

Seven

Dynamic Case Conceptualizations and Treatment Plans

Introduction to Dynamic Theory

You have just received a referral from the juvenile probation department due to your expertise in working with adolescents. Sergio, a 17-year-old Latino male, was recently arrested for selling marijuana to his high school classmates. He was sentenced to 1 year of probation and mandated into treatment. Sergio's parents, along with a large extended family, live in a rural farming community where there has been significant racial tension between the Mexican and non-Mexican populations. His siblings include Raoul (age 12), Ana (age 10), and Jose (age 8). Sergio's parents and extended family are migrant workers who originally came to the United States for the spring and summer months and then returned to Mexico for the rest of the year. Now, they have settled permanently in the United States. Their income is below the poverty level. Within his family, Sergio is described as a respectful son and responsible family member. At school, Sergio's academic performance has always been in the average range, and he has never been in trouble before now.

You practice a form of time-limited dynamic treatment that considers interpersonal relationships as primary to both adaptive and maladaptive functioning. The goals of treatment will be to improve Sergio's manner of relating to himself and others. Time-limited dynamic treatment has roots in object relations theory, interpersonal theory, and self psychology as well as other psychological theories (Levenson & Strupp, 2007). Sergio, like all people, has biologically programmed needs for human connections in which he will feel safe and loved (Bowlby, 1973; Levenson & Strupp, 2007). Sergio may come to treatment complaining about symptoms of anxiety, depression, or anger. However, it will be his interpersonal style, not these symptoms, that will be the focus of treatment. The following detailed description of time-limited dynamic treatment is taken predominately from the work of Levenson and Strupp (2007) and Strupp and Binder (1984).

How do dysfunctional interpersonal styles develop? They arise from faulty interpersonal relationships, particularly those of early childhood. Sergio will not be pathologized if he has developed a dysfunctional style of relating to others; it will have developed in his realistic attempts to get his basic needs for human connection met. These faulty patterns of relating may be modified or completely transformed based on new life experiences. An adult will only maintain rigid patterns learned in childhood if they are supported by current relationships.

How can Sergio's interpersonal problems be modified or resolved in treatment? The curative factors will develop within an effective treatment relationship. Sergio will inevitably re-create any cyclic maladaptive pattern(s) (CMP) of relating he has developed as he tries to relate to you. However, in the treatment relationship, he will (a) experience a new outcome when relating to you, as opposed to what he received from others, and (b) develop a new understanding of how he has been relating to others, including himself, in his current and possibly his past relationships.

While all clients in time-limited dynamic treatment will experience a new outcome and gain a more flexible pattern of relating to others, not all clients will be guided to experience insights into the development of their CMP(s). Sergio may benefit from insight because he is very intelligent and has shown the ability to reflect on both his motivations and the motivations of others. Some clients may not be capable of this, but they can still profit from time-limited dynamic treatment. For these clients, the clinician will help them develop a healthy interaction style within the treatment setting, and then they will be guided to generalize this to relationships outside of treatment.

Why might Sergio need treatment at this time? Although the focus of treatment will be on Sergio's current life functioning, his need for treatment will be embedded in his early development. In healthy development, Sergio's basic needs for intimacy (ability to relate to others, to form and maintain attachments, to give and gain affection, and to have emotional access) and autonomy (a sense of independence and self-regulation acquired through exploration of one's abilities) will have been met effectively and consistently in his relationships with caregivers (Bowlby, 1973; Strupp & Binder, 1984). Through these healthy interpersonal relationships, Sergio will have learned to accept limitations on his caregivers' ability to respond to him, and he will have learned to tolerate reasonable delays in getting his needs met. Through these age-appropriate and minimal frustrations, the young Sergio will have learned to soothe himself when necessary. As a result of these experiences, he will have a positive sense of self (trust in himself), realistic and adaptive expectations of himself and others, and a flexible way of relating to people. These healthy attitudes and patterns of relating will be internalized into a model of how the interpersonal world works.

In contrast, if Sergio's needs were not met consistently in his early interpersonal relationships, he will have developed one or more CMPs (Bowlby, 1973; Strupp & Binder, 1984). Sergio will have developed these faulty and rigid patterns of relating in an indirect attempt to get his needs met and avoid anxiety or depression. Sergio will have developed an internalized model of the interpersonal world that contains self-defeating expectations of himself and others. He will have poor self-esteem and low self-efficacy. Sergio's internal model of the interpersonal world represents his personal interpretation of reality and consists of the roles he casts for himself including his thoughts, feelings, and wishes in relationship to others; the roles he casts for others including his expectations and perceptions within interpersonal interactions; and his introjects about himself. These introjects will contain his thoughts, feelings, and wishes in relation to himself. Sergio's internalized model of the interpersonal world should contain many different interpersonal patterns of relating so that Sergio can respond flexibly to the situation he is in and the person he's relating to. However, if Sergio has a maladaptive model of the interpersonal world, he will have at least one CMP and possibly more. In this case, time-limited dynamic treatment will focus Sergio's attention on his most pervasive or problematic style of relating.

Will Sergio's early life experiences inevitably influence his present behavior? Environmental circumstances may change with age; however, Sergio's interpersonal behavior could still be guided by fantasies, fears, and misconceptions developed early in life. If this is so, Sergio's dysfunctional interpersonal patterns could be replicated in all of his current interpersonal relationships, including sibling or peer relationships, work or academic relationships, parental relationships, and the treatment relationship. However, his model of the interpersonal world is always open to change and will respond to changes within his ongoing relationships as a teenager. When he leaves home and engages in a fully adult life, Sergio's internal model of the interpersonal world will continue to be open to change based on interactions with new people in his life and any changes in their behavior. Thus, if Sergio developed a dysfunctional style of relating in early life, it will only be continued, unchanged, if the maladaptive patterns continue to be fostered in his current relationships.

How might current relationships foster dysfunctional styles of relating? One way would be for Sergio to enter into complementary maladaptive relationships with other individuals who also have dysfunctional interpersonal patterns. Assume that in Sergio's childhood, he was able to receive nurturance from his authoritarian parents only if he engaged in submissive behavior. Although he may have desired greater independence, he may have preferred to subvert this need to maintain a sense of emotional connection to his parents. As an adult, Sergio may now unintentionally seek out relationships with autocratic individuals because he understands how to get his needs for nurturance met through such individuals.

Another way his dysfunctional patterns could be reinforced would be if he unintentionally solicited from others exactly those reactions that he most fears or wants. For example, by his submissive behavior, Sergio may elicit authoritarian behavior from others. Finally, Sergio may interpret social interactions in a manner consistent with maladaptive expectations. For example, if a teacher asks him what project he would like to work on for class, Sergio might interpret this as a setup in which the teacher is looking for ways to criticize his behavior if he does not choose the "right" project. Thus, the behavior of others in Sergio's current relationships could inadvertently reinforce Sergio's maladaptive pattern of relating. A dysfunctional interpersonal episode that occurred once in response to an unusual circumstance in Sergio's life would not be a CMP. For example, if there is a tyrannical teacher at his high school around whom all of the students behave submissively, Sergio showing submission in reaction to this teacher is saying more about the teacher than Sergio. In addition, it will be important to examine whether some of his interpersonal patterns are typical for his cultural group and/or represent adaptations to cultural demands, rather than idiosyncratic interpersonal patterns of Sergio. Although Sergio is consciously aware of some aspects of his internal model of the interpersonal world, much of it is preconscious or unconscious (Strupp & Binder, 1984).

Role of the Clinician

In time-limited dynamic treatment, you are a participant/observer of interpersonal behavior who provides Sergio with a new model to identify with and who collaborates with Sergio, as a trustable and reliable ally, in the process of examining his interpersonal behavior. Broadly, there will be two treatment goals: (a) to create a new interpersonal experience within the therapeutic relationship and (b) to create a new understanding for Sergio of how he relates to himself and other people. You will need to be very aware of your thoughts and feelings as you relate to Sergio. These will provide key data for you to use in both figuring out the nature of his interpersonal problems and determining what to do differently to provide the new experience that Sergio needs to have within the treatment relationship.

Your first task is to determine if Sergio has one or more CMPs that, though they may be historically significant, can be clearly related to his present life struggles. In addition, if appropriate, this pattern will be explained to Sergio using terms that he can understand. If you determine that insight into the pattern is not in Sergio's best interests, you will discuss his relationship problems only in terms that are directly relevant to his specific presenting problems.

To evaluate Sergio's interpersonal relationships and determine if there is a rigid and dysfunctional pattern of relating, you seek to answer four questions:

1. What is Sergio's role for himself in interacting with others? This includes how he behaves toward other people as well as his feelings, thoughts, and intentions toward other people. Sergio may act in ways to evoke certain feared or wished-for reactions from others.

2. How does Sergio expect other people to respond to his interpersonal behavior? This includes all the thoughts Sergio has that anticipate how other people will respond to his interpersonal behavior.

3. What are the acts of others toward Sergio (how do others relate to him), and how does he perceive this interpersonal behavior? This includes how other people respond to Sergio's interpersonal behavior and how he interprets the meaning of their responses. Sergio may also misconstrue the behavior of others as meeting his prior expectations.

4. What is Sergio's role in relating to himself (his introjects)? This includes how he behaves toward himself (self-punishing, self-nurturing, and so forth) as well as his thoughts, feelings, and intentions toward himself. He is likely to treat himself in the same way he perceives significant others as treating him.

Trying to understand Sergio's interpersonal model, through organizing his interpersonal behavior into these four categories, is valuable because it helps reduce a large amount of information about his experiences into a concise format; it may also help you clarify Sergio's reactions to you and your reactions toward him.

At times it may be confusing to you to determine exactly which of Sergio's thoughts, feelings, and behaviors are directed at others or at himself. It may not be critical to make this discrimination if it won't interfere with you understanding his overall interpersonal style. The identified CMP represents your hypothesis for explaining Sergio's current interpersonal difficulties. It may need to be modified as more information about his relationships becomes available. You may also become aware that some of Sergio's interpersonal behavior represents flexible and adaptive patterns; these reflect his interpersonal strengths.

As Sergio is intelligent enough and reflective enough to benefit from it, once you have developed an understanding of Sergio's focused CMP, your second task will be to help Sergio develop insight into it as he relates to you within the treatment session. Once this is accomplished, your next task will be to help him explore the ramifications of it for his current life. Over the course of treatment, once Sergio begins to show signs of improved relating within the session and outside of it, it is important for you to comment on this and help Sergio value his interpersonal strengths (Levenson & Strupp, 2007).

How are these tasks accomplished? The clinician must create a good working relationship with Sergio through communicating interest in him, listening empathetically to him, and developing an understanding of his inner world. The clinician will also provide a new model for Sergio to identify with that is more adaptive than the models available to him in childhood. At first, Sergio may not be able to benefit fully from this good relationship. If conflicted, he will attempt to re-create his CMP with you. As a participant-observer of this interpersonal process, you will routinely step out of the process to observe and then comment to Sergio about what is happening within the treatment relationship in terms of transference and countertransference phenomena. Transference is Sergio's inevitable attempt to repeat his internalized interpersonal patterns (ideas and beliefs about self, others, and the interaction of self and others) with you. You need to be vigilant to, and comment on, Sergio's attempts to elicit a type of interpersonal response such as domination, control, manipulation, exploitation, criticism, and so forth in order to re-create his CMP.

You will also experience countertransference reactions to Sergio's behavior. Countertransference provides important clues to you as to what Sergio needs as a corrective experience. First you determine the pattern you have been pulled into and then you determine how you should start behaving, within your role as a clinician, to disrupt this rigid, interpersonal pattern. By choosing, from the many relationship-enhancing manners of responding to Sergio, what would be most valuable to him, you are individualizing treatment to his interpersonal needs. Perhaps he needs you to be matter-of-fact, not angry, when he engages in teasing behavior. Perhaps Sergio needs you to show respect for his desire to be treated as an adult male. If the countertransference you show is not parallel to how other significant others are relating to Sergio, then you need to examine whether the countertransference really relates to your own unique history rather than to Sergio.

Your interpretation of the interpersonal process provides Sergio with cognitive and experiential learning about his cyclic maladaptive patterns of relating to others. Whether the interpretations are concrete and very much tied to the presenting problem or reflect more insight-inducing comments about the interpersonal pattern depends on Sergio's abilities to think and reflect about himself and others. Interpretations in the here and now are emphasized more than those of early childhood relationships. Narrative truth to Sergio is considered more important than historical validity. Inferences should be kept to a minimum, and interpretations should be tied to a reality that he understands. The interpretation process can be damaging if you communicate too complexly and/or are rejecting. As Sergio lives through affectively painful and ingrained interpersonal scenarios yet receives a different reaction from you (different from what is expected based on past relationships), he will gain a greater ability to question his prior assumptions about his self-image and about the attitudes and intentions of others. As Sergio gains confidence in examining his own CMP, he will have an increased ability to confront his previously repressed emotions and fantasies associated with them. You are a reliable and trustworthy ally in this process. Through the context of a good relationship with a supportive and empathetic listener, Sergio can develop new patterns of thinking, feeling, and acting within relationships. Time limits must be set at the beginning of treatment and discussed on a continuing basis with Sergio. A planned termination is considered essential to solidifying treatment gains within short-term, dynamic treatment.

Case Application: Integrating the Domain of Race and Ethnicity

Sergio's case will now be examined in detail. There are many domains of complexity that might be appropriate to apply to him. The Domain of Race and Ethnicity has been selected to consider within a dynamic case conceptualization and treatment plan. As racism is an important issue in this case, assume the clinician has no Mexican heritage.

Interview With Sergio (S) From a Dynamic Perspective

C: Good afternoon, Sergio. As you know, your probation officer called me yesterday to set up this appointment. He selected me because I work a lot with teenagers. He told me that your family is from Mexico. I have never been there, but I have seen some pictures and it is a very beautiful country. (long pause) Would you mind telling me why you are here from your point of view? (long pause) I was told that your family speaks Spanish at home. Spanish is a powerful language for expressing yourself. (pause) I'm sorry that I don't speak it. Perhaps you would prefer to talk in Spanish?

S: (sullenly, looking down) I am here because I have to be here.

C: It has been forced on you. (pause) You have a lot of self-control to come here when you feel forced.

S: (starts calmly but gets sullen) Yes, I have control. Is that so surprising to you?

C: I was meaning to show respect for your point of view, but the meaning of it became garbled somehow and you feel insulted.

S: (angrily) I want to be treated with respect and not jerked around by you and everyone else.

C: Jerking people around is wrong. I don't ever intentionally do that. However, if you ever feel jerked around, I would appreciate you letting me know.

S: (pause, sincerely) If you mean it, (looks briefly up at C) that is good.

C: I do mean it. (pause) I read the court records on your case, and I saw that your entire family came to court with you.

S: (defiantly) My family is everything to me.

C: I wonder if you think I can't ever understand how much you love your family. (S nods and looks down, long pause) Would you tell me about them?

S: I live with my mother and father in a house next to my mother's parents. All over the neighborhood there are other Mexican families, many of whom are related to us or who lived near us in Mexico. My uncle Jose came here first. When his boss at the farm, Mr. Zuckerman, needed more help, we all began to come. We work very hard for this man on his farm during the summer. He is a good man. He isn't like the other Whites in this town.

C: You love your family, and you respect this man. You are dedicated to them.

S: I respect my parents and grandparents. (pause and then emphatically) Everyone should respect them. They have always worked hard. (pause, lovingly) They do everything for me, my brothers, and my sister.

C: Their role is to care for you, and they do it with love. (S nods) What do you do?

S: (sincerely) I try to help. We all help bring in crops over the summer, and my mother also sews in a factory during the other months when the farm doesn't need us. When she is working, I watch my younger brothers and sister a lot. I try to help them with their schoolwork and their duties at home.

C: How do your brothers and sister react to this?

S: (smiling down at his lap) They look up to me. I watch out for them.

C: You describe a very close-knit and caring family. Are there any problems?

S: (sullenly) We have no problems. We have a tight community—we stay together. We try to avoid the Whites, except at work, but they still cause us trouble.

C: What do you mean?

S: (disgustedly) Some of our neighbors are White, and they are always spying on us.

C: How are they spying?

S: (sarcastically) They come out on their porches to watch us doing yard work or playing ball, to listen to us talk.

C: How good are they at spying?

S: (with a chuckle) They don't understand Spanish. So, they don't know what we are saying. They just pretend to be busy, but they aren't doing much of anything.

C: Do you always speak Spanish at home?

S: (defensively) It's our language.

C: I didn't mean to insult you. I'm sorry. (pause) Have you wondered how your neighbors would react if they could understand what you say?

S: (calmly) It wouldn't be any different. (pause, angrily) They reported my parents last year to the police because I was out late at night.

C: It sounds like this made you very angry. (S nods) What happened?

S: (angrily) Some Child Protective Services worker investigated us. (pause) They were so disrespectful to my parents, but my father . . . he insisted we just answer their questions and then be quiet. They told him I had to be in the house by 11; that is the curfew for teenagers. He said OK to them, but (pause) my parents know what is right for me—not those ignorant people.

C: What do your parents expect from you?

S: (reflectively) On a weekday, I need to come home right after school ends to take care of my brothers Raoul and Jose and my sister Ana. On the weekend, my parents let me run around as much as I want with my *primos.* (C looks confused) Sorry, I mean my cousins. They don't expect me home until I get there.

C: So, you might come home really late at night.

S: (calmly) Sometimes not until morning. I can handle myself. We have a good time.

C: Your parents trust you and respect your decision about when you are ready to come home.

S: (calmly) They know I am a man now. They respect my judgment.

C: You expect this respect from them. They understand you can be trusted.

S: (smiling) Yes. (pause) Of course when I was little, they guided me, babied me. I don't need that now.

C: What are you doing when you are out with your cousins?

S: (smiling) We are just hanging out in someone's house or yard eating, listening to music, joking around, maybe cruising in a car. (pause) It's nobody else's business.

C: How are you feeling when you're with your cousins?

S: (smiling) Great. I always feel accepted by them. They know who I am. (S is silent)

C: What are you thinking about?

S: (tensely) Are you going to tell my probation officer that I'm out late sometimes past the stupid curfew he set for me?

C: I will not report you. But, I know the probation department is serious about its rules. If your probation officer finds out, he will come down hard on you.

S: (reflectively) My parents worry about this too.

C: They do? (S nods) What would it mean to you to come home earlier while you are on probation?

S: (emphatically) I don't want to be told what to do by that officer who doesn't know who I am and doesn't respect me.

C: When you feel respected, like by your parents, are you willing to listen?

S: (calmly) Of course. Elders are there to guide us, (angrily) but my probation officer knows nothing about me at all. He has no respect for me!

C: How do you know he doesn't respect you?

S: (tensely) I am not treated as a man and allowed to speak. He just tells me to sit, listen, and do what he says. It is only out of respect for my parents' wishes that I go to see him (pause) and come here—not because of him!

C: Even though you perceive this officer as disrespectful, you are still showing up for your appointment with him out of your deep respect for your parents.

S: (sincerely) I don't want to bring more trouble to my parents. I was trying to help them when I got into all this trouble to begin with.

C: With the marijuana?

S: (resignedly) The laws here on marijuana are just stupid. Many people smoke in Mexico just to relax. It is nothing. I know guys who bring it with them when they come across the border each summer. Money was tight at home, so I asked these guys if I could have some to sell to make money for my parents; some of those White kids at school have lots of money to spend.

C: Did your parents know what you were doing?

S: (sadly) No, and they were angry when they found out. They say it's against the law here and that I should respect the law.

C: Do your parents smoke?

S: (angrily) No, of course not!

C: I'm sorry, but you said "it was nothing" and that "many people smoke."

S: (sheepishly) My father thinks it is a waste of a life to smoke, and he has forbidden me to smoke. Still it is true that a lot of people I know do smoke. No one cares when a White person does it.

C: What makes you say that?

S: (frustratedly) I had seen a lot of drugs around the high school before. Some people have gotten caught, but I have seen only ME getting sent to the police.

C: Why would they pick you out?

S: (angrily) I'm Mexican, and they blame everything bad on us.

C: For you, racism is the issue, not selling marijuana.

S: (angrily) They are punishing me for being Mexican and going to their school. The people want us in the summer to work on their farms, but they don't want us staying in town afterward. We are supposed to go back to Mexico until the next summer. They don't care how hard it is to live without a permanent home.

C: How do you know all this?

S: (angrily) No one wanted to rent a house to my parents except in the crummy part of town. All the Mexican families live in these broken-down houses, while on the other side of town most Whites live in beautiful places. When we go shopping, they look at us funny, and they won't let their kids hang out with us at school.

C: You sound angry.

S: (reflectively) I don't know. I guess I am used to it, but Ana was in tears the other day because four other girls in her class were going to some birthday party she hadn't been invited to. I told her to forget those girls—they are bad. We don't need any of them. Our community has parties all the time, and those girls aren't invited. We have lots of good times. We don't need any of them.

C: You feel close to family members, and you enjoy your time with them. But why do you say those girls are bad? What do you know about them?

S: (emphatically) I asked Ana; they are all White. With a few exceptions, like Mr. Zuckerman and some of my teachers, the Whites here don't trust us.

C: Is it possible those four girls were friends before Ana even came along?

S: (pause, reflectively) I guess so. I didn't think about that. Some of the Whites are probably alright like Mr. Zuckerman, but most are racist.

C: You sound so sure. How do you know?

S: My parents don't speak English well and can't read the signs at stores or the labels on things. I shop for them because English came easily to me. At all the stores, I am followed around like I am a thief. At first, I didn't know what to do. Now I play some games with the employees. Sometimes I say, "I'm too busy to shoplift today. Maybe I'll come back tomorrow" and just leave the store without buying anything.

C: It hurts you to feel distrusted. (S nods) You sometimes respond by teasing people. How do they react?

S: (ironically) They get scared; they take it seriously. They are just stupid. My family works hard for the money I spend in their stupid stores. Everyone in our community works hard. We are honest people, and we deserve respect.

C: Hard work does deserve respect. When people follow you, you have a right to feel angry about it. You tease them; they get scared. (pause) Do you always do this?

S: (reflectively) Sometimes I just take a long time to find the money at the cash register.

C: Do they know you are teasing them?

S: (tensely) They just think I'm stupid and slow . . . like all Mexicans.

C: Mexicans aren't stupid or slow.

S: (angrily) I have heard them saying this when they think I can't hear them.

C: Their comments hurt you. (pause) Does part of you believe what they say?

S: (reflectively) Only when I am with them. Once I'm home, I know I am not stupid. I do well in school. My math teacher is trying to get me to work harder. He is one of the good teachers at school. He doesn't care about skin color; he just tries to help everyone. He has noticed I can follow everything he says in class—even when many others are lost. I could do better if I had more time to do my homework, but my brother Jose—he is 8—he has lots of trouble learning, and I have to spend a lot of time helping him; that must come first.

C: You are dedicated to all of them, but Jose—he particularly needs you. What do your parents think about your behavior at the stores?

S: (calmly) They don't want me to play these games, so I'm trying to break the habit. (pause) My father says it's childish. He's right. I am a man and shouldn't do it.

C: You are very focused on who you are as a man. What are your plans right now?

S: (emphatically) I need to decide how to help my parents. When I first heard about their money trouble, I told them I would drop out of school and work full-time, but they were against it. They are proud to think I could graduate from high school—I would be the first in the family. But my family needs more money.

C: Could anyone help you find a part-time job?

S: (earnestly) I asked Mr. Zuckerman if he could give me work. He says he doesn't need extra help in the winter and doesn't know anyone who does. He did say he would give me a good reference if I need one.

C: Can anyone in the Mexican community help you?

S: (calmly) No, we are all hungry in the winter.

C: It's painful to know your community doesn't get enough of basic things like food.

S: (sadly) It's the reality we live in. If the Whites were all like Zuckerman, we would be alright.

C: Mr. Zuckerman knows who you really are. How would he describe you as an employee?

S: (calmly) He would say I am always on time, I never take days off, and I work hard.

C: That sounds like the type of man anyone would want to hire. (S nods) You have confidence in this. Could your probation officer help you find work?

S: (uncertainly) Why would he help me? To him, I'm dirt. That's why he orders me around.

C: Could there be any other reason he acts that way?

S: (reflectively) He's White, so I assume he hates Mexicans. (pause) OK, I play stupid around him, and maybe that's not the right thing to do.

C: If you showed him who you really are, could something better happen? (S is silent) Is it possible he could learn to treat you with respect and maybe help get you a job?

S: (uncertainly) I don't know.

C: There is a lot of racism in this town. However, your expectations and perceptions of me and other people, both Mexican and White, are important to explore. Sometimes how you treat people has an important impact on how they treat you. We will talk more about this next week. I appreciate the respectful way you have treated me and my questions.

Dynamic Case Conceptualization of Sergio: Assumption-Based Style

Sergio comes from a close-knit, Mexican family in which his basic needs for nurturance, closeness, and emotional connection as well as his needs for autonomy and independence have been well met. He has identified strongly with his parents, whom he perceives as loving and self-sacrificing. As a result, he has developed a generally adaptive internal model for understanding himself, other people, and interpersonal relationships. This adaptive model is reflected in his predominately healthy narratives about himself and his family as reflected in his positive acts toward others, his realistic expectations of others, his accurate perceptions of the reactions of others to himself, and his constructive personal introjects. Sergio's parents have faced an intense, ongoing struggle to support their children financially within what appears to be a highly racist, White community. They have only other extended family (Mexicans) to turn to for help. This may have fostered an "us" versus "them" (Mexicans versus Whites) mentality. By his strong identification with his parents, Sergio may have internalized this tendency in the form of negative perceptions and expectations for Whites. This is not a true split of good versus bad as Sergio has been able to perceive differences among Whites or possibly non-Mexicans who aren't White (neighbors and storeowners versus teachers and the clinician). However, these negative expectations and perceptions are important factors in Sergio's recent conflicts with some White community members and the legal system.

How does Sergio act toward others? He is an active and socially outgoing individual who engages in positive interpersonal relationships with his parents, siblings, and extended family. His acts of self toward the Mexican community consist of socially outgoing and responsible behavior in which he values others, defers to the wishes of his elders, and is responsive to the needs of his younger siblings. His acts of self toward Whites range from flexible to rigid. Toward Whites or non-Mexicans whom he perceives as condescending to him, not respecting him, or reviling him (neighbors, school peers, storeowners), he responds with withdrawal, passive-aggressive behavior, or minor acts of verbal aggression. Toward Whites or non-Mexicans he perceives as relatively accepting (some teachers, Mr. Zuckerman, the clinician), he can be open, clear thinking, and assertive.

What are Sergio's expectations of others? He has positive expectations for how other Mexicans will react to him. He has a solid faith in his parents' love and respect for him as a growing man. He views them as trusting his ability to be independent and to make decisions about his own life. He is confident that his siblings love him and appreciate the time he takes to care for them and encourage their growth. His baseline expectations for the White community are negative. He expects the behavior of Whites in the neighborhood, schools, and stores to be disrespectful and demeaning; it is likely these oppressive behaviors are occurring. However, he is behaving in ways that can elicit the very negative behavior and stereotyping he most hates and fears from Whites or non-Mexicans who might not mistreat him without this evocative behavior. Sergio has shown the ability to test out his baseline expectations and take in clearly positive interpersonal feedback from Whites or non-Mexicans (some teachers, Mr. Zuckerman, the clinician) despite his overall negative perceptual set. Sergio's negative expectations have a foundation in reality as there have been racial incidents within his community.

How do other people respond to Sergio, and how does he perceive this interpersonal behavior? His Mexican family and friends enjoy his company and respect his judgment, and he perceives this positively. On the other hand, he has negative perceptions of most White people's behavior. He views many of them as distrusting and reviling him. While there have been racial incidents within the community, he may have misperceived or not perceived some ambiguous or nondiscriminatory community behavior. For example, the curiosity that all new neighbors tend to arouse in a neighborhood may have appeared to Sergio as antagonism. Similarly, the aloofness that a new student can arouse in a close-knit school group may have been misperceived by Sergio as racial antagonism. The report of neglect made against his family, while inappropriate within a culturally aware context, is not out of keeping with the reporting laws for abuse and neglect within the United States. However, the fact that White students were not arrested for bringing drugs to school but he was clearly suggests he was targeted because he is Mexican. Thus, while some of his perceptions of oppression are accurate, it is important for Sergio to recognize the role he sometimes plays in furthering or possibly initiating negative views of Mexicans by his intentionally irritating, provocative, or intimidating responses to White community members. Sergio has shown an openness to considering when his perceptions are and are not accurate.

What are Sergio's introjects? He views himself as a competent, loving, and responsible family member and believes that, if given the chance, he can be a successful worker. He is proud of his ability to care for his siblings. He primarily treats himself in a positive manner and appreciates and respects his capabilities. He experiences pride and self-respect when he considers the recommendation Mr. Zuckerman is willing to give him for his work on the farm. He experiences strong feelings of shame when he does things that are counter to his parents' values, such as his selling marijuana in the schools and teasing storeowners. There are some signs, in the comments he makes about his White peers and neighbors, that he may have taken in some negative Mexican stereotypes.

Sergio has learned how to get his intimacy and autonomy needs met effectively within his relationships with Mexicans. His fully adaptive functioning is presently inhibited by his rigid, but not inflexible, negative perceptions and expectations for Whites. These, added to what may be cultural confusion over the ethics of marijuana usage, have resulted in his current status as a drug offender. His drug dealing is not believed to reflect antisocial tendencies, and his conviction, which resulted in probation, may serve as a window of opportunity for challenging Sergio to reexamine his negative perceptions and beliefs about Whites within the treatment setting. Within a treatment relationship, Sergio can experience a reaction to any of his interpersonally distancing behavior such as teasing and acting stupid or showing hostility that is different from what he has experienced from the non-Mexicans in his town. Sergio can explore his unconscious struggle for acceptance from the White community and his tendency to use the defense of splitting (good/bad). He will recognize that his style of interacting with Whites is less effective than the one he uses with Mexican Americans. This insight will help ensure his probation ends satisfactorily and that his conviction does not have a continuing negative impact on his ability to succeed in the dominant culture of the United States. Sergio is highly motivated to gain employment, and an active approach in helping him do so will heighten his motivation for change, serve to further reinforce his interpersonal competencies within the White community, and support his positive identity as an adult male who provides emotionally and financially for his family.

Dynamic Treatment Plan: Assumption-Based Style

Treatment Plan Overview. The clinician needs to be sensitive to the likelihood that Sergio will experience further acts of overt or subtle racism during the course of treatment; otherwise these will create a barrier to treatment success. Treatment Goal 1 will focus on the treatment relationship and then expand as appropriate to other relationships (probation officer, teachers, neighbors, peers, parents). Treatment Goal 2 will be completed as part of the termination process. While helping Sergio find paid employment is not a typical goal from a dynamic perspective, it is considered a critical component of culturally sensitive treatment in Sergio's case as this is the goal he is most motivated to achieve in order to help his family. The competencies Sergio has shown in reflecting about his conflict-ridden interpersonal transactions with Whites suggest that short-term treatment will be effective. The treatment plan follows the *basic format.*

LONG-TERM GOAL 1: Sergio will use his experience within the treatment relationship to increase the flexibility of his internal model of the interpersonal world with Whites or non-Mexicans.

Short-Term Goals

1. Sergio will become aware of the role he has taken on within most White or non-Mexican relationships he is currently involved in; he will make a list of these individuals to facilitate this.

   a. Sergio will become aware of how he has acted within his relationship with Mr. Zuckerman and how this has increased the likelihood of Mr. Zuckerman maintaining or developing positive stereotypes of Mexicans.

   b. Sergio will become aware of how he has used eliciting maneuvers, such as teasing storeowners, that have increased the likelihood that some of these Whites or non-Mexicans will reject him and how his behaviors have supported their maintaining negative stereotypes of Mexicans.

   c. Sergio will become aware of his emotions, fantasies, and wishes involving each of these people and become aware of how his negatively cast ones may have led to his good/bad (Mexican White/non-Mexican) categorization.

2. Sergio will become aware of how he expects to be treated by specific Whites and the emotions that accompany these expectations.

   a. Sergio will become aware of his negative expectations for how each White person will treat him and how this has influenced his emotions during interactions with this person during the week.

   b. Sergio will become aware of his positive expectations for treatment by Mexicans and how this has influenced his emotions during interactions with specific Mexican people during the week.

3. Sergio will discuss his perceptions of the treatment he has received during the week from others and the evidence he has to support the accuracy of his perceptions toward specific Mexicans, Whites, or non-Mexicans.

   a. Sergio will discuss his positive perceptions and the evidence he has to support them for Mexicans, Whites, or non-Mexicans during the past week.

   b. Sergio will discuss his negative perceptions and the evidence he has to support them for Mexicans, Whites, or non-Mexicans during the past week.

4. Sergio will become more aware of his introjects as he takes on the role of a Mexican, son, brother, young adult, person on probation, and person in treatment.

   a. Sergio will more fully experience his feelings of anger and shame engendered by episodes of racism during the week within any of his roles and consider whether negative community stereotypes are influencing his introjects.

b. Sergio will more fully experience his feelings of pride, love, and respect that are engendered by positive interactions within any of his roles and consider how these interactions are influencing his introjects.

c. Sergio will more fully experience his needs as a young adult for emotional intimacy and independence and consider how well these needs are met within the roles he takes on and how these influence his introjects.

LONG-TERM GOAL 2: Sergio will increase his ability to meet his need for autonomy (being perceived by himself, his family, and others as an adult) through gaining paid employment to support his family's financial health.

Short-Term Goals

1. Sergio will become aware of the role he took on within his work for Mr. Zuckerman as well as his emotions, fantasies, and wishes for himself as an employee for someone else who is likely to be White or non-Mexican.

2. Sergio will explore, with the clinician, teachers, and the probation officer, the expectations of employers within the United States for their employees' behavior most particularly as it relates to on-the-job behavior as well as drug use.

3. Sergio will become aware of his own perceptions of his treatment by Mr. Zuckerman as well as his emotions, fantasies, and wishes for how White or non-Mexican employers may treat him when he first comes to work for them and what actions he could take to encourage a positive stereotype of Mexicans.

4. Sergio will become aware of his introjects about himself as a good employee and further explore any positive or negative emotions he has about his identity as a young adult seeking to help his family financially.

Practice Case for Student Conceptualization: Integrating the Domain of Gender

It is time to do a dynamic analysis of Steve. There are many domains of complexity that may be appropriate to him. You are asked to integrate the Domain of Gender into your dynamic case conceptualization and treatment plan.

Information Received From Brief Intake

Steve is a senior in college. He has majored in art. He describes himself as being in excellent health and a talented artist. He lives in an apartment off campus with several friends and periodically visits his parents who live in a city about 2 hours away. He comes from an upper-middle-class family, which has provided the financial support for his college attendance. He has referred himself because as he approaches graduation, now just 1 month away, he is becoming increasingly concerned about his ability to be financially independent after leaving college.

During a brief mental status exam, he demonstrated a moderate level of anxiety about his future; however, he showed no signs of suicidal or homicidal ideation or severe psychopathology He expressed a preference for a male clinician but is willing to take a female if that would give him an earlier appointment.

Interview With Steve (S) From a Dynamic Perspective

C: I understand from the phone intake that you have been feeling stressed for about a month.

S: (angrily) I feel really stupid being here. I should be able to handle this on my own.

C: You are angry about needing help from someone.

S: (confusedly) I don't really know why I came. I have always solved my problems on my own. (emphatically) All of my friends solve their own problems. I'm sorry that I have wasted your time.

C: Are you sure that asking for help is a waste of my time?

S: (with determination) Of course. If you can t take care of yourself, you are a loser. (pause) Why would anyone want to help a loser?

C: Might I have any other perceptions of you?

S: (dismissively) No. If any of my friends knew that I had come here, they would be laughing it up.

C: I will see you as a loser, and your friends will laugh.

S: (intently) You bet. They know how independent I am. (thoughtfully) At first, they would think I was kidding about coming here. Then, they would make fun of me and maybe call me "Mr. Psycho."

C: Your friends don't help you when you have a problem?

S: (derisively) Only losers have problems. All of my friends are artists; they are very self-sufficient. They talk of art, art theory, the stupidity of some of the art profs around here, or the moronic taste of most of the students here.

C: You belong to a group of young artists who keep separate from most of the other students here.

S: (calmly) Yes, we keep pretty much to ourselves; our goals are just on a different plane. We each have our own talent and work hard to develop it within ourselves.

C: It sounds like you are alone a lot.

S: (emphatically) Of course, you must be alone to create. (fervently) It's unbelievable to be on your own, creating something really important that maybe only a few people will ever truly appreciate.

C: You are alone with your art, your problems ... even with your friends. (pause) You keep changing your position. How are you feeling right now?

S: (with increasing stress) My back has been hurting a lot lately; it's been keeping me from doing my work.

C: The pain in your body has slowed you down and given you more time to think.

S: (intently) Yes, I have been thinking a lot, but these aren't the type of thoughts I share with my friends. (softly) They would just laugh and then find a reason to walk out.

C: What will happen if you tell me?

S: (reflectively) I guess it's your job to listen. (pause) I hear seniors talking all the time about their plans for after graduation. Some are getting married; some have jobs. All of them seem to be having parties or something to celebrate. I haven't been invited to any parties, and my parents haven't suggested I have one. (confused) Not that I need that kind of thing—it's really irrelevant.

C: But it feels strange not to be connected to friends the way most of the other students seem to be.

S: (nodding) Yeah, I never have been even as a child. I have always been self-sufficient, even from my folks. I only need my art.

C: Your art. (pause) What does it mean to you?

S: (sounding happy for the first time) I feel really free and expressive.

C: Has something changed? (pause) You don't look like you feel free.

S: (softly) It used to feel great, but now it doesn't. In the studio, I look over at my friends painting, and I wonder who they are.

C: Have you asked them?

S: (sarcastically) They would just laugh if I asked them something like that. We are always laughing at the boring lives most people lead, constantly fighting with each other and being jealous of each other. (anxiously) I'm not laughing now. I don't have anyone to be jealous of and yet . . .

C: You feel alone even when you're with your friends because you don't feel you can safely share your thoughts. Is there anyone you can turn to when you feel alone?

S: (firmly) No. My folks are very busy and very independent. They wouldn't understand at all. My father is still bent out of shape that I chose to major in art. He thinks I've wasted his money. He would really blow his top if he knew that I wasn't even sure about art anymore.

C: Why have you wasted his money?

S: (sarcastically) Well, he's the director of a bank. (pause) Since I was a kid, all that he's had time for is money. He can't understand why I chose art. He says since I am not Picasso, I am going to be dependent on him forever.

C: But (pause) you are so self-sufficient.

S: (anxiously) I don't need people. (pause) But, if I don't make money, I'll be under my father's control forever.

C: His control?

S: (intently) If I need his money to start an art studio, he'll make me grovel for it.

C: Grovel?

S: (impatiently) Spend time at the bank, go to his parties, try to suck up to his friends. (head in his hands, fearfully) I can't paint; I feel so pressured!

C: You can't express yourself with your parents, your friends, now even your art . . .

S: (desperately) I have to get out of this chair; my back is killing me.

C: This is the second time that, when discussing loneliness, you have shifted the conversation to your back. I wonder what role the pain is playing in your life.

S: (angrily) It's been building these past few months, ever since my last talk with my folks about money.

C: What happened?

S: (intently) I have to make money. I have always known that in the back of my mind. (pause) But art isn't about money and competition. It's about what's inside you. I have had this fight repeatedly with my dad. (angrily) He's a brick wall. He keeps saying, "You'll be like a kept woman."

C: He puts your manhood on the line.

S: (sarcastically) Ever since I was about 2.

C: Tell me more about this.

S: (furiously) I can still hear my dad's voice in my head saying "be a man" every time I asked for help.

C: Help with what?

S: (sarcastically) My shoes, my homework . . . I was a real pain to them as a kid, but I learned as fast as I could and tried not to ask for help with the same thing twice.

C: You wanted your parents' approval, and they didn't approve of you needing help.

S: (calmly) In our house, to ask for help is to be a loser. I heard it a thousand times: "Do it yourself, try harder, be a man, or you'll always be a loser!"

C: Who said that?

S: (angrily) They both did, but my dad was the loudest.

C: In your family independence was important; needing help was stupid. How did you experience that?

S: (with determination) I thought my parents were right. I was a loser.

C: You say demeaning things to yourself. Did you learn to treat yourself this way from your parents?

S: (matter-of-factly) Sure, but my friends call dependent people losers too. People need to take care of themselves. Don't you agree?

C: Your parents, your friends, and your inner voice all criticize you for needing help, and you assume I will. What else could it mean for children or adults to need help besides that they are losers?

S: (long pause, calmly) Maybe it's OK for children to need help; you aren't born knowing everything. But this is different—I'm an adult man.

C: You have said that men have to be competitive, make money, and not need anything. Is this really true?

S: (confusedly) Why am I still sitting here? What's the point?

C: Part of you is ready to go. Part of you wonders if it's OK for a man to get help.

S: (jumping up, angrily) I'm tired of your stupid comments. (shaking a fist toward C) Maybe you are the loser!

C: (very loud, angrily) I don't like being called a loser, and I don't like people shaking their fists at me!

S: (sitting down, defensively) I didn't mean . . . I just feel so edgy, and I can't create anything and . . . (hanging his head down)

C: (long pause, calmly) I apologize for yelling. I don't like being called a loser. You don't either. (S looks up, long pause) Have you ever noticed that when someone yells at you, something inside wants to make you yell back?

S: (reflectively) That's what always seems to happen with my dad, even when I tell myself ahead of time to stay cool.

C: I don't think you're a loser. (pause) What I do think is that it would be important for us to continue talking about your relationships with others next week.

Exercises for Developing a Case Conceptualization of Steve

Exercise 1 (4-page maximum)

GOAL: To verify that you have a clear understanding of time-limited dynamic treatment.

STYLE: Integrative essay addressing Parts A–C.

NEED HELP? Review this chapter (pages 226–233).

A. Develop a concise overview of the assumptions of dynamic theory (the theory's hypotheses about key dimensions in understanding a client's interpersonal functioning; think broadly, abstractly).

B. Develop a thorough description of how each of these assumptions is used to understand a client's relationship history (for each assumption provide specific examples).

C. Describe the role of the clinician in helping the client develop a new pattern(s) of relating to others (consultant, doctor, educator, helper; treatment approach; technique examples).

Exercise 2 (4-page maximum)

GOAL: To aid application of dynamic theory to Steve.

STYLE: A separate sentence outline for each section, A–C.

NEED HELP? Review this chapter (pages 226–233).

A. Assess how adaptively or maladaptively Steve is relating to his parents, his peers, and his teachers and analyze his interaction style within each type of relationship using either a CMP, an adaptive pattern of relating, or a mixed pattern with both adaptive and maladaptive features. Be sure to include in each interpersonal pattern his role for himself in relating to others, his expectations of others' attitudes and intentions toward him, his perceptions of the behavior of others toward him, and his role toward himself (introjects).

B. Overall, how well is Steve relating to the clinician at this time, considering (a) any signs of transference from Steve, (b) any signs of countertransference from the clinician, and (c) any signs of openness to interpretations of his interpersonal patterns?

C. Over all his relationships, what strengths (strong points, positive features, successes, skills, factors facilitating change) and weaknesses (concerns, issues, problems, symptoms, skill deficits, treatment barriers) does Steve bring to the interpersonal process, and how well is he getting his needs for intimacy and autonomy met across all these relationships?

D. Does Steve bring any strengths or weaknesses to treatment that are separate from his manner of relating to others? If so, how might these weaknesses affect the treatment process, and how might these strengths be used to support treatment success?

Exercise 3 (4-page maximum)

GOAL: To develop an understanding of the potential role of gender in Steve's life.

STYLE: A separate sentence outline for each section, A–D.

NEED HELP?   Review Chapter 2 (pages 39–47).

A. Assess the personal costs or benefits to Steve's current gender role in terms of self-image, emotional life, expectations, perceptions, behavior, and access to personal resources.

B. Assess the social costs or benefits to Steve's current gender role in terms of family relationships, social relationships, educational or work relationships, and access to social resources.

C. Overall, how much have Steve's view of masculinity and femininity, society's definition that they are opposites of each other, unrealistic societal expectations for males, and the devaluation of women and their values influenced his mental or physical health, and how aware is he of this?

D. Overall, how much power and choice does Steve have to live his life as a nongendered individual with unique needs and goals, and how strong are counterpressures on him to be a gendered male?

E. Consider whether the gender role you have taken on, your stereotypes of Steve's gender role, or gender biases within your treatment approach might lead to marginalization of Steve's point of view and/or Steve's current situation and consider what could be done to increase the likelihood of a positive treatment outcome.

Exercise 4 (6-page maximum)

GOAL:

To help you integrate your knowledge of dynamic theory and gender issues into an in-depth conceptualization of Steve (who he is and why he does what he does).

STYLE:

An integrated essay consisting of a premise, supportive details, and conclusions following a carefully planned organizational style (see Chapter 2).

NEED HELP?

Review Chapter 1 (pages 7–28) and Chapter 2 (pages 39–47).

STEP 1: Consider what style you could use for organizing your dynamic understanding of Steve that (a) would support you in giving a comprehensive and clear understanding of his dynamics and (b) would support language that Steve might find persuasive considering his fear that needing treatment means he's a loser.

STEP 2: Develop your concise premise (overview, preliminary or explanatory statements, proposition, thesis statement, theory-driven introduction, hypotheses, summary, concluding causal statements) that explains Steve's overall functioning as a young man fearful of his ability to succeed as an artist. If you are having trouble with Step 2, remember this should be an integration of the key ideas of Exercises 2 and 3 that might (a) provide a basis for Steve's long-term goals, (b) be grounded in dynamic theory and sensitive to gender issues, and (c) highlight the strengths Steve brings to dynamic treatment.

STEP 3: Develop your supporting material (detailed case analysis of strengths and weaknesses, supplying data to support an introductory premise) from a dynamic perspective that integrates within each paragraph a deep understanding of Steve and his struggles with society's definition of masculinity. If you need help with Step 3, consider the information you need to include in order to support the development of short-term goals that (a) are grounded in dynamic theory and sensitive to gender issues and (b) integrate an understanding of Steve's strengths in interpersonal relating whenever possible.

STEP 4: Develop your conclusions and broad treatment recommendations including (a) Steve's overall level of functioning, (b) anything facilitating or serving as a barrier to his changing his interpersonal patterns at this time, and (c) his basic needs in the interpersonal process at this time, being careful to consider what you said in Part E of Exercise 3 (be concise and general).

Exercise 5 (3-page maximum)

GOAL: To develop an individualized, theory-driven action plan for Steve that considers his strengths and is sensitive to gender issues.

STYLE: A sentence outline consisting of long- and short-term goals.

NEED HELP?   Review Chapter 1 (pages 8–28).

STEP 1: Develop your treatment plan overview, being careful to consider what you said in Part E of Exercise 3 to try and prevent any negative bias to your treatment plan.

STEP 2: Develop long-term (major, large, ambitious, comprehensive, broad) goals that *ideally* Steve would reach by the termination of treatment to have a flexible pattern of relating to others as an adult male. If you are having trouble with Step 2, reread your premise and support topic sentences for ideas to transform into goals to help give Steve insight into his interpersonal style and the ability to relate in a flexible manner to others (use *style* of Exercise 4).

STEP 3: Develop short-term (small, brief, encapsulated, specific, measurable) goals that Steve and the clinician could expect to see accomplished within a few weeks to chart Steve's progress in developing interpersonal insights and skills, instill hope for change, and plan time-effective treatment sessions. If you are having trouble with Step 3, reread your support paragraphs looking for ideas to transform into goals that (a) might help Steve gain a new experience within the interpersonal process with you, (b) might help him gain a new understanding of how he relates to others as a man, (c) might enhance factors facilitating or decrease barriers to him developing a flexible style of relating or getting his needs for autonomy and nurturance met, (d) utilize his strengths to build a flexible style of relating as an adult male whenever possible, and (e) are individualized to his interpersonal needs rather than generic.

Exercise 6

GOAL: To critique short-term dynamic treatment and the case of Steve.

STYLE: Answer each question in essay form or discuss them in a group format.

    A. What are the strengths and weaknesses of this model for helping Steve (a college student struggling with rigid gender role stereotypes)?

    B. Discuss the strengths and weaknesses of using emotion-focused treatment with Steve in comparison to dynamic treatment. Be sure to consider his goals for treatment (greater emotional intimacy, career direction) as well as his ability to be motivated to work within this approach.

    C. Discuss Steve considering the Domain of Socioeconomic Status. How might having been raised in a wealthy family have influenced his interpersonal style and contributed to his fears about the future? Compare the importance of class versus gender issues in guiding Steve's treatment. Overall, how big a difference would it make in your treatment plan?

    D. Steve is socially isolated, involved in serious family discord, and feeling hopeless about his future. Discuss whether supporting Steve, in departing from the gender role stereotypes of his family, would increase or decrease his risk for suicide. What more do you need to know from Steve in the next session to feel confident in your assessment of his risk?

    E. Dynamic treatment requires a great deal of self-awareness on your part along with strategic use of your own internal reactions to the client. Consider your internal reactions to Steve as you peruse the interview again, this time taking note of what comments from him evoked what reactions from you. Discuss these countertransference issues and how much you consider them to be a reaction to Steve's pattern of relating and how much they are a result of your own personal history.

Recommended Resources

American Psychological Association (Producer) & Freedheim, D. K. (Trainer). (n.d.). *Short-term dynamic therapy: Part of the Systems of Psychotherapy Video Series* [Motion picture, #4310833]. (Available from the American Psychological Association, 750 First Street, NE, Washington, DC 20002–4242)

Binder, J. L. (2004). *Key competencies in brief dynamic psychotherapy: Clinical practice beyond the manual.* New York: Guilford Press.

Levenson, H. Retrieved April 9, 2009, from http://www.hannalevenson.com/

Levenson, H., & Strupp, H. H. (2007). *Cyclic maladaptive patterns: Case formulation in time-limited dynamic psychotherapy.* In T. D. Eells (Ed.), *Handbook of psychotherapy case formulation* (2nd ed., pp. 164–197). New York: Guilford Press.

Eight

Family Systems Case Conceptualizations and Treatment Plans

Introduction to Family Systems Theory

You have just received a referral from Mrs. Walters, a third-grade teacher. She says a 9-year-old White girl named Alice has been a constant behavior problem; Alice is disrespectful and will not follow instructions in class. In addition, Alice is described as bossy and immature in relating to her peers. Alice is a new student in the school. She moved into the district when her mother (Katherine, age 30) and her father (Dave, age 32) were divorced this past summer. While Katherine has primary custody, Alice spends almost every weekend with her father and her paternal grandparents. Her father is using Alice as a confidant. He wants Katherine to return to the marriage, and his parents support him in this. He has asked Alice to spy on Katherine so that he can find a way to get their family back together. Katherine revealed all this information to Mrs. Walters during a parent-teacher conference; Mrs. Walters gave Katherine your phone number.

Your approach to Alice's situation will be based on the structural family approach of Salvador Minuchin. Alice might have an individually focused problem, such as a learning disability, that is leading her to misbehave in school. However, the power of your approach comes through its recognition that Alice's problems might be a reflection of family conflict. Much of the conflicts that Alice experiences in her life will involve her interactions with others. Considering her family a unit, determined by its interactional patterns, provides many new and nonblaming explanations for Alice's situation; she is an individual, doing her best to get her needs met within the context of her relationships—most particularly her family relationships.

Every family is a social group that has a structure. The purpose of the structure is to ensure that family tasks get done such as paying the bills, cleaning the house, helping children with homework, and caring for sick family members. The structure also determines how each family member's needs for independence and emotional closeness get met. For a family's structure to be functional, the tasks need to be coordinated, and personal needs must be met, in a dependable fashion.

The structure of a family can be analyzed in terms of its basic features. One important feature is its subsystems or the smaller units that make up the family system. Subsystems may develop around specific functions that need to be achieved in the family such as parenting children. Family subsystems may also develop around gender, generation, or both. Another important structural feature is the boundaries that develop between subsystems and between the family system as a whole and nonfamily members. Boundaries determine how much subsystems communicate with each other and how much family members are encouraged to individuate versus how much emotional closeness is encouraged. Family structure also carries within it a hierarchy that determines who is in charge of coordinating tasks and making decisions. This hierarchy of power and authority often has a spousal subsystem at the top.

If Alice's family is functioning well, it will be encouraging developmentally appropriate autonomy (individuation) and developmentally appropriate relatedness (a sense of belonging) for all family members. If Alice's family system is malfunctioning, treatment will intervene to help family members alter their interactional patterns and develop a structure that is more effective in meeting their needs as a unit and as individuals. The following more detailed paragraphs are based on the work of Salvador Minuchin and his colleagues (Minuchin, 1974; Minuchin & Fishman, 1981; Minuchin, Nichols, & Lee, 2007; Nichols, 2008).

When Katherine and Dave married and moved in together, they created a new family system. Their family had only two members (Katherine and Dave), but it had three smaller family groupings or subsystems: the

Katherine subsystem, the Dave subsystem, and the spousal subsystem. Each subsystem had tasks to accomplish, and members within each subsystem were likely to develop complementary roles to each other. At first, Dave and Katherine needed to adjust to, and negotiate with each other, who would do what tasks in the family. They also needed to develop rules related to how to communicate with each other and how to resolve conflicts. While Katherine and Dave needed to have loyalty to their couple as a unit (spousal subsystem), they still needed to maintain loyalty to themselves as individuals (Dave subsystem, Katherine subsystem). This personal loyalty helped ensure that while Katherine and Dave made some accommodation to each other, they continued to support their own autonomy needs.

As enduring patterns were developed between Dave and Katherine, they each began to use only a limited number of the behaviors they were capable of; this is because each had been delegated to engage in only certain family tasks. For example, at the beginning of the marriage, Dave may have initiated early social contacts between the family and extended family because his relations lived close by. However, as this continued to occur over time, he and Katherine may have developed the expectations that he would always be in charge of this, and an enduring pattern within their family was established; the longer this pattern endured, the more it seemed necessary rather than optional. Thus, a family rule may have developed that only Dave could set up social engagements. The family rules that develop over time may be explicit or implicit and govern the range of behaviors that are considered appropriate for each family member.

As more members enter a family, more subsystems develop. When Alice was born, two new subsystems formed. The parental subsystem was formed to be responsive to Alice's developing needs, and Alice formed her own subsystem. Alice and her mother could also form a subsystem of females. The parents interact with each other and with Alice to carry out socialization functions. Alice, in interacting with her parents, learns what to expect from people who have more strength and greater resources. She learns what brings rewards and what brings punishments. If other children enter the family system, then a sibling subsystem forms. Within a sibling subsystem, children learn important interpersonal skills such as how to accommodate and negotiate with peers and what to expect from individuals with power equal to theirs. If at first an older child stands up for a younger one in a fight with another child, this begins to develop an expectation, and then a family rule, that the older one will take care of the younger one; this may continue even after it is not functional because the "younger one" is now old enough to take care of him- or herself. If the older one remains the protector, the younger one may not learn to stand up for him- or herself. Thus, expectations between family members, if they continue to be met, establish family rules for how each member "should" behave.

What boundaries developed among the subsystems of Alice's family? Boundaries are invisible barriers that determine how frequently and in what manner subsystems interact with each other. A boundary also exists around the family system as a whole in interacting with the outside world. Minuchin describes boundaries as being clear, diffuse, or rigid. Clear subsystem boundaries exist when family members are supported, nurtured, and allowed to individuate. In this case, although the parental subsystem has the most power, the parents will modify the family rules to accommodate, for example, the growing needs of teenagers to make decisions and have control over aspects of their day-to-day lives. There is frequent communication among subsystems. Thus, subsystems can communicate and negotiate with one another, and family rules accommodate to situational and developmental challenges.

Diffuse boundaries exist when family members are supported and nurtured but not allowed to individuate. There is no clear hierarchy of authority, and family members negotiate and accommodate too much with each other. This may lead family members to being enmeshed (extremely dependent on one another emotionally). Enmeshed children are immature and rely too much on their parents and not enough on their own abilities. The growing children may need more personal control but fear either that individuation will be a rejection of family members or that they cannot successfully be independent. Parents may fear disastrous consequences if children have more autonomy. On the other hand, a child who is enmeshed with a parent may believe he or she has the right to interrupt this parent and demand attention even when the parent is engaged in a vital task or in an important communication with another person; the parent's authority in the family is not respected. In interacting with individuals outside of the family, enmeshed family members continue to expect to be cared for and will make unrealistic demands on others.

Rigid boundaries exist when family members are encouraged to individuate and master personal interests but needs for nurturance go unmet. Rigid boundaries restrict interpersonal contact between family members, leading to emotional disengagement (emotional isolation).

Family members have little room to negotiate and accommodate to each other. There is only restricted access between subsystems. As a result, each family member may be an island, facing successes and failures alone. It may be that some members of a family are disengaged from each other while others are enmeshed. For example, Katherine and Alice may have become emotionally overinvolved (enmeshed) with each other to make up for their feelings of loss following the divorce. On the other hand, Dave may have become emotionally distanced (disengaged) from Alice because his time with her was reduced following the divorce. Dave may have sought to get his needs met by his parents again, as he did as a child, becoming enmeshed with them. Boundaries between the entire family and the outside world can also be clear, diffuse, or rigid.

How have authority and power been distributed in Alice's family? A family's hierarchy refers to who in the family has the most power and authority to make rules and decisions. In a healthy family, parents have more power and authority than children, and older children may have more power and authority than younger children. For a well-functioning parental subsystem, Katherine and Dave should have a strong, positive coalition with each other so that they work as a team to raise Alice. This coalition reflects mutual respect and concern so that they do not undermine each other's authority as parents. In addition, members of the extended family, such as grandparents, should support the authority of parents. When a child is born, the child's needs for autonomy and nurturance are respected, but the child is not allowed to disrupt the parental coalition or make important family decisions. In a healthy family, it is the adults who have the ultimate authority, and all the children in the household have their dependency needs as children respected.

In a malfunctioning family, cross-generational alliances may have formed that disrupt the family hierarchy. For example, an alliance may have developed in which the paternal grandmother and the father exclude or demean the participation of the mother in the parenting subsystem. Another type of cross-generational alliance can occur when a child is brought into a coalition with one of the parents. Although the child may gain the benefit of additional authority within the family, the child's own developmental needs go unmet. The child may be expected to make decisions or to handle situations that he or she doesn't have the skills or experience to do; this puts the child under stress.

There are times when a family's structure remains stable (periods of homeostasis); however, all families go through periods of stress and growth resulting from internal or external demands for change (periods of disequilibrium). Internal demands for change can come from the birth or death of family members or through the changing needs of family members that come with age. If family members stay together, Minuchin considers them to progress through four stages: couple formation, families with young children, families with older or adolescent children, and families with grown children. External demands include employment changes, educational changes, and deaths of extended family members. Change requires the family to accommodate and negotiate (modify the family rules) so that the needs of family members are still met.

All families have problems, but healthy families have functional strategies for dealing with these problems. While a healthy family may struggle at first in times of change, it will be able to accommodate to these changed circumstances. Unhealthy periods of homeostasis occur when there are legitimate pressures for change but the family is attempting to maintain its past structure and not adapt. Unhealthy periods of disequilibrium represent a disintegration of the family structure when it is under pressure to change.

As a result of divorce, Alice is no longer part of a nuclear family system. Family systems come in many other configurations, including extended families, single-parent households, divorced couples, and stepfamilies. It is not the configuration of a family per se that determines its health but the ability of the system to balance the needs of its members for nurturance and autonomy in times of homeostasis and disequilibrium. You will assume that her family is basically healthy but is in need of reorganizing itself so that it can solve its own problems; the goal of treatment is to alter the family structure.

To help Alice's family you will progress through a four-step intervention model (Minuchin et al., 2007). The first step will be to discuss the family's point of view on the presenting complaint and then open up alternative explanations for it for their consideration. The second step will be to highlight how current family interactions are maintaining the presenting complaint. The third step will be to explore the past, from a structural perspective, to give adult family members some cognitive insight into how their childhood experiences are related to the current problem within their family. The final step will be to help the family members explore alternative ways of relating to each other and determine how they will use their strengths and resources to overcome their problems and develop a more functional family structure.

During this treatment process, you and Alice's family members will not discover the "truth" about what caused their current problems and the "right way" for the family to be structured. Rather, each family member will participate in a construction of the family's current reality or story and will be involved in any reconstructions that may help the family function within a created family story they find more satisfying and adaptive.

Role of the Clinician

How will you help Alice? You are an expert, a coach, a collaborator, and a helper.

Your first task will be to understand the family. You will join with it in a collaborative stance to help understand how each person experiences the family, and you will experience this reality with each of them; this is called joining the family. You will convey an understanding for, and respect for, every family member. The family usually locates the problem within one individual. You have an alternative view, or a reframing of the problem, that there are complementary roles played by family members and that the problems are located within the family structure rather than within an individual.

The family is the context for understanding its members. Thus, to help them develop an understanding of their structural problems, all of them will need to attend at least the initial sessions. Later on it may be valuable to have meetings with just subsystems or even individuals. Within sessions, you will encourage family members to communicate directly with one another and thus bring their patterns and processes of interacting into the treatment session; when family members interact in their normal manner, it is called an enactment. You will alternate between observing these interactions and participating in them.

Once you develop an understanding of the dysfunctional family structure, you'll develop a new formulation of the identified problem that explains how, rather than residing in one person, it really encompasses the interactions of all family members. There are many techniques you could use to widen the family's view of the presenting complaint. One is to have each family member articulate a strength he or she sees in the symptom bearer (the person who is supposed to be the problem). The strengths and weaknesses of all family members may also be highlighted. This helps take the identified patient off the hot seat of being the "trouble" in the family. The role each family member plays in maintaining the problem will be underscored in a nonblaming and nonjudgmental manner, and alternative conceptualizations, or reframes of the problem, will be discussed that may open up alternative interaction patterns within the family. There is no one "true" reframing" of the problem. If a reframe helps the family reorganize in a constructive manner, then it is a successful one for the family.

The third step in treatment will be to help adult family members develop cognitive insight into the unproductive family assumptions that are limiting their view of themselves and others. In the early history of structural theory, insight was not considered important—the goal was to just change family interactions until a functional structure developed. However, recent work suggests that helping adult family members develop cognitive insight into how their past childhood experiences are related to their current family interactional struggles serves to increase their willingness to see themselves and their family members in more flexible ways and maintain changed interaction patterns in the long run (Minuchin et al., 2007).

These discussions of the past will always be tied clearly to the presenting concerns of the family members so that they can understand why the family is "stuck" in dysfunctional patterns. This will lead into the fourth step of treatment where you help the family members consider ways of getting "unstuck" that involve trying out a variety of different ways of relating to each other; the goal is to expand their choices in developing a new family structure. Each family member who would need to do something different will be asked to consider what he or she would and would not do to get his or her family moving into a new pattern of interactions; you ask for such willingness because you cannot force a family member to interact differently. You want to build collaboration between family members to try new things; if any family members change their interaction style, it will have an influence on the entire family system. Within each session, you will help family members actively experience a new way of relating to each other. This new way of functioning as a family is based on the reframing of those difficulties you developed together; this represents a constructed truth about the family. If this new construction opens up more satisfying interactions than the old one, the family may choose to keep using it.

How will you provide Alice's family members with new experiences in relating to each other? Your overall plan will be to disrupt the old structure. This may involve adjusting boundaries and realigning subsystems in a manner that will be more functional for the family at its current stage of development. How will you begin? You will actively disrupt the old subgroups as they are interacting within the immediacy of the session; you will respond to what you see and experience within the session while still treating with respect family members' own descriptions of what is happening within their family at home.

You may increase the experienced intensity of the family member's conflicts so that they will need to question their manner of interaction and search for alternative behaviors, cognitions, and affective responses to the ones they have been currently using. Structural treatment offers many techniques for raising intensity. For example, Katherine and Dave could be asked to discuss their conflicts with each other while seated facing each other with their knees touching; this is a method of raising intensity through manipulating physical proximity. As another example, if Katherine said, "I feel sad about my marriage failing," you could say, "You feel tortured by your marriage failing"; this method raises intensity through manipulating language.

Treatment is individualized to each family, and a variety of techniques exist for helping family members interact more productively with each other. A few common ones will be discussed including strengthening appropriate coalitions and developing clear boundaries. While you will be sensitive to the needs of individual families, you consider that a healthy family with children needs to have a cohesive parental subsystem. Thus, you will work to create a strong parental coalition between Dave and Katherine and support the authority of the parental subsystem over the child subsystem of Alice despite the divorce. Second, if there are enmeshed subsystems, you will strengthen boundaries and encourage individuation of family members when needed. Third, if there are disengaged subsystems, you will increase direct communication among family members to strengthen their emotional connections with each other. For example, Dave may have limited his contact with Alice (become disengaged) because he sees the divorce from Katherine as requiring his being "divorced" from Alice. You could provide Dave with a renaming or reinterpretation of this divorce context, such as "Now that you don't have to fight daily with Katherine, you can have the freedom to really enjoy your time with Alice." This reframing of Dave's divorced family reality will be successful if it frees Dave to reestablish his emotional connection to Alice. You could build on Dave's strengths by pointing out relationships where he has maintained emotional connection and show faith in Dave's ability to reconnect with Alice. Shaping competence (building on strengths) encourages Dave to use constructive behaviors in his interactions with Alice and Katherine that are alternatives to those he is currently using.

Another important technique is called boundary making. If a child is interrupting a parent, you will encourage the parent to tell the child to stop; this helps the parent take on a higher level of parental authority and strengthens the boundary between the parent and child subsystems. The child may have previously been a "parentified child." This is a child who has been allowed to take on some of the power of a parent. While this gives the child added freedom and power, it also puts him or her in a position where he or she is making decisions that he or she isn't developmentally ready to make. If a parent keeps interfering when two siblings fight, this person will be told to stay out of it so that the siblings can learn how to solve their own problems.

In the technique of "unbalancing," you change the relationship between members of a subsystem. For example, a family can be stalemated in problem solving when two people, holding opposing views, are not able to reach a compromise; fear of change is often behind this. You could take the side of one member of the power struggle, shifting power to this person. The intent is to shake both of them out of the stalemate so that they can work toward a solution of balance and fairness. During the course of treatment, you will align with every family member, in turn, as is needed to aid problem solving.

How much do you need to do? Each family has within it the ability to move itself toward an adaptive structure. You will keep trying different techniques until you facilitate family members' moving beyond their presenting concerns to develop a functional structure that supports the welfare of all of them. It is not the techniques themselves that are critical to change; it is your being able to help the family develop a new and more satisfying way of carrying out family tasks that supports the needs of each member to age-appropriate autonomy and nurturance.

Case Application: Integrating the Domain of Age

Alice's case will now be examined in detail. There are many domains of complexity that might be relevant to her case. The Domain of Age has been chosen to examine within a family systems case conceptualization and treatment plan.

Interview With Alice (A) and Katherine (K) From a Family Systems Perspective

C: Hello, Katherine, Alice. Can you tell me why you are here?

K: (calmly) Alice is having trouble adjusting to a new . . . (Alice interrupts)

A: (accusatorily) Everyone at school is mean to me.

C: What were you going to say, Katherine?

K: (calmly looking at C) The teacher thinks that Alice doesn't know how to cooperate and share with the other children.

C: Look at Alice and tell her what you think.

A: (venomously) I hate that Mrs. Walters. She is always telling me what to do, and she will never help me!

C: Alice, your mother has something important to tell you.

K: (turning to Alice, calmly) I want you to have friends.

A: (angrily) I don't want to be friends with any of them. They are selfish. We do all these projects in class. They never give me the stuff I want to use. They always say, "Wait. It's not your turn." (K tries to stroke A's hand, but A jerks it away) Then, if I grab it from their grubby hands, Mrs. Walters takes ME away from the group!

C: You feel angry and treated unfairly. Ask your mom what you could do about it.

A: (dismissively) She can't help me. People always push her around.

K: (looking at C, calmly) Dave has always bossed me around. I don't like to boss people. The teacher says Alice is very bossy at school; she learned this from Dave.

C: You seemed to cringe, Alice.

A: (angrily) She is saying bad things about Dad again. They both do it. (Stomping her feet) I HATE IT! Why do they have to say mean things?

C: Tell your mom what you want her to do.

A: (glaring at K, yelling) Mom, stop talking to me about Dad and stop fighting with Dad in front of me. (turning to C) They are so loud, they just scream at each other in front of me all the time.

C: Keep looking at your mom. She needs to know how you feel.

A: (shaking her fist at her mom and yelling) I HATE THIS! If you would just move back home, these fights could end!

K: (calmly but squirmingly) Alice, your dad and I are divorced. I am never going to move back. Our home is here now.

A: (condescendingly) Dad says you will come home when you come to your senses.

K: Don't talk to me like that, Alice. (Alice interrupts)

A: (condescendingly) He says you have forgotten your promises to him. You went out and got a job instead of staying home to care for me like you should. Grandma and Dad BOTH say so!

C: Katherine, Alice interrupts you a lot. Is this OK with you?

K: (concernedly) Well, this divorce hurt her a lot. She has always been close to her dad. I don't want to disrupt that. I tried for a long time to work things out with her dad. I'm not surprised his mother is still blaming me. She always did that.

C: You're a good mom. You are aware of her feelings about the divorce and you realize her dad is important to her. But, is it OK that she interrupts you all the time? YOU are the MOTHER.

K: (reflectively) I think Alice wants to be the boss. She doesn't listen to me, and the teacher says Alice doesn't listen at school.

C: What do you think Alice needs?

K: (firmly) She needs to be able to listen to her teacher and learn from her, and she needs to have friends her own age.

C: You have a good grasp of her academic and social needs. What about her adjustment to the divorce?

K: (calmly) I don't mean to complain to her about Dave. He is still so angry at me that he picks a fight with ME whenever he comes to get her. I used to let Dave and his mother push me around. Now, I stand up for myself; the fights do get loud.

C: The fight is between you and Dave. So, Alice shouldn't be drawn into it. Look at her and tell her what she needs to hear from you.

K: (Looking at A) I'm sorry that I let you get in the middle of my fights with your dad. We are going to keep fighting for a while until we work some problems out. I will try not to do it in front of you.

C: (A is looking down) Alice, can you look at your mom? (A looks at K)

K: (sincerely) I am going to try, Alice, but I need YOU to try too.

A: (dismissively) I'm not going to follow those stupid rules! I've told Dad, and he says I don't have to follow them.

K: (angrily) He has no . . . (C interrupts)

C: Katherine, you are forgetting not to complain about Dave. Tell Alice what you think about the rules and say it in a voice that tells her you mean it.

K: (firmly) The teacher told me you are more impatient, share less, and are less helpful than the other kids at school. You are really smart and sweet, Alice. You could be the teacher's favorite student. It's my fault. Before the divorce, I did all the housework and organized your homework. I didn't see that you were growing up.

A: (looking at K, whiningly) I hate cleaning up. I don't want to do it.

C: You are setting a good example for your mother, Alice. You looked right at her and told her what was on your mind without blaming anyone.

A: (looking at K, whiningly) Mom, I like it when you do everything.

C: OK, that was simple and clear—but only babies have their moms do everything. You are 9. Find out what 9-year-old goodies you might get if you take on the responsibilities of a 9-year-old.

A: (aggressively) Mom, if I do the stupid cleanup, are you going to give me something fun?

K: Alice, your teacher says . . . (C interrupts by whispering in K's ear, "Tell her what YOU think") Alice, if you are responsible and do your chores and homework, I could let you invite a friend to stay overnight.

A: (excitedly and loudly) TONIGHT?

K: I don't know. (looks at C) Alice, I am not ready to have a friend come over tonight. We need to work out the chores first. Let's think about who you could have over next week if you act responsibly.

A: (sadly) All the kids at school hate me.

K: (sadly) I don't really know how to start with that problem.

C: Alice can do a lot of things for herself that she isn't aware of yet—like making friends at school. Alice, who were your friends before you moved here?

A: (calmly) My dad's farm is way out in the country. I mostly played with my older cousins. They were neat to play with. They always let me choose what to do. They weren't pushy like the kids here.

C: Do you see your cousins now?

A: (angrily) Only if I am with my dad. They are all from his side of the family, and none of them are speaking to my mom.

C: Why not?

A: (angrily) They say my mom is bad for leaving my dad.

C: They put you in the middle of the fight again. What would happen if you told them that it made you feel bad to be in the middle of the fight?

A: (anxiously) Maybe they would hate me like they hate Mom.

C: That would hurt, and no one wants that to happen.

A: (whiningly and demandingly) So, how am I going to make friends?

C: Let's see if your mother could be a good example for you to learn from. Katherine, are there any grown-ups helping you with your own hurt?

K: (sadly) My parents died before Alice was born. I was an only child.

C: Friends?

K: (reflectively) The farm was isolated. We socialized with Dave's family. I have met some new people, but I don't know them well.

C: Katherine, what is going on with Alice as we talk?

K: (calmly) She looks very sad.

C: Can you help her?

K: (calmly) It's hard for me to make friends too, Alice, but I am going to find a way to help you. I know you need friends.

C: You are a perceptive mother, Katherine. Is there something you can do right now to help Alice? (K goes over and hugs A)

A: (crawls into K's lap and cuddles; K cuddles back, and they both smile)

C: You are both smiling now and look happy. Families can't be happy all the time, but we need to make your family happy for as much of the time as we can. We know that Alice needs friends. She also needs to be responsible for kids' stuff like homework, and NOT grown-up stuff like the divorce.

K: (still cuddling A but twisting to look her in the face) Alice, we will keep coming back here until we have worked these problems out. I really love you.

A: (sweetly) I love you too, Mommy.

Family Systems Case Conceptualization of Alice: Symptom-Based Style

Alice has been referred for treatment by the school system because she is bossy, immature, and sad. Although she appears to be a bright and verbal 9-year-old, she behaves immaturely for her age and engages in disruptive behavior with adults and peers. At her age, she should be developing significant peer friendships. Instead, she is struggling with the earlier developmental tasks of learning to cooperate and share. While still being connected strongly to her parents, a 9-year-old should be turning to teachers and other adults as additional role models. Instead, Alice does not seek to acquire her teacher's approval or recognize the teacher's authority. Alice is also feeling sad and stressed by her parents' postdivorce conflicts. These symptoms can be viewed as reflections of a malfunctioning family system. Structural dysfunctions within Alice's nuclear family resulted in Alice not acquiring a realistic view of her own power vis-à-vis adults and not developing the ability to accommodate and negotiate with peers. These skill deficits became more problematic for Alice as her nuclear family dissolved and her divorced family began the struggle of creating new subsystems and boundaries. Family strengths that are emerging during this period of disequilibrium include Katherine's commitment to her role as a parent, her ability to recognize and respond to Alice's needs for emotional support, and both Katherine's and Alice's willingness to explore new patterns of relating.

Why is Alice bossy with adults? Within her nuclear family, Katherine and Dave did not have a strong parental coalition. Dave had the final authority for making decisions in the family, and he allowed both his own mother and his daughter to devalue Katherine's role as a mother. Katherine, having developed a complementary pattern to her husband and daughter of submitting to avoid conflict, unintentionally delegated her authority as a parent to Alice. Katherine's submissive behavior also made it unnecessary for Alice to develop the negotiation and accommodation skills she needs to develop constructive relationships with adults. Brought into a pseudoparental role, Alice developed a false sense of her power within child-adult relationships. Alice tried to bring this increased power into the school setting. While seeing that other children in school follow the teacher's rules, she does not think that the rules apply to her. At the present time, Alice is struggling to retain her pseudoadult role; Katherine recognizes it is healthier for Alice to act her age and follow rules both at home and at school.

Why is Alice immature in her peer relationships? As an only child, Alice socialized primarily with adults and older cousins. These older individuals accommodated to her wishes. Because they always yielded to Alice, the egocentric play style that would be expected of a preschool-age Alice has in many ways been maintained, unintentionally, within Alice's family and extended family system. Thus, when she interacts in school with peers and needs to alter her style to fit relationships of equal power, she does not know how. She responds by escalating her bossy, controlling behavior to try to force these other individuals into her familiar pattern of relating where others have always submitted to her demands. Alice sees her conflicts with other children at school as their fault. Katherine recognizes that Alice needs to learn to share, compromise, and make friends her own age.

Why is Alice sad? Katherine and Dave were both highly committed to their role as parents. They were loving and attentive to Alice. Although this led to emotional connections, these connections are now disrupted. The divorce has substantially decreased Alice's time with her father, and his anger over the divorce has interfered with his ability to recognize and respond to Alice's developmental needs. Katherine and Dave unintentionally have placed Alice in the middle of their conflicts by fighting in front of her and by complaining about each other to her. Dave's family has supported this. Alice feels torn between her parents, responsible for helping them reconcile, but unsure of what her role should be; no 9-year-old would have these skills or should be put in this position. With the clinician's support, Alice was able to ask her mother to stop putting her in this role; she is willing to try to do the same thing with her father and grandparents. Katherine has taken responsibility for blurring the parent-child boundary in the past; she is open to support from the clinician in taking on a fully adult role in her new family with Alice.

Alice, Katherine, and Dave are in a period of disequilibrium in which prior family roles have been disrupted and a new homeostasis has not yet emerged. Dave may be trying to reinstate the old family structure and boundaries. Katherine, with Alice, is trying to establish a new family system. Within this new system, Katherine needs to increase her authority as a parent, and Alice needs to take on age-appropriate responsibilities and learn how to accommodate and negotiate with people of greater authority (parents, teachers) as well as with people of equal authority (peers). Alice is at a stage in development in which she has the cognitive abilities to understand cause-and-effect relationships and can understand the needs of others if they are presented in concrete terms. These competencies will serve her well as she seeks to expand her repertoire of interpersonal behavior to fit the multiple systems in which she is a member (Mom's family, Dad's family, the school system). Katherine is highly motivated to be an effective parent for Alice. However, Dave and his family may be more focused on postdivorce conflicts than Alice's needs to grow and develop at this time; if so, their behavior may serve as a barrier to treatment success.

Family Systems Treatment Plan: Symptom-Based Style

Treatment Plan Overview. Alice's difficulties in school have developed within the context of disturbed family relationships. The most helpful plan for Alice would be if all the adults who are parenting her would attend treatment. However, while Dave and his parents will be asked to participate, few goals have been developed for them because Katherine believes that they will reject the idea of treatment. The clinician will invite them in, emphasizing Alice's problems as a hook for them to consider establishing coparenting strategies despite their anger over the divorce. Goals 1 and 2 will be introduced at the same time. The treatment plan follows the *basic format.*

LONG-TERM GOAL 1: Alice will decrease her sadness and level of stress concerning her parents' divorce.

Short-Term Goals

Katherine and Alice Family System Appointments

1. Katherine will ensure that Alice is out of the room and not listening when she has discussions with Dave about parenting before and after visitation.

2. Katherine will learn not to talk to Alice about her problems with Dave.

3. Katherine and Alice will talk about fun memories of their family when it was together and look at family albums in session.

4. Alice will sit on her mother's lap while Katherine tells her things she likes about Dave and expresses regret that their old family system had to change (giving Alice hugs for emotional support when needed).

5. Katherine will clearly tell Alice that the divorce is final despite what she hears at her dad's house but that she wants Alice to continue loving her dad with all her heart and hopes someday Dave won't be mad anymore about the divorce.

6. Katherine will talk to Alice about fun memories they have together as a new family, and the clinician will take fun photos of them together during the session for them to put in a new family album.

7. Other goals will be developed as appropriate to help Alice feel loved by Katherine and clearly allowed to continue loving Dave as her father.

   Dave, Grandparents, and Alice Family System Appointments If Possible (otherwise Alice will be given homework assignments to do this on visitation)

8. Alice will ask her dad not to talk about his problems with her mom and explain that it makes her sad.

9. Alice will ask her dad to help her tell her grandparents that it makes her sad to hear them criticize her mom.

10. Dave and his parents will discuss how to parent Alice without criticizing Katherine while Alice listens but isn't allowed to interrupt this adult discussion.

Katherine and Dave Divorced Family System Appointments

11. Katherine and Dave will discuss how they can continue parenting Alice, for her benefit, and keep their own disagreements with each other out of it.

12. Other goals will be developed as appropriate for strengthening these new family systems in their ability to parent a happy Alice who can love her parents and grandparents.

LONG-TERM GOAL 2: Alice will decrease her immature and bossy behavior.

Short-Term Goals

Katherine and Alice Family System Appointments

1. Katherine will develop age-appropriate rules for Alice's behavior (home, neighborhood, school) and consequences if these rules are not followed.

2. Katherine will discuss with Alice her responsibility for her schoolwork and her room at home and tell her that, when she is acting like a 9-year-old, she will be able to stay up 15 minutes longer at night or, if she is not being responsible, she will go to sleep 15 minutes earlier.

3. Katherine will discuss with the clinician possible adults she could try to be friends with and how she might start a friendship. Alice will be allowed to listen but not interrupt this adult conversation so that her mom can role-model friend-seeking behavior for her.

4. Katherine will invite one of these potential friends out to lunch, bringing Alice along so that Katherine can model the good friend behavior of cooperating, listening, and sharing. If Alice acts like a 9-year-old, she will get dessert at lunch. If she doesn't act like a 9-year-old, she will not get dessert at lunch, and she won't get it at dinner either.

5. Katherine and Alice will watch appropriate movies and TV shows together where Katherine can point out good friendship behaviors between kids Alice's age.

6. Katherine will coach Alice to play a board game with the clinician where Alice cooperates, shares, and is a good sport.

7. Katherine will help Alice pick out a person from her class to invite over for a play date along with this person's mother or father. Katherine will call the mother and pick the day and time first and then coach Alice to very nicely ask this person over on the phone.

8. While maintaining an appropriate adult-child boundary, Katherine will help Alice make this a fun play date so that this person will want to come back over.

9. Other goals will be developed as appropriate to help Alice socialize appropriately with peers.

Practice Case for Student Conceptualization: Integrating the Domain of Race and Ethnicity

It is time to do a family systems conceptualization and treatment plan for Tanisha and Marcus, an African American couple. Although many domains of complexity may have relevance for them, you are asked to try to integrate the Domain of Race and Ethnicity into your case conceptualization and treatment plan. As a conflict between the clinician and the clients over race and ethnicity is critical to the interview, assume that the clinician is not African American.

Information Received From Brief Intake

Tanisha, a 30-year-old African American, and Marcus, a 32-year-old African American, have been married for 7 years. They moved to western Pennsylvania about 2 years ago from a suburb of Detroit, Michigan. Tanisha indicated her marriage was generally happy but that she and Marcus needed help dealing with the death of their infant daughter Latisha. Tanisha was referred to treatment by a close friend who was very happy with the outcome of her own marital treatment with this clinician. Marcus doesn't know that Tanisha is making this appointment, but she is confident he will come.

During a brief mental status exam, Tanisha showed signs of clinical depression but had no signs of suicidal or homicidal ideation or other serious psychopathology. Tanisha's description of Marcus suggested he was not depressed or showing signs of significant psychopathology.

Interview With Tanisha and Marcus From a Family Systems Perspective

C: Tanisha, Marcus. Thank you for coming in. I had a chance to talk with Tanisha earlier and explain how I generally conduct treatment sessions and the ethical and legal rules of privacy that I follow. Marcus, are there any questions you have about any of this before we start?

M: (tensely) No. Tanisha filled me in and showed me those pamphlets you gave her.

C: Great. If you have any questions about what I'm doing or the treatment process itself, please don't hesitate to ask. (pause) Could we start with one of you telling me about your family?

T: (tensely) Marcus and I are the only members of our family living here. (T looks at M who is looking down) Awhile back, (pause) we decided we needed a fresh start, and Marcus accepted a promotion that led us to move here. We both have a lot of family back in Detroit, Michigan. We try to get back there to see them four to five times a year. We still talk regularly by phone and write with e-mail. It was hard to move far away, but Marcus and I have always emphasized our careers.

C: So, the family back in Detroit is very important to you. (pause) Is anyone else living with you, or around you, right now? (long pause)

T: (looking briefly at M, regretfully) No. Marcus's younger sister did live with us last summer to take some courses at the university near us—we were the only ones really encouraging her to get a college degree and would have liked her to stay with us. But, she's at Wright State now, and it has the advantage of being around the corner from where her mom and our other relatives live.

C: Both getting an education and being around family were important to her.

T: (tentatively) Yes . . . (Marcus breaks in on this)

M: (angrily) What is the point of this? The family in Detroit is fine, so talking about them is a waste of time.

C: Marcus, I don't mean to waste your time. Knowing who is in your family is a part of the process of my understanding what you need from me. (M and T are glaring at each other; T's fists are clenched)

C: Look at your fists, Tanisha. (T relaxes her hands) You need to say something. Why don't you turn your chair toward Marcus, rather than me, so that the two of you can discuss together how you want to tell me what your family needs right now. (T turns her chair toward M and then looks up at C, who nods)

T: (hesitantly, looking at C) I guess (pause) I'll start by telling you . . . (C interrupts)

C: I apologize for interrupting. I need you to discuss it with Marcus. I'll listen.

T: (hesitantly, looking at M) I know we came here to get a new start, but I still can't stop thinking about our little girl dying 5 years ago. (pause) I just can't stop crying over her. You've been able to get on with things. (pause) I feel I have gone on at work but not at home. (pause) You want another child, and I love children but I don't think I . . . (long pause, T leans forward with her face in her hands. M leans toward her and pats her knee softly)

C: It's devastating to lose a child. (long pause) What happened?

M: (speaking calmly but emphatically) I think it's better if we don't go into all of those details. It's just going to make Tanisha cry, and it's not going to change anything.

C: It's a very painful topic.

M: (with an edge to his voice) And, the topic is closed.

T: (tearfully) Marcus, this is what we're here for. This is what I came here for. Our baby, Latisha, was born with some kind of birth defect; they don't know why. My pregnancy was healthy. There were no problems in delivery, but as soon as she was born, (pause) it was clear something was wrong. She had heart and lung defects. They transferred her to the Cleveland Clinic because they had a specialty unit there for babies like her. She never left that hospital. I went to visit her every weekend for a year. My poor little darling had tubes up her nose. Never got to play, rarely got to see her family outside of me because the hospital was so far away. My dad is in really bad health, and my mom was always afraid to leave him and drive out with me. My mother-in-law came with me a few times. (T starts to cry softly)

M: (angrily) I told you this was a bad idea. (glaring at C) Let's just go home, sweetheart; this isn't going to help us. (M stands up and gently pulls on T's hand)

T: (fiercely) No, I'm staying. I know you don't like talking about it, Marcus. But what we've been doing isn't working, and I need help. We need help. (M sits back down)

M: (glowering at C) Talking about Latisha is not going to help.

C: I can see that I've made you angry. I didn't mean to do that. Of course, you know Tanisha a lot better than me, but my eyes tell me that she needs to work this through.

M: (accusingly) You don't know what she needs.

C: My goal would be to help you two figure it out together. (pause) I can see what a strong couple you are. Could you give me a chance to try and help you deal with the traumatic death of your Latisha?

M: (sinking into his chair, tiredly) Look, I have nothing against you, but Tanisha has to let go of this. I'd like to have another child, but if she doesn't want to try again—I'll live with that. We have a good life as it is. (M begins to move forward in the chair as if to stand up again)

C: I can see you don't want to talk about your daughter, but would you be willing to talk more with Tanisha about the good life you have together?

M: (looking away from C and back at T, who sits back against her chair, tiredly) OK, I'll talk about that. (looking at C) I'm a postmaster in a town about 20 minutes from here. I make a good living. So does Tanisha. She's the regional manager for Rite Aid. Together, we have made enough money to buy a really nice home and fill it with beautiful things. We take a great vacation every year. Last year, we went to Mexico, and the year before that we went on an Alaskan cruise. (Looking at T, emphatically) Tanisha, you've got to admit we're living the good life.

T: (sadly) I never said we weren't. I'm grateful for the good things we have. But I wanted our little girl to grow up. I had a plan. I was going to stop working and have a big family like my mother did. I loved growing up in a house full of kids. (wistfully) I didn't care that we would be giving up a lot of money if I stayed home.

M: (softly) I wanted that too. We could still do that.

T: (shaking her head, sadly) You just don't get it. Our Latisha is dead. I don't want another child. I want HER. (long pause where T is holding her face in her hands)

C: Try and look at Marcus, Tanisha. He wants to remind you what a beautiful life you have together despite the terrible loss of your daughter. He wants to remind you how much strength and love you have together even without her. (T looks up at M and gives him a little smile) The two of you love each other but are in a different phase of family life. He has finished grieving over the tremendous loss of his Latisha, and what he has left is his love for you and a desire to try and be a father to another child. Tanisha, you are still deeply in grief. The pain and suffering have been so heavy that you feel mired in the horror of her death. You can't consider, right now, even the idea of another child. (pause) Can you take Marcus's hands and just experience his strength to help you pull back from some of this pain?

M: (M pushes his chair backward, as T begins to take his hands. Glaring at C and yelling) I WON'T STAND ANY MORE OF THIS! WE ARE NOT PUPPETS. STOP ORDERING US AROUND!

C: You're both strong people and nothing like puppets. (long pause) Is it the techniques I'm using, to try to help the two of you talk, that's the problem, or am I the problem?

M: (firmly) You just can't get what we're going through, and so you should stay out of it.

T: (angrily) Marcus, stop taking your anger out on her. She's right about me. I think about our girl every day, but you don't want to hear that. This is what you always do. I need to talk about it, but you just get mad and walk away. Well, you're not the only one who gets mad. I've kept more than my pain about our little girl in my heart for so long. I have to tell you how mad I am that you never went with me to visit our girl.

M: (defensively) There was no point going there. She couldn't see us, and she couldn't hear us—the doctors said so.

T: (loudly) I held her hand. She might have been able to feel that. She was ours. She needed us.

C: The two of you understood what the doctor said in different ways. Tanisha heard that she couldn't help Latisha by talking. So, she tried touching. You, Marcus, heard that there was no hope, and you began to grieve for her even before she actually died.

M: (angrily) Don't try to manipulate me. I told you I wasn't going to discuss Latisha. Tanisha, we need each other, but we don't need this. Look at yourself; you're more depressed now than you were when we began driving here.

T: (tiredly) I'm just letting out what I've had inside. I want to be here. If you don't want to be here, (long pause) you can leave. (long pause)

C: Marcus, I know that being here is not what you want, but could you consider staying, because it feels like the right place for Tanisha to be right now?

M: (M shakes his head no, long pause) I don't feel comfortable with you or with this situation.

C: It's strange to be talking about such private things with someone you just met. (pause) Marcus, you feel manipulated. I'm sorry you feel that way. My way of helping couples talk through problems is very directive. I'm honestly trying to help you two talk about Latisha in a way that's different from what you two have done before. I heard Tanisha say she needs help working through the reality of Latisha's death. I was trying to help set up a conversation that might help Tanisha with this—not because I want to force something on you. If this doesn't help, my plan would be to suggest we try something else. I am willing to keep trying until we find something that works for both you and Tanisha that feels right. (pause) What do you think?

M: (intently) I look at you and can tell you can't get me and you can't get what we've been through.

C: You're right that we look different from each other. What you are going through is your struggle, not mine. Any problems or oppression you have faced is part of your life.

M: (jumping on this) Then, we agree this was a mistake.

C: You are right: I am not African American, and this difference between us might represent a barrier to our working together successfully. But, on the other hand, something I noticed that we do share is we are hardworking and ambitious without forgetting the importance of loving connections to family. I don't want to make you live "my way." I want to help you find a way to relate to Latisha as parents that allows you to continue this wonderful and strong couple of Marcus and Tanisha.

T: (demandingly) Marcus, you are not helping me with this. I want to drop this racial thing and talk about our girl.

M: (angrily) No. We can't just drop it. (long pause)

C: My not being African American is clearly a big issue. Why don't I go into the next room and give you two time alone to discuss what it means to each of you to work with me? You can come and get me once you decide if we should work further together or if I should give you the names of other clinicians and tell you about their cultural affiliations and strengths.

T: (emphatically) No. I don't want to talk about that. Marcus, focusing on race is just another way to not talk about Latisha. I want to talk about her.

M: (compellingly) Tanisha, someone who isn't African American can't understand and will make things worse even with the best intentions.

C: That would be terrible if instead of helping I made things worse. I can understand why you would want to prevent that. (long pause) My goal in being here is to support the strength within you two, not to try to transform your marriage into my image of what a marriage should be. There are lots of things I won't understand about what you need unless you help me understand. (Tanisha starts to cry again)

M: (emphatically) Can't you see how you are hurting her with this? I can't allow that.

C: You love her. You want to protect her from pain. But, is it possible to protect her from the pain of your daughter's birth defects and death?

T: (T leans over and takes M's hand, calmly) He's a good man, and he does a lot to take care of me. But, you are right. He doesn't understand that I can't just go on and forget about our Latisha. We bought our house outside of Detroit so she would have a backyard to play in. (painfully) That's one of the reasons we moved away from Detroit. What was the point of that house, especially after Marcus gave away our Latisha's things—leaving me with nothing but memories? He couldn't take those away.

M: (frustratedly) I didn't just give the stuff away. Your sister needed it for her son. She didn't have the money to buy her own. It wasn't doing any good, locked away in that room. It was better for you to get it out of the house.

T: (calmly) I guess we spent our first 3 years of marriage with him being the big boss you can see now. But you can't boss me out of this. (moving her chair farther away from M) I want to be here. I need to be here. I can't be silent about it anymore. I've tried that. It doesn't work for me.

M: Why here? If we have to do this, let's find someone else.

T: Someone I trust got help here. Marcus, please give this a chance.

M: (torn) I'll give in to this for 1 more week. But, I still don't buy it that this will help.

C: Your wife's been crying for 5 years; 1 week isn't enough time. How about 3 weeks? Then, if you two talk and decide I'm the problem, I'll try to help you find someone else. But, if you think maybe it could be working, you keep coming.

M: (firmly) OK, you've got 3 weeks. (sardonically) You've got a fast mouth; I'll give you that.

C: I can't argue with that.

Exercises for Developing a Case Conceptualization of Tanisha and Marcus

Exercise 1 (4-page maximum)

GOAL: To verify that you have a clear understanding of a family systems approach.

STYLE: An integrative essay addressing Parts A–C.

NEED HELP? Review this chapter (pages 257–266).

    A. Develop a concise overview of the assumptions of family systems theory (the theory's hypotheses about key dimensions in understanding families; think abstractly, broadly).

    B. Develop a detailed description of how each of these assumptions is used to understand a family's functioning (for each assumption, provide specifics, concrete details).

    C. Describe the role of the clinician in aiding a family in developing an adaptive structure (consultant, doctor, educator, helper; treatment approach; technique examples).

Exercise 2 (4-page maximum)

GOAL: To aid application of family systems theory to Tanisha and Marcus.

STYLE: A separate sentence outline for each section, A–E.

NEED HELP?   Review this chapter (pages 257–266).

   A. What are the strengths (strong points, positive features, resources) that you see in Tanisha and Marcus, both as individuals and as a couple, at this time?

   B. What are the weaknesses (concerns, issues, symptoms, problems, treatment barriers) that you see in Tanisha and Marcus, both as individuals and as a couple, at this time?

   C. Provide a detailed analysis of how these strengths and weaknesses could be understood within a family context by describing the following:

      1. Who do Marcus and Tanisha consider to be members of their family, and do they agree or disagree about this?

      2. What are the family subsystems, and what is the composition and function of each?

      3. What type of boundaries exist between subsystems, between the family and extended family, and between the family and other social systems?

      4. Who has the power in the family to do what, what are the family rules, and is this a change from the past (issues of hierarchy and alignments)?

      5. How well are the needs of each family member, and the system as a whole, being met in terms of emotional intimacy and independence?

      6. What role does Latisha play in the family system at this time?

      7. Do Tanisha and Marcus have the same perceptions of the impact of Latisha's birth defects on their family system, and how has this influenced their expectations and behaviors within their current family system?

   D. What stage of development is the family in now, is the family in a period of homeostasis or disequilibrium, and how well is the family functioning overall?

   E. What changes in family structure might be beneficial at this time, what strengths does the family bring to the process of treatment, and are there any factors facilitating or inhibiting structural change at this time?

Exercise 3 (3-page maximum)

GOAL: To develop an understanding of the potential role of the African American culture in Tanisha and Marcus's marriage and current situation.

STYLE: A separate sentence outline for each section, A–E.

NEED HELP?   Review Chapter 2 (pages 50–55).

   A. Assess the role of their African American heritage in the lives of Tanisha and Marcus in terms of the strengths, resources, and power it may be bringing to them within personal, family, social, vocational, and political spheres.

   B. Consider how current or historical events have influenced the African American people and assess if any of Tanisha and Marcus's current problem(s) could be a result of direct or indirect oppression or trauma, their responses to this oppression, assimilation stress, and/or a mismatch in values with the dominant society and its institutions.

   C. Assess how well the couple is functioning at this time, including a comparison of Tanisha and Marcus's functioning through the lens of their African American heritage with that through the lens of the dominant cultural group. Consider if there are realistic constraints influencing them within the dominant culture at this time and if any of Tanisha and Marcus's behavior within the dominant society might represent a healthy adaptation to injustice that would be supported by the African American community.

   D. Assess Tanisha and Marcus's personal worldviews and the role of their African American heritage within them and consider if there are any culturally specific resources, treatment strategies, or helpers they would value at this time and how these might be used within your treatment plan.

   E. Assess whether any aspects of your identity and cultural conditioning or any implicit bias within your treatment approach could lead to communication problems, values conflict, difficulty understanding the couple's lifestyle or experiences, or invalidation of the couple's strengths and consider how treatment could be modified to increase the likelihood of a positive outcome.

Exercise 4 (6-page maximum)

GOAL: To help you integrate your knowledge of family systems theory and racial and ethnic issues into an in-depth conceptualization of Tanisha and Marcus (who they are and why they do what they do).

STYLE: An integrated essay consisting of a premise, supportive details, and conclusions following a carefully planned organizational style.

NEED HELP? Review Chapter 1 (pages 7–28) and Chapter 2 (pages 50–55).

STEP 1: Consider what style you could use for organizing your family systems understanding of this couple that (a) would support you in providing a comprehensive and clear understanding of the family's structure and how it is functioning and (b) would support language Tanisha and Marcus might find persuasive considering their disagreement over the need to get help outside of their family and the African American community.

STEP 2: Develop your concise premise (overview, preliminary or explanatory statements, proposition, thesis statement, theory-driven introduction, hypotheses, summary, concluding causal statements) that explains Tanisha and Marcus's issues as a couple whose child died and who disagree about whether they need to process this loss further than they already have. If you're having trouble with Step 2, remember it should be an integration of the key ideas of Exercises 2 and 3 that (a) provides a basis for the family's long-term goals, (b) is grounded in family systems theory and is sensitive to Tanisha and Marcus's African American heritage, and (c) highlights the strengths the family brings to family systems treatment.

STEP 3: Develop your supporting material (detailed case analysis of strengths and weaknesses, supplying data to support an introductory premise) from a family systems perspective that integrates within each paragraph a deep understanding of Tanisha and Marcus as an African American couple. If you're having trouble with Step 3, consider the information you'll need to include in order to (a) support the development of short-term goals, (b) be grounded in family systems theory and sensitive to racial and ethnic issues, and (c) integrate an understanding of the structural strengths within Tanisha and Marcus's family whenever possible.

STEP 4: Develop your conclusions and broad treatment recommendations including (a) the couple's overall level of functioning, (b) anything facilitating or serving as a barrier to the couple's developing a new family structure at this time, and (c) the couple's basic needs as a family system at this time, being careful to consider what you said in Part E of Exercise 3 (be concise and to the point).

Exercise 5 (3-page maximum)

GOAL: To develop an individualized, theory-driven action plan for Tanisha and Marcus that considers their strengths and is sensitive to their African American heritage.

STYLE: A sentence outline consisting of long- and short-term goals.

NEED HELP?   Review Chapter 1 (pages 8–28).

STEP 1: Develop your treatment plan overview, being careful to consider what you said in Part E of Exercise 3 to try and prevent any negative bias to your treatment plan.

STEP 2: Develop long-term (major, large, ambitious, comprehensive, broad) goals that *ideally* Tanisha and Marcus would reach by the termination of treatment that would lead them to reach an adaptive homeostasis in their marriage that acknowledges the role of Latisha in their lives. If you are having trouble with Step 2, reread your premise and support topic sentences for ideas, paying careful attention to how they could be transformed into structural goals (use the *style* of Exercise 4).

STEP 3: Develop short-term (small, brief, encapsulated, specific, measurable) goals that Tanisha, Marcus, and you could expect to see accomplished within a few weeks in the family's structure to chart its progress, instill hope for change, and plan time-effective treatment sessions. If you are having trouble with Step 3, reread your support paragraphs looking for ideas to transform into goals that (a) might enhance cognitive insight into the different family expectations Tanisha and Marcus brought into their marriage based on their childhood families; (b) might support structural change; (c) might enhance factors facilitating or decrease barriers to their effectively dealing with the death of their daughter; (d) might utilize their individual, relationship, and extended family strengths whenever possible; and (e) are individualized to their needs as an African American couple rather than generic.

Exercise 6

GOAL: To critique family treatment and the case of Tanisha and Marcus.

STYLE: Answer Questions A–E in essay form or discuss them in a group format.

A. What are the strengths and weaknesses of family systems theory for helping Tanisha and Marcus (an African American couple in grief, separated by a large distance from extended family, who have experienced cultural oppression)?

B. Discuss the pros and cons of feminist treatment for Marcus as a member of a minority group and an *individual* for whom issues of oppression may be very salient. Discuss how important it is to integrate gender issues in this couple's treatment.

C. Discuss the validity of Marcus's concerns that a White clinician would not be able to understand him, Tanisha, and their situation. What might or might not change if the clinician was a person of color but not African American? What might or might not change if the couple was White but the clinician was African American?

D. What ethical issues are raised once Marcus expresses concerns about the clinician being culturally different from his own family and therefore unable to provide competent treatment? What needs to be assessed further before deciding whether to try and treat this family yourself or refer Tanisha and Marcus elsewhere?

E. How did you react personally to Marcus's challenging comments to the clinician, and how might you handle the situation if it happened to you? (If you are African American, assume the couple is White and the husband raised the same concerns.) If you are culturally different from a family, in one or more ways, what could you do to try and foster a strong treatment relationship and a positive outcome? Consider how you would prepare yourself prior to treatment, how you might handle the structure of the sessions differently, and what differences might need to occur in the process of the sessions.

Recommended Resources

American Association for Marriage and Family Therapy. http://www.aamft.org/

Family Institute of Kansas City, Missouri (Producer), & Corales, R. (Trainer). (1986). *The major theories of family therapy teaching tapes: VT 112 structural* [Motion picture]. (DVD #7AQ3717 available from Insight Media, 2162 Broadway, New York, NY 10024, 1-800-233-9910)

Minuchin, S., Nichols, M. P., & Lee., W.-Y. (2007) *Assessing couples and families: From symptom to system.* Boston: Allyn & Bacon.

Nichols, M. P. (2008). *Family therapy concepts and methods* (8th ed.). Boston: Pearson Education, Inc.

Nine

Constructivist Case Conceptualizations and Treatment Plans

Introduction to Constructivist Theory

Zechariah arrives at an appointment made for him by the disciplinary board of a midsized, rural university. He is a 19-year-old African American freshman. He has a 17-year-old sister and two younger brothers aged 15 and 13. They have been raised by his mother and his grand-mother in a large northeastern city that is about 4 hours away from the university. The Christian religion plays an important role in Zechariah's family's life, and he was named after the Prophet Zechariah, whose teach-ings were repeatedly quoted to him during his childhood. Zechariah has been referred for anger management. He disagrees with the referral, believing it reflects a racist university system. However, he plans to coop-erate. He is determined to succeed academically and become the first member of his family to graduate from a university.

The postmodern tradition encompasses many different viewpoints rather than providing a unified theory for clinicians to follow. What these diverse approaches have in common include the beliefs that individuals are motivated to impose order on the phenomena they experience, that this imposed structure helps individuals understand their experiences and derive meaning from them, and that these represent socially constructed realities rather than an objective reality that holds true for an individual across time, across different individuals, within a culture, or across cultures. You also believe that it is the conversational exchanges people have with themselves or others that serves as the medium for imposing order on experience so that meaning construction can take place; this last addition is what makes your treatment orientation "relational constructivism." This approach "emphasizes the primacy of interpersonal relationships and conversational exchanges in human life" (Neimeyer, 2000, p. 216) and seeks to explain that all-important concept, "the self."

You believe that Zechariah maintains a coherent sense of himself through the stories he tells about his past. These "storied selves" are always open to revision as he explores and elaborates on his experiences within conversational exchanges. His stories contain first-person narration in order to (a) integrate his disparate experiences together into a coherent whole, (b) position him in relation to others, and (c) temporarily provide him with fictional coherence for understanding himself; it is fictional because while it is functional for him in the moment, it is not "objectively" or "reality based."

Zechariah is the protagonist within the story of his life, and in order to understand it, Zechariah must talk about it with you. This dyadic dialogue is the process that allows him to construct knowledge for understanding himself, you, and his situation; this meaning creation is mediated by the language used in the dialogue. As he tells you what he is going through at the university, he is engaged in a social performance that is, by its nature, a relational act. You will take a very ideographic approach to helping him. Until Zechariah comes to his appointment, you'll have no plan about how you will proceed beyond encouraging him to tell his story and intending to fully participate with him in cocreating a healing experience. It is a cocreated experience, because who (Zechariah) tells what (his problems with his roommate) to whom (you) when (after a disciplinary board hearing) is highly influential in what story unfolds and the meaning that Zechariah draws from it (Neimeyer, 1995, 2000).

Who in fact is Zechariah? A university student? An African American male? An eldest son? An angry young man? Zechariah does not have a true self that is knowable or that is real as an entity. Zechariah has multiple selves within him that each say something about his life and his relational exchanges and that open up more or less resilient constructions of the world for use in guiding him in the future. Who he is in the moment will change based on who he is dialoguing with. This is because his immediate sense of himself is a process under construction within every interpersonal exchange. Thus, he can be viewed as having a "storied self," a sense of himself as whole or coherent that is based on the stories he tells himself and others about his past experiences; these stories are always open to revision (Neimeyer, 2000).

Zechariah is continuously in the process of trying to make meaning from his experiences through exploring and elaborating on them. The past experiences Zechariah is attempting to incorporate within his self-understanding are in fact heterogeneous, complex, and at times contradictory. Thus, many different stories are possible, and no one is more objectively true than another. How will a dialogue proceed? As Zechariah relates his life to you, he will organize his experiences into units that seem meaningful to him in the moment. He may perceive patterns or themes within these experiences as he does so. For example, he may remember many instances in which he helped his younger siblings. The meaning he creates/draws from these stories about himself could include that he is a loving older brother (who he is) who actively seeks to help his siblings (what he does). This understanding of himself, or self-theory, can be considered functional for him if it is plausible within the constraints of his current day-to-day life, if it offers opportunities for expansion or revision so that it can integrate new experiences, and if it leads to positive mood states.

Does Zechariah need treatment? It depends on whether he has a coherent and life-enhancing narrative guiding him in the moment. To determine if this is the case, consider the following questions: Is he experiencing a lot of positive emotions? Does his current narrative give him an adaptive and coherent view of himself? Is he relating effectively to others? Is he taking actions that support adaptive goals within family, school and/or work environments? Is he able to adaptively accommodate new experiences into his ongoing narrative? If so, then his narrative is life enhancing, and he doesn't need treatment. On the other hand, if he is experiencing a lot of negative emotions; if he is experiencing a disorganized, negative, incoherent, or overly rigid view of himself; if he is struggling within dysfunctional relationships; if he is unable to take adaptive actions; or if he is unable to be responsive to new experiences, then the answer is yes.

At this moment in time, Zechariah is defining his identity using a problem-saturated narrative; the problems he has faced as a new student, his roommate's accusation that he is violent, the behavior of the disciplinary board, and his feelings of oppression and invisibility within society are dominating Zechariah's view of himself and his world. Other aspects of his experiences, such as his success in his coursework, his happiness at finding African American friends, and the love and respect he receives from his family members, are thin (not well-elaborated) stories that are not experienced as potently at this time as this thick (well-elaborated) story of oppression. If he chooses to participate in treatment, his awareness of these positive experiences, and the emotions they evoke, could be enhanced through further exploration and elaboration so that they could form powerful counternarratives to the painful one that is currently dominating his constructions. Zechariah would be in charge of any meaning he draws from these treatment experiences, but through attending to his emotional responses (verbal and nonverbal), you would guide him to develop a more life-enhancing narrative (Neimeyer, 1995, 2000).

Role of the Clinician

Treatment starts with a conversation between Zechariah and you. While his words and actions are going to define how treatment starts, you are not a passive participant in his reality. As you intervene in his narrative process by asking questions, reflecting on what he's said, and encouraging him to experience his emotions and bodily sensations more deeply, you and Zechariah are temporarily creating segments of his experience (subplots). These have an assumed beginning and end that punctuate a seemingly linear event, even though no objective linear cause-effect relationships are actually possible (Kelly, 1955).

For example, Zechariah may have found an experience in his morning psychology class confusing. You will encourage him to explore this experience more deeply by helping him recall further details of the class to enable him to consider his actions, thoughts, feelings, and interactions with others from multiple perspectives. Through this process, he will gain deeper meaning from what he experienced. In the moment, he says that a particular statement made by the professor was subtly insulting and "caused" him to feel rejected. Zechariah has worked hard in this class and doesn't understand why the professor would mistreat him. Fully processing negative emotions plays an integral part in the meaning-making experience of treatment, so Zechariah's emotion of rejection will be explored fully. He defines the beginning of this experience with the professor's comment and the end of it as his feeling of rejection. However, if a different segment of time was chosen, a different interpretation of cause and effect might have enfolded. For example, based on your questions, you determine that, due to a faulty alarm clock, Zechariah rushed into class late. This entry disrupted the class discussion. The professor responded by criticizing Zechariah for coming in late. In this way, "the lateness" is now the cause of the rejection, not the professor's comments. Thus, there is no true linearity that can be used to determine cause and effect, only a perceived linearity.

As Zechariah tells his story, you will try to achieve narrative empathy—where you are attuned to his feelings and thoughts and are engaged in reflecting and validating his identity as it unfolds. You will be curious and encourage exploration rather than being directive or didactic. His emotions always carry important meaning, and they will be actively explored whenever signs of them, either verbal or nonverbal, emerge in the session. To process his experiences and support meaning construction, you will engage him in three basic processes: articulating his story as fully as possible; elaborating any aspects of it that might be confusing, incomplete, or problematical; and negotiating interpersonal meanings from his experiences that support understanding his world and his place in it, with a sense of coherence and optimism, and that support an adaptive lifestyle.

Both of you are bound in some ways by the language you use while conversing. Treatment can turn its attention to this language, within which the assumptions of the dominant culture are embedded, along with the family, or cultural assumptions behind Zechariah's self-theories; some of these may be guiding him in adaptive ways, but others may be problematic and need to be challenged. For example, a son involved in an incestuous relationship with his father could be labeled an "incest victim," an "incest survivor," or a "thriver despite incest." Subtle and not-so-subtle changes in language could have a potent impact on the son's view of himself in relation to others.

How will you encourage adaptive meaning construction? The overall process will start with you and Zechariah deconstructing his story (taking it from one whole into many parts such as the setting, characters, and plot) and then elaborating further aspects of it that he may not have fully attended to. This allows him to draw more meaning from his past experiences. There are many techniques you could use in this process. While you listen actively, you will suggest techniques that might resonate with his needs in the moment. As the treatment process is highly collaborative, a technique will never be imposed on Zechariah; he will be asked about whether he wants to try something or not. Techniques developed from many different schools of treatment may prove useful within the spontaneous interactions that unfold during the session. However, the storied-self metaphor can be used to provide practical guidance for encouraging Zechariah in the meaning construction process. This metaphor can be explored and elaborated along three dimensions including its (a) narrative form and features, (b) points of view and voice, and (c) issues of authorship and audience. Each dimension offers ideas for how your conversation with Zechariah could intervene in the meaning construction process to make more narrative possibilities available. Narratives that don't open up opportunities for new meaning construction are considered thin and in need of further exploration and expansion; this is called thickening the narrative. The following descriptions for how to use these dimensions in opening up new narrative possibilities for Zechariah, the "author-protagonist," come from Neimeyer (2000).

Narrative form and features is a structure for understanding Zechariah's autobiographical account that includes articulating details of the setting (where), the characterization (who), the plot (what), the themes (why), and the goals (purpose) of the narrative. The setting emerges from a step-by-step account of what is going on during a particular aspect of his history and indicates the where and when of a segment of experience. You will help Zechariah recall as many details of the setting as possible, and you will accent the meaning he is attaching to them so that Zechariah can explore his constructions more thoroughly.

Characterization refers to defining who the actors are within the story as well as the hypothetical intentions of these individuals as told by the narrator. While Zechariah may be sure he understands his roommate's motivation, you may help him explore alternative possibilities. Individuals often have complex intentions. By considering these possibilities, Zechariah's story gains greater psychological depth. This process may leave Zechariah with a deeper insight into other people. Zechariah's own intentions can also be examined in this way, and you may offer metaphors or other methods for helping him understand his own complex internal experiences. Finally, this work will help Zechariah see how his "self" and "other" constructions are interrelated within his story.

Helping Zechariah articulate the plot of his story, or what happened in a certain episode (or subplot) of his story, is used to increase his awareness of all the actions that occurred within the order of occurrence. Inadequate understanding of events will interfere with Zechariah having a coherent sense of his identity. If he is having trouble recalling details of a subplot, you will help him vividly reexperience it. Through this, he will be guided to fill in gaps in the story. For example, Zechariah may have aspects of himself that he has kept secret from others in an attempt to separate himself from trauma, negative experiences, or some disliked or disowned behavior on his part. You will help him clarify the *meaning* of these parts of himself in a more self-affirming and accepting way. Similarly, he may be confused because aspects of his experience are directing him to behave in contradictory ways. You will help him clarify these confusing experiences, negotiate meaning that takes all of them into account, and develop a plan of action that directs him in a life-affirming way. You will then help him consider how each part of the experience helps him understand what has happened.

The wherefore of the narrative is the well-defined, if fictional, goals that you will help Zechariah set for himself. These goals are future oriented and will reflect positive actions that he could take to sustain himself in living within a coherent self-understanding, while he relates adaptively to others. While in fact no particular goal represents the reality of how he "should" be, these goals represent possibilities that are open to him. They may also include attempts to seek social validation for his new positive self-constructions. While these goals may be satisfying to him or designed to satisfy the university's disciplinary board, success in treatment is never based on goal attainment per se as his life is an ongoing process of construction without a knowable endpoint. Goals are successful if they set Zechariah on a forward-moving narrative into the future.

As Zechariah relates his narrative to you, there is both an intrapersonal and an interpersonal focus. The intrapersonal focus is highlighted by the point of view and voice of the narrative. Zechariah can choose from five different points of view in telling his story. In the first, he can be engaged in an interior monologue where he is providing an uncensored, free-flowing description of his experiences as they spontaneously occur to him. Second, he may be engaged in a dramatic monologue where he is attempting to explicitly persuade the listener of his point of view. Third, he may be engaged in a letter narrative, which like the internal monologue is a form of self-exploration. However, in writing the letter, it is more organized and less free floating. The writer assumes that the reader of the letter will form a response to it; therefore the narrative needs to be made clear to this potential other. Fourth, Zechariah could relate his narrative in the style of a detached autobiography where he tries to show objectivity in examining his life. Finally, in anonymous narration,

Zechariah could articulate the viewpoints of more than one character within the story. In this way, the story wouldn't have an "I" focus.

In telling the story, the voice Zechariah chooses to use may provide clues to the meaning he has been drawing from it. For example, does he use a pleading voice as if telling himself that he has done the best he could? Does he use a condemning tone of voice where he blames himself for what has happened? Zechariah has many voices within himself. If only one can be heard, he risks ignoring important aspects of himself in constructing his identity.

Why is Zechariah choosing to mention some details of his story but not others? How is this intended to influence you? Storytelling is an interactive process with reciprocal influence between the teller (author) and the listener (audience). From this perspective, it has an interpersonal focus. Zechariah is implicitly or explicitly bringing you in as a listener and participant in how he decides to tell you his story and in how he decides which of his heterogeneous experiences to share with you. In addition, the very language he uses in talking about himself is influenced by his social context. The culture Zechariah lives in provides the language that he can use to try to understand his experiences and that he can use to reshape his experiences. You will help Zechariah understand how languaging (the using of words to describe experience) is a process that occurs in the context of one person communicating to another. The language an individual uses implicitly or explicitly punctuates experience and thus can bias the individual's construction of meaning from a story. Zechariah may need new words to use in developing a more functional meaning from aspects of his story or to use in plotting an alternative narrative.

In summary, many techniques can orally or in writing help Zechariah deconstruct a problem-saturated narrative and begin creating a more life-enhancing one. The process of deconstruction provides Zechariah with new possibilities for how he could think, feel, or behave as he reconstructs a new life story. At the end of treatment, Zechariah will be telling his story in a more life-enhancing manner. What will that reflect? His stories about himself will include self-acceptance, validation, and continuity. He will have positioned himself in a positive way in relation to others. He will have active, positive ways of connecting to the social world that receive positive validation from others. His new story will be able to guide him toward achieving his goals as a student and loving family member. You will have validated any constructive changes Zechariah made in how he sees himself, how he sees his place in the world, and how he interacts with others. However, strong, health-seeking identities are best validated by significant others in his life beyond the treatment setting. Thus, you will have helped him determine if, how, and when he will document any new aspects of himself in his interactions with other people. You will have supported Zechariah in developing his own idiosyncratic meanings from the patterns he has punctuated in his life. The healthy meanings he has constructed will lead him to goal-directed and health-discovering behavior, thoughts, and emotions. How long will treatment be? Each session will end with a consideration of its value and whether the client feels another consultation would be of value (Neimeyer, 1995, 2000).

Case Application: Integrating the Domain of Socioeconomic Status

Zechariah's case will now be examined in more detail. While there are many domains of human complexity that could provide insights into his behavior, the Domain of Socioeconomic Status has been selected to integrate within a constructivist case conceptualization and treatment plan.

Interview With Zechariah (Z) From a Constructivist Perspective

C: (handing Z a copy of the report) Here is the disciplinary board report. I thought you would want to see it. (long pause while Z reads through document) I found it very confusing. You've got an outstanding academic record for your first semester here—a 4.0. To me, this means you must be a disciplined, high-achieving young man. Yet, the board describes you as impulsive and angry.

Z: (tightly gripping the report, calmly but with intensity) This is all racist bullshit. What's wrong with everybody here? (speaking loudly and firmly) I got angry a few times at the hearing because my roommate was lying about me. That doesn't make me an angry person. (pause) I could tell the moment I walked in that the board had prejudged me and found me guilty.

C: What told you that?

Z: (matter-of-factly) There were 10 of them all sitting across from me and just staring at me throughout the hearing—all wearing fancy suits. I was wearing my church clothes, but they were from Kmart; I doubt those people ever needed to shop at Kmart.

C: You felt their clothes set them apart from you. It was hard to imagine that people who were so much wealthier than you would treat you fairly. Was there anything else?

Z: (angrily) I was separated by a stupid screen from my roommate. My lawyer warned me about this in advance . . . but, I . . . (he is choked up)

C: The screen hit you hard. What did it mean to you?

Z: (angrily) It was saying I was set apart—invisible. He was free to accuse me of anything, and (pause) Henry—my roommate—told the board that he was so scared of me, he couldn't testify if he saw me, (pause, hands on chair, knuckles white) and they let him get away with it.

C: It was an ordeal, painful, and it felt rigged against you.

Z: (intently) I had to sit there and listen to all this testimony where he insisted I'd been threatening him from Day 1. I could see his hands on the table because the screen wasn't very large. He was clutching a Bible like he was some pious man. The panel questioned him gently as if he was on the brink of a breakdown. When it was my turn, I asked him if it wasn't true that I tried over and over to befriend him; he just kept muttering I was just trying to intimidate him. (voice getting louder) I asked him if it wasn't true that I was hardly ever in the room except to sleep. He said that was because I was always off drinking. (fists pounding the side of the chair) I wasn't out drinking. I was in the library studying, but he assumes everything bad he can about me.

C: Why does he do that?

Z: (intently, looking down) He's a racist, pure and simple. (looking up and saying sarcastically) Are you one of those people who believes racism is a thing of the past?

C: The world, including this campus, is still filled with stories of oppression, pain, and suffering. (pause) I'm sorry these stories are still being created. Every student has a right to feel welcomed and respected here.

Z: (quietly) I dreamed of a university being like that, ever since I was little. I can still remember my mother taking me downtown to walk around the public library every Saturday—it was huge. She would say that universities were full of buildings like this and, one day, I could go if I worked hard enough. I was so excited. I did work hard, and I got here. That first day started out joyfully. But, now . . . (pause)

C: Thinking of a university was exhilarating, (pause) but something went seriously wrong.

Z: (intently) I knew I was headed for a challenge coming here.

C: (pause) What do you mean by "challenge"?

Z: (ironically) I've grown up around African Americans. Looking at the brochures this school sent me, I saw nothing but White faces. I knew I would be an outsider here. I wanted to go to Hampton University in Virginia. It's a private school for African Americans . . . but this is a public school, and the tuition is much lower. I could see the look in my mom's eyes as we sat at the kitchen table looking at my acceptance to both schools. She didn't have to say anything; there was pride, but there was . . . (tearing up)

C: (softly) You needed . . . (pause) your family needed to put the cost first?

Z: Yeah . . . this place gave me the most money, and I really needed to go where the money was. (long pause where he is looking at his hands thoughtfully) I knew it wouldn't be easy, but I was not prepared for that fool Henry. When I first saw this skinny White kid moving into my room I honestly just couldn't believe it. I assumed I'd be rooming with a brother. Henry couldn't even look at me when I greeted him. He had these two heavy suitcases. They looked too heavy for him; he's such a small guy. I came over and took one and swung it up on his bed. I wasted my breath all weekend being friendly.

C: You tried to help him and reach out, but he didn't understand the meaning of what you were trying to do even though you did obvious things like helping with his suitcase.

Z: (softly) He barely answered me when I asked him questions, but I was cool with it. I told myself he was shy and kept trying. On Sunday morning, I saw he was reading the Bible. Being a regular churchgoer myself, I tried to talk with him about Jesus, but (pause) he was so rigid. I'm a Baptist Christian, and he doesn't think I'm going to Heaven. He thinks only people from his church hear the true word of

God and the rest of us are damned. (pause, intently) Jesus saved us all, (pause) but I was respectful and just waved as I left. I prayed hard on it in church, but I just couldn't feel any spiritual connection to him. (sounding sad and looking up at C)

C: You still sound sad about it. You kept reaching out to him. You tried hard to build the foundation for a friendship, but there was nothing to build. Even talking about God left the room feeling empty of understanding.

Z: (sadly) Yeah, it was an empty room, and I felt lonely so I wrote letters to my sister and brothers to help myself. It all slammed down fast the next day. I came back in the room, just out of the shower, and saw him hiding his money underneath his mattress. This really hurt. The day before I was talking about God with him and telling him how much Jesus was in my life, yet he thought I'd steal. I was so mad I walked out as soon as I could grab my clothes.

C: You tried to share your soul with him, but he rejected the chance to know you, holding on fast to his false image of you.

Z: I didn't come back until 5 p.m. By then I was chilled out and tried another time to get through to him. (pause) The Prophet Zechariah had a tough job trying to get the tribe of Israelites back to the word of God after they lost their way, so I thought surely I had the strength to move this one White boy. I decided not to tell him what I saw. I just invited him to go to dinner. He said no, not even looking up from the computer screen. At that moment, I wanted to just move out to an apartment, but I had no money for it. (shaking his head) That would have settled the whole thing. But, I had to stay.

C: Lack of money kept you feeling trapped.

Z: (sadly) Yeah, you got it. No matter what I said, he couldn't hear me. I was raised to speak the truth to my neighbor—that's from Zechariah 8:16. It's a tough standard to always speak the truth, but I work at it every day. I told the truth to the disciplinary board, but they were deaf to me. Henry is the problem. (emphatically) Not me. Henry. I have never been, and never will be, violent. I am following the path of Jesus Christ.

C: Violence has no place in your story. It's crafted around a deep and sincere faith in God. I can hear your strength of purpose.

Z: (intently) Thank you for understanding that violence thing is a lie. (pause) I decided I would forgive my roommate for his ignorance but stay away from him. I set out to find some brothers. It's a big place; they had to be somewhere.

C: You were looking for friends so you persisted, like you persist with your schoolwork. You recognized Henry wasn't going to be a friend, and you moved on.

Z: (smiling) I was lucky and found a group of brothers hanging out in the cafeteria. They've been on campus since last year—they got it right away what was happening.

C: I can see that it was a relief to find people who understood what was happening.

Z: (emphatically) They understood how bad I felt inside and reached out to help. It started with a party to welcome me. Then, we went to the mall, and they helped me buy some posters to hang in my room. I didn't bring anything but my clothes. Henry had signs of himself everywhere. The posters would rid my side of its emptiness. They would make ME visible.

C: That's a really important theme to your life, wanting to be visible, to leave your mark.

Z: (intently) I was tired of feeling ignored, like the space only belonged to him and he could decide if I was in the room or not. To be fair, he never told me to get out.

C: The way he talked to you and the way he didn't talk to you seemed to say, "Stay out."

Z: (softly) You got it. (smiling) Well, we hung the posters when I knew Henry would be in class. (seriously) I'll give him that . . . (pause) he does go to class.

C: He's really hurt you, but you still try to be fair to him. (pause) In the report, Henry accused you of hanging up posters to scare him out of the room.

Z: (seriously) They were pictures of my heroes—Reverend Martin Luther King, W. E. B. Du Bois, and Malcolm X. I figured that seeing those posters every day would remind me to be strong and fight injustice in my own way. I did wonder how Henry would react to my being visible—I pretended to read when he walked in. He just flipped out and ran. I started laughing . . . (pause) it was just so crazy, but I'm not laughing now.

C: I'm puzzled by why you were watching for his reaction. (pause) Did you expect something to go wrong?

Z: (sheepishly) I knew that Henry was ignorant and wouldn't understand the words on the posters. (long pause)

C: What did they say?

Z: (intently) Dr. King was saying, "A man can't ride your back unless it's bent."

C: What did that mean to you?

Z: (seriously) That my roommate, or other people, could insult me and try to degrade me but they couldn't succeed if I didn't let them.

C: That's a powerful message. It's self-affirming that others can't take away who you are. (long pause) What about the others?

Z: (forcefully) W. E. B. Du Bois was saying, "Now is the accepted time, not tomorrow, not some more convenient season . . ."

C: What does that mean to you?

Z: (calmly) I needed to study and listen hard and learn as much as I could as this was my time. (pause) It was the Malcolm X poster I was watching his face about. I knew, in my heart, that I should have bought a different one. (looking up sheepishly) Malcolm X has his fist raised high. (pause) I guess my anger took over and left the forgiveness behind when I picked that poster.

C: He rejected you in a lot of painful ways. You had a right to feel angry. But, the quote?

Z: (intently) "Be peaceful, be courteous, obey the law, respect everyone; but if someone puts his hand on you, send him to the cemetery."

C: Maybe it was the cemetery part that (both Z and C are chuckling here) bothered him.

Z: (serious again) Malcolm has inspired me my whole life. I regret using him that way to scare my roommate. It was just supposed to shock him for a second. It made me feel sick inside when I saw, at the hearing, that the fool's hand was actually shaking. He really is scared of me, and it hurts. I am NOT dangerous.

C: You have many parts of yourself, (pause) but they all seem to contain religious convictions and following the path of peace, not violence. Your interactions with Henry have contained anger because his constructions of you involve preconceived, negative beliefs. Henry knows very little of the Zechariah you have striven to be all your life. That particular poster carried with it potent negative meaning for Henry because his constructions of African Americans appeared full of fear.

Z: (angrily) He thinks we're all violent. To me, the poster meant I should continue living my life as my family taught me to live it and, if someone tried to keep me down, I should fight for my right to live as I choose; I was strong, not invisible.

C: The report said something about you threatening to kill him.

Z: (sadly) That night, the brothers and I were going out for dinner, but I realized I left my wallet, so I rushed back upstairs and found Henry looking through my chest of drawers. I told him off the same way I've told my younger brothers and sister anytime they got into my stuff. (angrily) Sure, I used a strong voice and strong words, but he had no business going through my drawers. My lawyer pointed that out at the hearing.

C: Did he say what he was up to?

Z: (snorting) He was looking for guns and drugs. He decided my friends and I were some kind of gang, and he was looking for evidence to bring to the police.

C: Did he admit this at the hearing?

Z: (angrily) Yes, but he justified it saying he didn't know where else I could get the money to be here. I got a presidential scholarship, and I got it from my hard work all through school. I earned my way here, and it wasn't easy. I'm buying all my books used so I can send part of my scholarship money home to help my sick grandmother. (looking down tearfully)

C: Even though you worked hard to get here and need the money, you send some of it to those you love.

Z: (firmly) My family would do anything for me, and I would do anything for them.

C: When you began talking of your family, love was shining in your face, but then the light went out.

Z: (sadly) His accusation that I didn't earn my way really hurt. My family didn't have much. But, what we have we earned through hard work. My mother works two jobs, one cleaning an apartment building during the day and one cleaning a department store at night. She comes home exhausted, but she always found time to ask me about my schoolwork. My grandmother should have retired, but we just can't afford for her to stop working. It hurts me to know she's working when her arthritis is so bad.

C: Your family story is full of self-sacrifice and love. (pause) When you talked about your grandmother's arthritis, I could see the pain in your face.

Z: (looking down) My grandmother should be seeing a doctor now. My mom says she's so worried about me that she can't sleep. She can't go to the doctor because we owe him too much money. My sister told me the emergency room was really rude to my mom last weekend, saying my grandmother wasn't an emergency case and shouldn't be there. Nobody wants to help us. Most folks just don't have the time for us or care what happens to us. We don't count to them. (firmly) I say we do count.

C: Your grandmother, such a wonderful and self-sacrificing individual, needs health care, and she's not getting it. That's an ugly theme that keeps resurfacing, that the world is treating your family like they are invisible even though they are good, hardworking people who deserve everyone's respect.

Z: (firmly) I wasn't going to be invisible at that board hearing. My lawyer told me not to say much, but I just couldn't sit there and say nothing—maybe I did yell. I have rights like everyone else. (softly) That's what the student handbook says anyway.

C: I understand why you didn't want to be invisible. How would the board be able to tell you had the righteous anger of a wrongly accused person rather than the anger of a young man who was out of control?

Z: (strongly) Shouldn't my record in my classes count for anything? This report has only one line about my good grades. Everything else is how they're judging me based on one night. Yes, I lost my cool that night and yelled my lungs out at him. Still, I never touched Henry and had no intention of ever touching him. (sadly) He claims to be a man of God, yet he lied about me. (reading from the report) "He threatened to kill me." Maybe I said those words, but he took it all wrong. How could he not get that?

C: You were both there and heard the same words, yet you each took very different meaning from them.

Z: (frustratedly) I've said those same words to my friends, my brothers, and my sister all the time. Man, why did he make such a big deal about it? I was staying out of his face. Why couldn't he stay out of mine? All they need to do is give me a new roommate. I don't need anything else. I don't need to be here.

C: I hear you, and I have to say that I agree. I have to write a report to the board about whether I think you're a danger to others or not. (Z frowns) I will be saying that you're a credit to the university and we're very lucky to have you here.

Z: (long pause) Thank you, I appreciate that.

C: I don't know what they will do in response. They might just drop their demand you come here. They might not. Would an appointment next week be useful to you?

Z: (firmly) I don't think so. But, I need this degree, so I'll come back if they insist. (pause) It has been a relief in a way to talk to you. I don't want to worry my family about this.

C: You talked a number of times of having rights like everyone else. I just want you to know that you have the same right as every other student on this campus to come here and talk about racism on this campus, the stress of worrying about your grandmother, or wanting to figure out a career for yourself after graduation. The Counseling Center is free to all students here.

Z: (calmly) I'll definitely be back if the disciplinary board tells me it's required. If they don't, (pause) I'll think about what you said and let you know. I like the idea of taking advantage of a service that's free to me, especially when at home every service comes at such a high price.

C: I'll be here if you decide to talk some more.

Constructivist Case Conceptualization of Zechariah: Symptom-Based Style

Zechariah is feeling depressed, confused, angry, and alienated as a result of negative experiences he has had at the university—particularly the discrimination and oppression he's experienced in interacting with his roommate and the university disciplinary board. He came to the university filled with excitement and hope that, in this setting, he could achieve academic success and begin his family's journey out of poverty. His self-constructions were filled with the love of his family, strong spiritual beliefs, and pride in his African American heritage. Now, he is prey to strongly contrasting emotions that flicker back and forth in his self-constructions as he attempts to adjust his dreams of university life with his perceived reality of the recent past. Zechariah is currently relating a problem-saturated narrative in a voice of rejection. Dominating his story are constructions of himself as an "other" functioning on the margins of dominant society. While his negative emotions are running painfully deep at this time, he has a contemplative voice that allows him to easily attune to alternative aspects of his experience; this voice can serve as a powerful ally within a treatment relationship. In addition, Zechariah has found positive and adaptive meaning from his religion, his family, and his academic achievements in the past. This bodes well for him being able to coconstruct a new and more life-enhancing narrative to propel him toward an adaptive future free of poverty.

Zechariah feels depressed; however, this reflects a profound change in his emotional state. His narrative of life at the university began with exhilaration at being the first member of his family to study at the university level. As a young child, his mother had started him on a future-oriented narrative in which, through educational achievement, he could enter a world filled with large buildings and books; it was to be a way out of poverty for himself and his younger siblings. Zechariah began working hard then, and continues to work hard now, on his goal of becoming well educated so that he will be prepared to succeed financially. While poverty and racism had served as anchors dragging his family down in the past, the voice that predominated after he gained the prestigious presidential scholarship was confident and hopeful that he was finally on the road out of poverty and invisibility and that he would be able to bring his family along with him.

Zechariah became increasingly confused and disappointed as interactions with his roommate indicated they would not be "brothers" interacting within an evolving, joint subplot of academic success. Rather, Henry seemed determined to coconstruct a stable narrative that was replete with negative racial stereotypes and that actively ignored counternarratives presented by Zechariah's open and friendly behavior and deeply expressed religious beliefs. None of his efforts, such as his reaching out for Henry's suitcase, inviting him to meals, and engaging him in discussions of scriptures, showed any sign of influencing Henry's constructions of their relationship; Zechariah's narrative voice began to lack confidence. Throughout his life, Zechariah has been forced to interact within oppressive relationships, and these have always left him with feelings of invisibility and marginalization. He had hoped to escape into a more uplifting reality when he went off to school. Given a free choice, he would have gone to Hampton University, a private school for African Americans; in this context he would have had the freedom to be surrounded by people of his own race and to not have "race" made an issue throughout his day-to-day life. However, poverty served to deny him this context of acceptance. He needed to put his personal desires aside and take the larger scholarship offered by a primarily White, public university. Here, he expected to continue facing invisibility as an African American. However, in a voice of dejection, he relates that he hadn't expected to face it in his new home—his dormitory room; in past constructions, home had always been a context of acceptance and love.

Zechariah struggled with deep feelings of anger and disappointment as Henry continued to reject his overtures of friendship. He had assumed his interactions as a roommate would fit the pattern of his interactions as a loving son, grandson, and older brother. Thus, what he was experiencing was doubly upsetting to him. However, Zechariah tried to find meaning from these experiences that could hold angry constructions at bay. He explained Henry's behavior to himself through a lens of forgiveness and kindness; he assumed that Henry's behavior was the result of shyness or poor social skills. Zechariah had wanted to be like his namesake, the Prophet Zechariah, and lead Henry out of ignorance and into friendship. Such a self-construction became untenable once Henry's behavior deteriorated from subtly rejecting to overtly insulting. The day Henry hid money underneath his mattress and seemed, from Zechariah's perspective, to be degrading his spiritual beliefs was the day that a plot of oppression and racism seemed fully formed between them; Zechariah's constructions of their relationship now came through only with voices of anger and disappointment.

However, Zechariah did not want to passively accept a stable story dominated by these negative emotions. He sought out other African American students, hoping that in finding support for his past constructions of pride in his African American heritage, acts of racism would stop dominating his university constructions. When Zechariah was able to share his feelings of anger and disappointment with these students, they reciprocated with their own stories of racism on campus; Zechariah's sense of invisibility as an individual was lessened. They actively sought to help Zechariah regain his feelings of hope and optimism. They helped him purchase, and hang in his dorm room, posters with inspirational messages from W. E. B. Du Bois, Malcolm X, and the Reverend Martin Luther King. The meaning Zechariah drew from this experience was of loyalty from his friends and strength and persistence from strong African American heroes who had faced their own oppression head-on. In addition, the posters served to make him feel visible in his room and to have a sense of ownership of it; his experienced value as a human being increased. However, a voice of anger continued to exert some influence on Zechariah, and he chose a poster of Malcolm X that was intended to disturb Henry.

Zechariah was satisfied with the changes his posters brought to the dorm room, but this mood quickly shifted back to anger once he experienced the poisonous construction Henry drew from all of them. Ignorant of African American culture, and perhaps with a determination to maintain a stable sense of reality for himself, Henry appeared to draw meaning from these posters that reinforced and deepened his negative stereotypes of African Americans. Within this reality, the posters represented threats to his safety, and he became highly fearful of Zechariah. Henry then took actions that seemed justified to him—he searched through Zechariah's belongings in search of illegal drugs and weapons. Zechariah caught Henry in the act. Responding in the justifiable anger of the moment, Zechariah threatened Henry using the same strong language and nonverbal behavior that he had often used before in dealing with his own friends and siblings. However, having grown up in an extremely restricted religious community and seeming to have no positive constructions of African Americans, Henry took this outburst of anger as representing a serious intent to harm him; he reported Zechariah to the disciplinary board. Poverty continued to exert a powerful influence on the plot of this story. With more money, Zechariah could have moved out of the dorm room. However, he was trapped by his straitened circumstances within a stable and hostile reality with Henry.

The themes of poverty and racism once again dominated Zechariah's narratives of himself, his family, and the world; the voice of discouragement predominated within his storytelling.

Zechariah's constructions of reality were dominated by feelings of fear as he faced the disciplinary board. He feared that his grandmother's health was in serious jeopardy, as money she needed for medicine was being spent on his defense. He was also fearful that his dream of a future free from poverty would end if he was expelled from the university. While his family emphasized spirituality and loving relationships as more important than worldly goods, Zechariah was deeply conscious of the benefits affluence could bring in terms of access to higher-quality medical care, housing, and educational resources for his family. This made the personal sacrifice of having to suppress his anger and accommodate to the disciplinary board's view of reality one he was willing to try and make. However, the harshness of the setting and the behavior of his roommate and the board members served to make the plot seem stacked against him. Based on Zechariah's story, it appears as if his roommate's White privilege did carry weight at the university, as most roommate disputes are settled at the residence hall level. This same privilege may have been in Henry's favor at the hearing. Despite his fears, Zechariah made some attempts to defend his view of reality, and this may have made some positive impact as, while the board seemed supportive of Henry, Zechariah was mandated into treatment rather than expelled.

Zechariah attended his appointment at the Counseling Center feeling very alienated by his referral for anger management. Despite this, Zechariah has within him a voice of rationality that allows him to easily become aware of possibilities for more positive meaning construction. At this time, Zechariah's life narrative as an African American, freshman male is heterogeneous and full of conflicting positive and negative emotions. He has segmented his university experiences in a manner that highlights themes of invisibility and racism; past experiences, since childhood, have supported the strength of these themes in his meaning construction. However, he has shown significant resilience in building narratives that are future-oriented, hope-enhancing, and filled with themes of family love and religious conviction, despite the often desperate financial circumstances in which he and his family find themselves. Zechariah doesn't need anger management. However, he might profit from support in navigating the prejudices and stereotypes of others who might serve as barriers to his educational success. His willingness to consider appointments at the

Counseling Center as a resource open to all students, rather than as a place he is mandated to go, may provide a window of opportunity for him to profit from treatment at this time. While a coconstructed treatment narrative may still contain racist or oppressive segments within it, the meanings that he draws from them would hopefully no longer be destructive to his continued pursuit of achieving a bachelor's degree, supporting his siblings in attending a university and using the money he makes as a university graduate to help his family out of poverty. The disciplinary board holds a lot of power over Zechariah. The treatment relationship might be a powerful tool for removing this barrier to Zechariah's achievement of his life-enhancing goals.

Constructivist Treatment Plan: Symptom-Based Style

Treatment Plan Overview. Zechariah was sent to the Counseling Center for help with anger management. He does not need help in this regard as he has a deep well of positive emotions, adaptive thoughts, and behaviors that he has drawn on in continuing to construct his life story as a successful student. However, the Counseling Center and the treatment relationship might be a resource that he could use, without negative impact to his family, for support in being successful within an environment where he has experienced oppression for his lack of financial resources and his African American heritage. These goals will be offered to Zechariah within a collaborative framework, and if they represent what is meaningful to him, they will be worked on simultaneously. The plan follows the *problem format.*

PROBLEM: Zechariah has developed a problem-saturated narrative based on negative interactions he had with his roommate and the university disciplinary board.

LONG-TERM GOAL 1: Zechariah will explore the reality he could construct within the treatment setting as an emotionally supportive context for processing any confusing, stressful, or offensive experiences he has as he relates to others at the university.

Short-Term Goals

1. Zechariah will use his relationship with the clinician to find counterexamples to experiences he finds oppressive on a day-to-day basis at the university.

2. Zechariah will use his relationship with the clinician to consider what meaning he could draw from his university experiences that might prove of value to him as he helps his siblings move toward academic success.

LONG-TERM GOAL 2: Zechariah will reach out to form deeper relationships with other students and faculty who are White, to help him develop counternarratives to feeling invisible when relating to individuals from the dominant, White culture.

Short-Term Goals

1. Zechariah will look for opportunities to have conversations with professors after class and during office hours to establish his visibility as their student and to create meaningful interchanges that deepen their relationship with him.

2. Zechariah will ask questions and respond to faculty questions during class to establish for the other students the reality that he is a well-prepared and articulate young man who is visible and deserving of their respect.

3. Zechariah will learn about the educational, vocational, and personal resources that are available to him as a student at the university that might support his life-enhancing goals.

Practice Case for Student Conceptualization: Integrating the Domain of Violence

It is time to do a constructivist analysis of Josephina. There are many domains of complexity that might provide insights into her behavior. You're asked to integrate the Domain of Violence into your constructivist conceptualization and treatment plan.

Information Received From Brief Intake

Josephina is a 17-year-old, Mexican American mother; she was born in the United States. She has been married to Roberto, a 25-year-old Mexican male, for 13 months; they met 3 months before their marriage. He is a distant relative who had just emigrated, illegally, from Mexico. They have a son, Carlos, who is 16 months old. The family has been living in a small home in a rural area for the past year. They moved to this area from New Mexico, where Josephina's father owns a small store, due to the promise of agricultural work. Both Josephina and Roberto had worked picking a variety of crops on a local farm until Carlos was born. At this point, Josephina stayed home to care for him. Josephina was referred for treatment by Child Protective Services (CPS) following her physical abuse of Carlos. Roberto suddenly left the family and has not yet been heard from since CPS began its investigation 2 weeks ago. At this time, Carlos is in foster care.

During a brief mental status exam, Josephina showed signs of significant depression and anxiety although there were no indications of suicidal or homicidal ideation or severe psychopathology. Josephina became completely overcome as the clinician reviewed the limits of confidentiality and said that CPS would be expecting regular reports on her progress in treatment to determine when and if it was safe to return Carlos to her care. CPS selected Josephina's clinician; she had no say in the matter.

Interview With Josephina (J)
From a Constructivist Perspective

C: Welcome to my office. (pause) As you know, your CPS caseworker thinks that you need help with your parenting skills. (long pause) I would appreciate it if you would tell me about yourself and what you consider it important for us to talk about. (J is looking down and clutching something hanging from her neck) I see that something important is hanging from your neck.

J: (looking up and down quickly, softly) Yes, it is important.

C: (long pause) Can you tell me what meaning it holds for you?

J: (whispering) It helps to protect me. (tearing up) You will think I'm bad like those other people do.

C: What people?

J: (hopelessly) Those people at CPS who say how dangerous I am to my son. But this rosary brings me close to the Virgin, Guadalupe—I need to be a mother like her. I pray to her every day asking for help.

C: Your Catholic faith is very important to you. (she nods) Can you tell me how the Virgin is helping you?

J: (tears are flowing down her face, whispering) I am praying to her, but since I've been condemned as a child abuser, I haven't felt her presence.

C: "Child abuser." (pause) Those are harsh words.

J: (anxiously) It's my duty to be a good mother. I do try, but Carlos cries and cries no matter how tired I am. (pause) He doesn't want to stop. Carlos was a small baby, and the doctor explained that this is why he cries so much. I don't really understand it exactly because my little cousins didn't cry so much. (very anxiously) The doctors and nurses were very cold and rude to me, so I was afraid to ask them any more questions.

C: You want to understand why Carlos seems so difficult to take care of, but you feel alone in figuring it out.

J: (deadpan) His crying makes Roberto very angry because he needs his sleep after working hard all day. Roberto told me only a terrible mother could make her son so unhappy.

C: Your face looks very pale and sad as you say this. (long pause)

J: (painfully) I was just remembering . . . (pause, deadpan) Never mind; it isn't important.

C: I can see in your face that it is important. (long pause) Could you tell me?

J: (whispering) Roberto hits me for being a bad mother and making his son cry.

C: You make him cry?

J: Roberto thinks a good mother keeps her son happy, so it's my fault that Carlos cries. (desperately) I always tried hard to get Carlos to sleep before Roberto came home, but (sadly) Roberto drinks after work and then makes so much noise he always wakes Carlos up. I tried so many things that didn't work. (whispering) A few weeks ago, my hairbrush was close by. I thought it couldn't hurt Carlos if I just took my hairbrush and struck him lightly on his feet—just as a sign of my disapproval, not to hurt him. His eyes went very wide, and he quieted down quickly. I thought it was a safe way to handle him.

C: How often did you strike him?

J: (whispering) At first, just at night to keep him quiet if Roberto was drunk. But then last week I noticed Carlos was beginning to look like Roberto, especially when his face got red from crying. (deadpan)

I knew I would have to be strict, or he would grow to be a bad man like his father.

C: Since Carlos looked like Roberto, you feared he might hurt others, like his father hurt you, if you didn't raise him properly. (pause) Is a mother supposed to be strict?

J: (emphatically) No, my mother was loving—and the Virgin was too. (whispering) I am so ashamed. (pause) But, I was desperate. I did try to ask the doctor once what to do, but he was in a big hurry, and he said Carlos was just teething. (pause) He had no time to help me; others were waiting.

C: You realized you needed help. You asked the doctor, but he didn't give you as much help as you needed. (J is crying) Did you try reaching out to your parents for advice?

J: (sadly) I did try once to call my mother when I first came back from the hospital. I was so tired, and Carlos seemed to do nothing but cry. My father answered the phone and asked so coldly what I wanted . . . I tried to explain that I didn't know what to do. He hung up saying, "Go ask your husband." But I can't ask him. He would just get mad.

C: What about another relative?

J: (listlessly) I know my godmother would help, but she doesn't have a phone. I wrote her a letter, but it was so hard to write down what was happening. She misunderstood me. She just wrote back saying my parents really miss me and if I can just act like a good woman they will forgive me. (sadly) They won't forgive. They will hear about me being a child abuser, and that will be the end.

C: The end? What does that mean?

J: (sadly) They will be done with me. I've really hurt Carlos. My father would be so angry. What kind of a mother hurts her child? (J is staring blindly ahead)

C: You look lost. (she nods) Has there been a time when you were not lost and people weren't calling you a child abuser?

J: (whispering) The day of my *quinceañera*, last year—that was my last day as a good person. (long pause) I was so excited. All my teachers noticed me smiling. I worked hard in school but was always quiet. I tried so hard to be a humble and sweet girl like my mother. But, on that day, I couldn't keep my mind on my schoolwork. I kept thinking about all the food I helped my mother prepare and all the relatives who were coming to see me.

C: You were feeling excited. What did you think of yourself?

J: (calmly) I was a good girl. I know that. I always helped my mother and any relatives who needed me. I helped a lot of my cousins with their schoolwork. I wanted to be just like my mother, but . . . (long pause)

C: But . . . (pause)

J: (softly) I wanted to be as warm and kind as her. I learned all of her special recipes. But, ever since I was very little, I was interested in healing. We had a female healer, a *curandera*, in our town who everyone used instead of the doctors at the hospital who were very cold and disrespectful to us. (smiling) Whenever anyone in the family was sick, she would come with candles and a special cross she would put over the head of the sick person. She would use herbs to brew special medicine and pray to God with special invocations. (earnestly) I wanted to be like her. I felt like God had chosen me to be a healer, but I also wanted to go on to medical school to learn everything else I could. I wouldn't have been like the doctors at the hospital. (her voice like a thread) I would have treated my people with respect like the *curandera*. I would have known her healing, and . . . (sobbing into her hands while still clutching her rosary)

C: (long pause) That rosary must have tremendous meaning for you. Your knuckles are white from your painful grip on it.

J: (softly) It is the special rosary I got at my *quinceañera*. I use it to pray to God and call out to Guadalupe to help me.

C: Before your *quinceañera* you had images of yourself as a good woman like your mother—kind, caring—and you were going to take this caring even further to become a *curandera* and help your people when they were sick. (pause) How did God choose you?

J: (confidently) I could feel it. When I was with the *curandera*, she would look me in the eyes, and I felt a strong pulse coming into me. I would dream of being a healer that night. This was God's message to me. I worked so hard in school to try to make it come true. But instead, I . . . (looks desperately at C)

C: Pain is overwhelming you. (she nods) You feel you had a destiny that you and your family would have been proud of, one in which you would help your people. The self you see now you define as a bad woman. That self doesn't make sense to me because I have heard your deep commitment to helping others.

J: (painfully, choking) Quick, so quick, everything changed. (pause) While the priest was blessing me, I knelt on a pillow with my name on it. My godmother knew of my dream to be a healer, and she had embroidered my name and special symbols she had created herself to give more power to my dreams. As I knelt there, with this rosary on for the first time, I was surrounded by God and the love of my family. (softly) My father changed my shoes to show the family I was now a woman. He had tears in his eyes, tears of pride. (pause) He looked like a thundercloud as he said goodbye after I married Roberto. All pride was gone.

C: Quickly, so quickly, things changed. (long pause) How did it happen?

J: (in a tight, high-pitched voice) I think the party went to my head. I had nothing to drink, but I felt giddy with all the attention I got. I was wearing a tiara in my hair, a fancy necklace, and earrings to go with the beautiful gown my mother had sewn for me. (pause, sadly) I sound so selfish.

C: It was a very important day full of meaning. It made sense to be excited.

J: (intently) My father was supposed to lead me in a dance, but some children spilled punch all over him. He was laughing and saying he must change when Roberto strode over, took my hand, and said he would dance with me. I was so surprised he wanted to dance with me. He was a cousin from Mexico who had just arrived in the USA. My father had a letter from his father that he was coming, and so of course he was invited to my party. He was so tall and so attractive. (long pause) My hand tingled in his. At the end of the dance, he whispered in my ear to meet him outside the house. (long pause, painfully) I said no, but he just laughed.

C: Why did he laugh?

J: (sadly) He could tell what kind of a woman I was. (pause, intently) I really just thought about a romantic walk outside and (pause) maybe a kiss goodnight. I have some friends at school who date. I knew dating wasn't for me, but their stories excited me.

C: You knew you shouldn't go on a date, but he danced with you at your *quinceañera*. He was family, so you believed he was a good man.

J: (intently) I did think that. My father let him take my hand. I just assumed he was good.

C: What would your father have said if he heard Roberto whispering to you?

J: (emphatically) He would have sent him out of the house. He would've been angry. I knew it was a little bit wrong, but I never expected . . . (long pause, whispering) It is all my fault. I shouldn't have let it happen.

C: What was your fault?

J: (long pause, tearfully) I had sex with Roberto like a bad woman.

C: You look confused. (she nods and looks blankly, long pause) What happened?

J: (fearfully) I got scared right away. Roberto smelled of alcohol. I knew he was older than me and would be offered a drink, but I had never seen a man drunk before. I tried to pull away from him, but he was much stronger. I can't . . . (wracked with sobs)

C: It is very traumatic for you to remember this.

J: I was supposed to be pure until I married. On that first night of being a woman, I lost my chastity. (pause) I have no excuse for my immoral behavior.

C: Roberto was so much older than you. He had been a man for years. He should have known better. He should have treated you with respect.

J: (long pause) Now that you say that . . . yes, he should have listened to me. I told him I wanted to go back in the house as soon as I smelled the alcohol, but he ignored this and my trying to push him away. He pulled my clothes up. (long pause, woefully) It is still my fault.

C: The meaning that comes through for me is different. This was your special night and your first night as a woman. You didn't have experience making adult decisions. You made a mistake by trusting your honor to a relative you didn't know well.

J: (sincerely) He looked so handsome I assumed he was good.

C: A young woman mistake. (long pause) Did you tell your family what happened?

J: (desperately) How could I? I would have taken away all their pride in me. It happened anyway, but at least they had 3 more months to love me.

C: What happened when they found out?

J: (whispering) They were deeply ashamed. My father is a gentle man, but he struck me. He had never done it before. Then, he left the house for a few days. When he came back, he would not talk to me. My mother prayed with me every day. Then, the letter came from Roberto's father in Mexico; my father had written him about me. They both agreed that we must marry. Roberto did not want to, but it was that or return to Mexico. He only had a counterfeit work visa, and my father knew that. (J is weeping)

C: Your pain is so intense—the meaning of the events so destructive—that you stopped viewing yourself as a good person, even though you have done so many good things.

J: (softly) I don't seem like such a wicked person when I hear my story from your lips. But, nothing can change the evil of what I have done to my son.

C: The good is still in you, despite the mistakes you have made. You did hurt Carlos; the injuries were serious.

J: (sadly) I know. I am ashamed that I let things go that way.

C: Under the law you did abuse him. Yet, you are a young mother, whose husband beats her, whose family lives far away, whose young son needs a lot of care. This is a reality where many things can go wrong.

J: (sadly) I will keep praying.

C: Your deep faith and your prayers to the Virgin are all important starting points. But, an important part of your story is your deep attachment to family. You need other people to help you with being a good mother. If your father knew that you did not consent to have sex with Roberto, if he knew that Roberto beats you, might he change his view of how you fit in his family? (long pause) Might he at least forgive you enough to take you back home where your family can help you with Carlos?

J: (anxiously) I don't know. I would be afraid to ask. What if he says no? (long pause) I don't know how to start, but I want my son back home. I want to be his mother.

C: Would you like to come back tomorrow and talk more about this?

J: (softly) I will keep praying, (pause) and yes, I will come back tomorrow.

Exercises for Developing a Case Conceptualization of Josephina

Exercise 1 (4-page maximum)

GOAL: To verify that you have a clear understanding of constructivist theory.

STYLE: An integrative essay addressing Parts A–C.

NEED HELP?   Review this chapter (pages 290–298).

A. Develop a concise overview of the assumptions of constructivist theory (the theory's hypotheses about key dimensions in understanding clients; think abstractly, broadly).

B. Develop a thorough description of how each of these assumptions is used to understand a client's narrative (for each assumption provide specific examples).

C. Describe the role of the clinician in coconstructing a life-enhancing narrative with the client (consultant, doctor, educator, helper; treatment approach; technique examples).

Exercise 2 (5-page maximum)

GOAL: To aid the application of constructivist theory to Josephina.

STYLE: A separate sentence outline for each section, A–E.

NEED HELP?   Review this chapter (pages 290–298).

   A. Create a list of Josephina's weaknesses (concerns, issues, problems, symptoms, skill deficits, treatment barriers).

   B. Create a list of Josephina's strengths (strong points, positive features, successes, skills, factors facilitating change).

   C. Write a brief synopsis for each of Josephina's main life stories.

   1. For each synopsis, illustrate each component of the narrative including the setting (where), the characterization (who), the plot (what), the themes (why), the goals (purpose) of the narrative, and the voice in which the story is told.

   2. For each synopsis, highlight areas of the story that are confusing, incomplete, problematical, and/or tied to negative emotion.

   a. Discuss how this might be related to one or more of Josephina's weaknesses

   b. What types of deconstruction of the story might be valuable to aid Josephina in developing more adaptive meaning from these troubling experiences?

   3. For each synopsis, highlight areas of the story that are complete, tied to positive emotions, and/or related to positive meaning construction.

   a. Discuss how this might be related to one or more of Josephina's strengths.

   b. What type of further attention to, or elaboration of, these positive aspects of her story might open up possibilities for new interpersonal meanings within the development of a life-enhancing narrative?

   D. Discuss how problem saturated Josephina's life narrative is at this time considering her storied self, her relationships to others, her view of her situation/past trauma, any negative emotions, any maladaptive goals, and her level of rigidity/difficulty in accommodating and integrating new experiences into her ongoing narrative.

   E. Discuss how resilient Josephina's life narrative is at this time considering her storied self, her relationships to others, her view of her situation/positive experiences, any positive emotions, any adaptive goals, and her level of flexibility/ease in accommodating and integrating new experiences into her ongoing narrative.

Exercise 3 (5-page maximum)

GOAL: To develop an understanding of Josephina, her family, and her situation using the Domain of Violence.

STYLE: A separate sentence outline for each section, A–D.

NEED HELP?   Refer to Chapter 2 (pages 84–91).

A. Assess the risk factors for engaging in violence and the protective factors discouraging violence that are currently in place for Josephina, considering:

1. The *internal* factors within her such as her ability to control impulses, regulate emotions, set limits on her own behavior, engage in reflective problem solving, and understand the emotions and behaviors of others.

2. Josephina's *long-term* social network and environment during her childhood and whether they supported or constrained violence such as the existence of any traumatic, ambivalent, or nonexistent emotional bonds; any positive emotional bonds; any family violence; any level of family toleration for violence as a problem-solving strategy; a positive or negative school or neighborhood experience; and religious influences.

3. The *current* environmental supports or constraints on violence from family relationships, peer relationships, educational attainment, vocation, current neighborhood, and current religious beliefs.

4. Any *immediate* eliciting or triggering factors that might serve to justify and/or make a violent or prosocial response more likely such as presence or absence of a weapon, level of alcohol or drug use, level of frustration/anger, and encouragement or discouragement of violence from others.

5. Josephina's worldview including a consideration of how generalized or circumscribed a role violence plays in it and whether Josephina is currently generating/promoting violence or generating/promoting prosocial behavior.

B. Assess Josephina's and Carlos's safety at this time and if and how safety could be enhanced in both the immediate and the longer term including a careful consideration of the *characteristics* of both Josephina and Roberto as perpetrators of violence.

    C. Assess the overall psychological and physical impact of violence on Josephina and others, whether there are more forces supporting violence or supporting nonviolence, and the prognosis for Josephina living a life free of violence at this time.

    D. Assess whether your past experiences with violence, your stereotypes of Josephina's violent lifestyle, or biases embedded in your treatment approach might lead to negative bias, marginalization of Josephina's point of view, or an increase in danger to her or Carlos and consider what you might do to modify your approach to increase the likelihood of a positive outcome (be thoughtful and detailed).

Exercise 4 (7-page maximum)

GOAL: Integrate your knowledge of Josephina gained from constructivist theory and violence issues into an in-depth conceptualization of Josephina (who she is and why she does what she does).

STYLE: An integrated essay consisting of a premise, supportive details, and conclusions following a carefully planned organizational style.

NEED HELP?   Review Chapter 1 (pages 7–28) and Chapter 2 (pages 84–91).

STEP 1: Consider what style you could use for organizing your constructivist understanding of Josephina that (a) would support you in providing a comprehensive and clear understanding of her story and how life enhancing it is and (b) would support language she might find persuasive as a mandated referral for child abuse.

STEP 2: Develop your concise premise (overview, preliminary or explanatory statements, proposition, thesis statement, theory-driven introduction, hypotheses, summary, concluding causal statements) that explains Josephina's story as a wife and new mother who has lost a sense of who she is. If you're having trouble with Step 2, remember it should be an integration of the key ideas of Exercises 2 and 3 that (a) provides a basis for Josephina's long-term goals, (b) is grounded in constructivist theory and is sensitive to issues of violence, and (c) highlights the strengths Josephina brings to constructivist treatment.

STEP 3: Develop your supporting material (detailed case analysis of strengths and weaknesses, supplying data to support an introductory premise) from a constructivist perspective that integrates within each paragraph a deep understanding of Josephina whose storied self includes being both a victim and a perpetrator of violence. If you are having trouble with Step 3, consider the information you'll need to include in order to (a) support the development of short-term goals, (b) be grounded in a constructivist perspective and sensitive to violence issues, and (c) integrate an understanding of the strengths Josephina brings to the coconstruction of a new and coherent storied self.

STEP 4: Develop your conclusions and broad treatment recommendations including (a) Josephina's overall level of functioning, (b) anything facilitating or serving as a barrier to her constructing a more life-enhancing narrative at this time, and (c) her basic needs in the construction of a life-enhancing narrative, being careful to consider what you said in Part D of Exercise 3 (be concise and general).

Exercise 5 (4-page maximum)

GOAL: To develop an individualized, theory-driven action plan for Josephina that considers her strengths and is sensitive to issues of violence.

STYLE: A sentence outline consisting of long- and short-term goals.

NEED HELP?   Review Chapter 1 (pages 8–28).

STEP 1: Develop your treatment plan overview, being careful to consider what you said in Part D of Exercise 3 to try and prevent any negative bias to your treatment plan.

STEP 2: Develop long-term (major, large, ambitious, comprehensive, broad) goals that *ideally* Josephina would reach by the termination of treatment that would create an adaptive narrative for herself and Carlos free of violence. If you are having trouble with Step 2, reread your premise and support topic sentences for ideas to transform into goals to deconstruct or reconstruct Josephina's stories (use the *style* of Exercise 4).

STEP 3: Develop short-term (small, brief, encapsulated, specific, measurable) goals that Josephina and you could expect to see accomplished within a few weeks to chart Josephina's progress in integrating new experiences into her prior stories of herself, instill hope for change, and plan time-effective treatment sessions. If you are having trouble with Step 3, reread your support paragraphs looking for goals that (a) might help her in the deconstruction and then reconstruction of her storied self and that are sensitive to violence issues, (b) would enhance factors facilitating or decrease barriers to her parenting effectively at this time, (c) utilize her strengths in developing new adaptive meaning from her life stories whenever possible, and (d) are individualized to her situation as being both a victim and a perpetrator of violence rather than generic.

Exercise 6

GOAL: To critique constructivist treatment and the case of Josephina.

STYLE: Answer Questions A–E in essay form or discuss them in a group format.

A. What are the strengths and weaknesses of constructivist treatment for Josephina (a young mother cut off from extended family who is both a victim and a perpetrator of violence)?

B. Discuss the pros and cons of using family systems treatment with Josephina and her family of origin. Comparing this approach to your constructivist one, which do you believe has the most utility for helping Josephina at this moment, considering the facts of this case? How and in what way would it alter your decision if you entered Josephina's story when she first recognized she was pregnant?

C. What role does Josephina's Mexican American heritage play in her current situation? Discuss in detail how it might be adding risk factors for violence and/or protective factors that support a nonviolent outcome.

D. You have an ethical responsibility as a mandated reporter to do your utmost to ensure Carlos's safety, and you do not have a parallel responsibility to Josephina. Considering this, discuss how safe Carlos would be, in the short run, if you used constructivist treatment with his mother. Do the risks increase or decrease in the long run, and why or why not? How might you tailor your treatment plan to assess safety issues, session by session, within a constructivist framework?

E. What would be your personal challenges in providing effective treatment to someone who has abused an infant? Do the facts of Josephina's case change these challenges in any way? Is there anything about this case that might make it difficult for you considering her gender, Mexican American heritage, and religious background?

Recommended Resources

American Psychological Association (Producer) & Neimeyer, R. (Trainer). (n.d.). *Constructivist therapy: Part of the Systems of Psychotherapy Video Series* [Motion picture, #4310704]. (Available from the American Psychological Association, 750 First Street, NE, Washington, DC 20002–4242)

Neimeyer, R. A. (2000). Frameworks for psychotherapy. In R. A. Neimeyer & J. D. Raskin (Eds.), *Constructions of disorder: Meaning-making* (pp. 207–242.) Washington, DC: American Psychological Association.

Neimeyer, R. A. (2004, February 15). *Constructivist psychotherapies.* Retrieved April 13, 2008, from the Internet Encyclopaedia of Personal Construct Psychology Web site at http://www.pcp-net.org/encyclopaedia/const-psther.html?new_sess=1

Society for Constructivism in the Human Sciences. (2008) http://constructing worlds.googlepages.com/?popup=1

Ten

Transtheoretical Case Conceptualizations and Treatment Plans

Introduction to Transtheoretical Theory

Jake is a 25-year-old White male. He is married to Jennifer, who is a 24-year-old White female. They have one son, Jamie, age 6. The family lives in a small Midwestern city in a blue-collar neighborhood. Jake earns his living driving a truck for a large food distribution company. Because he gets paid a bonus for "getting there fast," he frequently drives for several days at a time without sleeping. His wife is a homemaker. They have no contact with extended family members and no friendship network. Jamie has been removed from the home for the last week because of a report of child physical abuse. Jake's participation in treatment has been required by the court system as a prerequisite to Child Protective Services (CPS) returning Jamie to his home. CPS will be making weekly home visits to monitor the home environment.

You are a proponent of the Transtheoretical Model, a systematically eclectic approach developed through research on the change process (Prochaska & DiClemente, 1984, 1986). Will Jake change to get his son back home? The answer is not a simple yes or no, as you view change as an ongoing process rather than a static state. In addition, you believe that

Jake will be most motivated to change something that he himself views as a problem. Thus, although Jake may not be ready to modify his violent behavior immediately (a change from the court's viewpoint), he may be ready to think about his behavior and what it means in his life (a stage in the process of changing). The following summary of the Transtheoretical Model is drawn from the work of Pro-change Behavior Systems (2008), Prochaska (2005), Prochaska and DiClemente (1984, 1986), and Prochaska and Norcross (2009).

How could you define what Jake needs to change? The Transtheoretical Model posits that there are five equally valid *levels of change* at which Jake could define, perceive, or understand each of his problems: symptom/situational (Level 1), maladaptive cognitions (Level 2), current interpersonal conflicts (Level 3), family/systems conflicts (Level 4), and intrapersonal conflicts (Level 5). All behavioral models of treatment intervene at Level 1. All cognitive models intervene at Level 2. All interpersonal models intervene at Level 3. All family systems models intervene at Level 4. Constructivist, dynamic, emotion-focused, and feminist treatment are examples of intrapsychic/intrapersonal Level 5 interventions. Although defining his problems at any of these levels is legitimate, as the problem definition moves from symptom/situational toward intrapersonal conflicts, Jake will be less and less aware of the causes of his problems, the antecedents of these problems will be deeper and deeper in his past history, and the length of treatment needed to resolve these problems will become longer and longer. The Transtheoretical Model both respects the value of the diverse set of theoretical perspectives available for guiding treatment and provides a set of guidelines for choosing among these perspectives to maximize the likelihood that Jake will both attend (versus drop out of treatment) and change (versus just show up).

Jake may define his problems at only one level of change; however, the levels of change are distinct only on theoretical grounds. Jake is always thinking, feeling, and being influenced by his past history and present relationships, and thus his symptoms and life problems occur in an interrelated, multilevel context. For example, Jake has been referred to treatment because of his abusive behavior toward his son. On the symptom/situational level, he may be likely to lose control in situations in which he feels angry or threatened, and this tendency to lose control may be increased if he is drinking or unable to perceive negative consequences to his acting out. At the maladaptive cognitions level, Jake may think, in hearing a request, "I can never be safe if someone has power over me." At the current interpersonal conflicts level, Jake may be struggling with issues of control in his relationship with his wife that are accentuated by any attempts at "control" from others.

When Jake was growing up, he witnessed his father beating his mother, and he was abused by both his parents. Thus, at the family systems level, Jake considers violence a natural part of family life. At the intrapersonal level, Jake now feels helpless, out of control, and fearful unless he is in a position of domination over others. His experiences of pleasure and self-esteem are all tied to his ability to exert his will over others. Only in these situations does he feel he is acting like a man. When a spouse or another adult tries to develop a give-and-take relationship with Jake, he may react with violence because of unconscious and profound fears of dependence. From a transtheoretical perspective, it is legitimate to view Jake's problem with anger at any of these five levels, and interventions on any of these levels could help him continue in the process of constructive change. If he has more than one problem, you will analyze each one at each level of change. Then, you will need to select a level or levels to use in defining each problem during treatment; Jake will be most motivated to change a problem if you define it at a level that makes sense to him.

Jake's motivation to change can be viewed as being represented by one of five possible *stages of change*. These stages reflect a sequence of increasing motivation to make a change, including Jake's attitude toward the problem behavior as well as any actions he may have taken in regard to it. If Jake is in the first stage of change for his abusive behavior, *precontemplation*, he is unaware or underaware that it is a problem and he has no intention of changing his behavior in the foreseeable future. He sees more benefits to continuing his violence than disadvantages that come from it. If Jake is in the second stage of change, *contemplation*, he is aware that a problem exists and is considering what to do about it. He is considering the pros and cons of making a change; however, he has no commitment to take action and is highly ambivalent about doing so. If he is in the third stage of change, *preparation*, Jake plans to take action to change in the next month, and he may have taken small steps to change or have unsuccessfully tried to take action to change in the past year; he might tell others of his plan to change.

If he is in the fourth stage of change, *action*, Jake is actively modifying his behavior and trying to overcome his violent tendencies. Action involves the most overt behavioral signs of change; however, Jake needs to go through the thoughtfulness of the earlier stages to be prepared to take effective action. To be in this stage, Jake must have successfully altered his violent behavior for at least one day. His changes may last for 6 months; Jake's challenge is to not slip back into violence. If Jake has reached the fifth stage of change, *maintenance,* he is working hard to prevent relapses into violent behavior and working to consolidate the effective changes that he has made. This stage lasts from 6 months to an indeterminate period of time past the initial action to change. If Jake goes beyond maintenance into *termination,* he has absolute confidence (100% self-efficacy) that he has overcome his violent tendencies, and he is experiencing no temptation to relapse. It is unusual for anyone to reach termination; most people continue to experience temptation to relapse (Prochaska, 1999).

When Jake comes into treatment, what stage of change will he likely be in for his violent behavior? The vast majority of clients (80%) come to treatment in the early stages of change and will resist a treatment plan that requires immediate action. Treatment will need to provide Jake with experiences that change his "decisional balance" so that the pros of moving to the next stage of change outweigh the cons of not doing so (Prochange Behavior Systems, 2008). Thus, for treatment to be effective, you must correctly identify which stage of change Jake is in for a problem and then design treatment goals to move him forward to the next stage of change for this problem. Jake could be at a different stage of change for each of his problems.

While you prefer Jake to progress in a linear manner through the stages of change, his progression is more likely to follow a spiral. Individuals often start a pattern of change, relapse, and then progress forward again. Each time Jake moves toward action and maintenance, he will grow stronger and more effectively committed to the change process. Jake will develop increased confidence (self-efficacy) that he can maintain change despite temptations to relapse.

What will facilitate Jake's progression in the change process? There are 10 *processes of change* that Jake uses or can potentially learn to use to be able to change. A process of change is a type of activity that Jake can use to modify thinking, behavior, or affect related to a particular problem. Research with populations both in and out of treatment suggests that successful changers have used similar processes of change. Transtheoretical theory labels these change processes as helping relationships, consciousness raising, self-liberation, self-reevaluation, counterconditioning, stimulus control, reinforcement management, dramatic relief, environmental reevaluation, and social liberation.

If Jake makes use of a helping relationship, he is being open and trusting about his problems with someone who cares. If he is involved in consciousness raising, he is increasing his information about himself and his problems. Jake's self-liberation would involve him increasing his commitment to change and believing in his own ability to do so. Self-reevaluation would involve Jake assessing how he feels and thinks about himself with respect to his problems and recognizing that adaptive replacements for violence are what he wants for himself. Counterconditioning would involve Jake in substituting alternative behaviors and cognitions for his problematic ones. Stimulus control would consist of Jake avoiding or countering stimuli that elicit his problem behaviors and increasing his exposure to cues and reinforcements that support his adaptive behavior. In reinforcement management, Jake would reward himself or be rewarded by others for making changes; in addition, the negative consequences that result from his violence would be increased. Dramatic relief would involve Jake deeply experiencing and expressing his feelings about his problems as well as the feelings that can come from potential solutions to them. In environmental reevaluation, Jake would assess how both his problems and his adaptive behaviors could affect his relationships with others and his environment. Finally, in social liberation, Jake would recognize that society is much more supportive of nonviolent than violent behavior; thus, if he changed, he would have more alternatives for how to live his life that wouldn't include social control agencies such as Child Protective Services.

Research indicates that individuals within the precontemplative, contemplative, and preparation stages of change are helped the most by insight-provoking treatment interventions, although the preparation stage can also involve small action steps. In contrast, individuals in the action and maintenance stages are most helped by action-oriented treatment interventions. Thus, you will help Jake use the processes of change that are most appropriate to help him progress forward from his current position in the change process. It may not be a smooth progression. Jake might reach an impasse through the overuse, misuse, or neglect of an important process of change. Your role will be to determine what has impeded change and then provide Jake with a strategy to resume the change process.

Role of the Clinician

Treatment is a collaborative, interpersonal endeavor. You will serve as a consultant or coach facilitating Jake's ability to initiate constructive change. The first step in treatment will be for you to teach Jake about the stages of change, processes of change, and levels of change. This educational effort will serve to empower Jake because it allows him to see himself as involved with the change process whether he is presently in precontemplation or action.

The second step in treatment will be to assess each of Jake's problems at all five levels of change. Which level will be selected? While interventions at any level of change have value for Jake, whenever possible you should help Jake change at the level at which he could change most quickly; this is often the symptom/situational level because clients' level of awareness of their problems is usually greatest at this level. If Jake can succeed in reaching maintenance at the symptom/situational level, then no further treatment will be needed. If he is most motivated to change at a different level, you will attempt to "meet Jake" at his definition of the problem unless you have a very compelling reason for not doing so. For your definition to help him change, you will need to persuade Jake that your reason is valid; you can't impose change—he must be an active participant in the process.

The third step in treatment will be to assess Jake's stage of change for each problem he is currently experiencing. A basic strategy for selecting the level of change at which to plan treatment is to be guided by the level where Jake is already furthest along in the change process. For example, if Jake is precontemplative at Levels 4 and 5, contemplative at Levels 1 and 2, and in preparation at Level 3, you will select Level 3 for intervention unless for some reason Jake is against it.

Finally, you will help Jake implement the processes of change that will help him move through the stages of change, at the level of change that has been selected for intervention for each problem. This matching is critical for a positive treatment outcome. A precontemplative Jake is in need of insight-oriented processes. If, instead, you try to engage Jake in action-oriented processes when he is precontemplative, it will disrupt the treatment alliance, and he may drop out. Before implementing new processes of change focused on his violent behavior, you will assess what, if anything, Jake currently is doing to control his violent behavior himself and what, if any, processes he has tried in the past. You will attempt to maximize Jake's self-change efforts by facilitating neglected processes, deemphasizing overused processes, correcting inappropriately used processes, and teaching new processes that may be more appropriate to Jake's stage and level of change. Jake's insights will be treated with respect, and you will actively seek out Jake's strengths to use in the treatment process. An example of how you would assess Jake's violence using the levels, stages, and processes of change is provided in Table 10.1.

There are three treatment strategies to consider using to support Jake in the change process for his violent behavior. The first is called the *shifting levels strategy*. First, you bring Jake through as many stages of change as you can at the symptom/situational level. If Jake can reach maintenance at this level, then treatment ends. If he gets stuck in the change process before reaching maintenance, you shift to the cognitive level of change and again work to bring Jake to the maintenance stage at this level. If you are successful, then treatment will end. If Jake once again becomes stuck in the change process, treatment will shift down to the interpersonal level, and so on, until Jake successfully reaches the maintenance stage for his violence.

Table 10.1	How Jake's Violence Might Be Assessed Using Levels, Stages, and Processes of Change	
Levels of Change	**Stages of Change**	**Processes of Change That Are Appropriate**
1. Symptom/situational Jake is violent.	Precontemplative	Insight-oriented[a]
2. Maladaptive cognitions Jake has violent thoughts.	Precontemplative	Insight-oriented
3. Current interpersonal Jake is in conflict with his wife and son.	Preparation	Insight- and action-oriented
4. Family/systems Jake was raised in a violent family.	Precontemplative	Insight-oriented
5. Intrapersonal Jake has a profound, unconscious fear of dependence.	Precontemplative	Insight-oriented

NOTE: a. Processes of change that promote insight include consciousness raising, dramatic relief, social liberation, and environmental reevaluation. Processes of change that promote action include reinforcement management, helping relationships, counterconditioning, and stimulus control.

A second approach is the *key level strategy*. Treatment can begin at the level of change identified by Jake and/or you as particularly relevant to the problem that is the focus of change. If Jake indicates he wants to work on his relationship with his son at the current interpersonal level, you can follow his lead and use techniques (processes of change) specialized to his stage of change at that level. However, you might disagree with Jake. Based on your assessment, you might consider interventions at the intrapersonal level to be most critical to his being successful at changing. You cannot impose work at a particular level of change on Jake. Change will not be possible at this "key" level unless you can motivate Jake to define his difficulty at this level.

A final treatment strategy is the *maximum impact strategy*. This strategy involves intervening at up to all five levels simultaneously. This approach may be appropriate in complex clinical cases in which it is evident that multiple levels are actively involved in the etiology or maintenance of a client's problem. Intervening at multiple levels will be challenging for you and is most appropriate when a client, like Jake, has complex problems that will require lengthy treatment.

Case Application: Integrating the Domain of Violence

Jake's case will now be examined in detail. There are many domains of complexity that might be relevant to his case. The Domain of Violence has been chosen to examine within a transtheoretical case conceptualization and treatment plan.

Interview With Jake (J) From a Transtheoretical Perspective

C: I understand that Ms. Newton from Child Protective Services recommended that you come here.

J: (angrily) It wasn't a recommendation. It was blackmail. I come here, or they won't consider bringing Jamie home from foster care.

C: Why did they take Jamie away?

J: (angrily) They say I'm a dangerous man.

C: You sound very angry.

J: (rigidly) This is nothing; this is calm.

C: This is what you sound like when you're calm?

J: (ironically) Sure, am I scaring you? My caseworker says I'm scary.

C: I'm sure you could scare me. But I'm not scared now. I'm curious about how you are feeling now. You sound angry to me, your face looks angry, your body looks tense, but you say you're calm.

J: (tensely) Let's talk about my son; that's why I'm here. He's scared of me. I don't want that. I was scared of my old man, and I don't want that for my kid!

C: He's important to you.

J: (furiously) OF COURSE HE'S IMPORTANT TO ME. HE IS MMMYYYY KID.

C: Are you angry with me?

J: (tensely) Not exactly but . . . Jamie freaked out last week and ran to the neighbors. They called Child Protective Services. That's why I have to talk to you.

C: He freaked out?

J: (confusedly) He was gibbering, so I hit him a few times to calm him down, but he ran right through the glass door in the kitchen to get away from me.

C: He must have been terrified. What happened?

J: (matter-of-factly) I chased him to the neighbor's house, put him on my motorcycle, and took him to the hospital. The glass from the door had cut him up. Riding my bike calmed me down. It always does. But he was still trembling. I had to drag him off my bike to get him into the emergency room. While we were waiting for the doctor, the Child Protective Services jerks showed up. I told them to leave Jamie alone. (pause) Then the weird thing happened.

C: What was that?

J: (confusedly) He went with them right away. I told him to stay with me. He went with THEM. He had this funny, kind of familiar look on his face. Riding home on my bike I remembered that it was the look on my face when I saw my old man.

C: You don't want him to look at you that way.

J: (angrily) No. I am not like my old man. I hated him. I am not him.

C: What was he like?

J: (deadpan) He wasn't even human. He hated anything that lived— people, animals, plants. He was a destroyer. He tried to destroy me, but I outsmarted him.

C: How did you do that?

J: (proudly) I lived. Trying to snuff me out was a habit with him. He couldn't do it. I was too strong for him.

C: Were you always too strong for him?

J: (tensely) When I was real little, he had the upper hand. He did me in plenty of times, and I was really scared of him. But then it all changed when I was 8. I will never forget the day it happened. I had a bad cold. I woke up screaming from some dream. I had wet the bed. I tried to clean it up before he could find out. He caught me, shoved my face into the sheets, and beat me black and blue. Then, he made me sit with the wet sheets around my head. Even a dog shouldn't be treated like that. I stopped being scared and started to plan.

C: Plan?

J: (with satisfaction) Plan how I would get even. I started that very night. He got drunk and crashed on the living room sofa. I went out in the yard, let in the dog, and put dog shit all over my dad's back.

C: What happened?

J: (half laughing) When he woke up, he shot that poor stupid dog to bits. He was wrong. That dumb dog didn't do it. *I did it.* He never even suspected.

C: How did your mom fit into this?

J: (dismissively) She was the invisible woman.

C: Invisible?

J: (dismissively) She was there but not there. She was terrified of him.

C: Why?

J: (calmly) For every beating I got, she got TWO. Periodically, after beating her up, my dad would dump her at some hospital. Later, he would get her out, and she would be real quiet for a while. He knew how to control her.

C: Control?

J: (matter-of-factly) Keep her from interfering, make her jump to it.

C: Was there anyone who tried to help you or your mom?

J: (tensely) In this world, you have to save yourself. I learned that early in life. I was 14 when I saved myself and my mom. I had finally grown to be as big as my dad. I picked my moment. He was drunk. But he still fought back. I threw him out the back door a bleeding wreck. In the morning, he was gone. He never came back.

C: You were finally safe. He was gone.

J: (thoughtfully) Not exactly gone. He's in my head a lot.

C: What do you mean?

J: (angrily) If anything goes wrong, his voice screams abuse inside my head. Only a bike ride helps. If I gun the engine, if I really go fast, his stupid voice shuts off.

C: How long have you been hearing his voice?

J: (angrily) It seems like my whole life.

C: How do you know it's his?

J: (furiously) It's his words, not him. I heard them day and night for 14 years. They're IMPRINTED on my brain!

C: The words are his, but the voice comes from you.

J: (furiously) OF COURSE.

C: You sound really angry with me again.

J: (glaringly, loudly) How many times do I have to say that I'm not angry?

C: I'm sorry that you feel contradicted. I just want you to know that if I make you angry, I want you to tell me about it.

J: (glaringly) Fine. Let's just get on with this.

C: What's important is to build a relationship with Jamie, where you're confident he's not scared of you. You also don't want to be like your old man.

J: (emphatically) I'm not anything like him! (pause) Jamie should like me.

C: Tell me about what you like to do with Jamie.

J: (thoughtfully) I've taken him on bike rides. I figure it is something we could do together. When he's older, I would get him a bike, and we could rev off together.

C: Does Jamie like to go with you?

J: (frustratedly) He cries. My wife says he's terrified of the bike because I go so fast. That's stupid. You need to go fast. The kid will have to get used to it.

C: You want him to enjoy it, but he gets scared of you instead.

J: (emphatically) He's scared of the bike!

C: How often do you take him out?

J: (tensely) Maybe once a week. I can't take him more because his mother interferes.

C: Your wife stops you?

J: (uncertainly) Yeah, she thinks he's too young to ride on a bike; she says he should be home learning to read.

C: Does that make sense to you?

J: (tensely) Well, she's a good mother. She pays attention to the kid. I want Jamie to survive. It's a tough world. (thoughtfully) It's good she pays attention to him. (pause) She pays attention to me, too.

C: Your wife cares for you.

J: (long pause) We're having problems, but I think it will work out.

C: What problems?

J: (angrily) It's this child abuse crap. Protective Services said if I didn't come to see you, I would have to leave the house, or Jamie would stay for at least 6 months in foster care. My wife begged me to come here or get out because she wants Jamie back as soon as possible.

C: So, you chose to come here?

J: (furiously) I had no choice! I want to keep my wife and kid. I can live with coming here. (pause) I am not going to disappear like my dad.

C: Are there any other problems in your marriage?

J: (pause, calmly) She pretty much does just what I tell her to do. She is always waiting for me to come home. She talks a lot. Like you, she always asks a lot of questions. I'm usually OK with it.

C: Your wife and son are really important to you, and you want to keep things going the way they were before the abuse report.

J: (firmly) Yeah.

C: Have you ever beaten anyone else besides your dad and Jamie?

J: (angrily) I didn't beat Jamie. I hit him a few times.

C: Have you ever hit anyone else?

J: (angrily) Sometimes people need to meet force before they back off. It's no big deal.

C: There are times when you feel you have to hit people?

J: (tensely) Nothing serious. Maybe one time a few years ago, things got out of hand at a football game, and I had to spend the weekend in jail. I have lost a few jobs because I had to get physical with some people on the job.

C: You had to?

J: (furiously) You bet I had to. Since my dad, I vowed to never let another guy slam me down ever again. No boss, no one on this earth.

C: It sounds like you have gotten into a lot of physical fights.

J: (dismissively) It's a tough world. People are always looking to see you screw up. There are a lot of people like my old man out there. But I get the drop on them fast so I don't get slammed.

C: Does your wife get a drop on you?

J: (dismissively) No, she's OK.

C: Do you ever hit her?

J: (tensely) No, I told you I am not like my dad!

C: Is there anyone out there now you need to get a drop on?

J: (angrily) CPS is full of jerks, but I can't touch them.

C: Why not?

J: (furiously) Don't act stupid. I'd lose my wife and kid.

C: You can keep yourself from slamming them to save your family?

J: (tensely) Yeah, I'm in control.

C: Am I out to get a drop on you?

J: (ironically) You seem more of a talker than a fighter.

C: You're right. (pause) It seems like the most important thing for us to talk about is what you could do besides bike riding to help Jamie like you.

J: (tensely) That's what I want.

Transtheoretical Case Conceptualization of Jake: Theme-Based Style

"To be safe I must be violent." This is Jake's code. He sees violence as his only protection against a hostile world. At the symptom/situational level, Jake has been precontemplative about whether he could be safe without violence or if he should care about the negative consequences his violent behavior brings to others; his violence has been an integral part of himself. Despite losing several jobs and spending time in jail, he has never before been motivated to reexamine his code. Recently, he has developed some openness to change at the current interpersonal level. His son is terrified of him, and he does not like this. The environmental demands from his wife Jennifer and Child Protective Services that he change his violent behavior, coupled with the failure of his only strategy for having fun with Jamie, have put him in the preparation stage of change about his father-son relationship. Jake's strengths lie in his current greater openness to improving his relationship with Jamie, his willingness to talk about how to build a positive relationship with him, his desire to maintain his marriage, and his ability to reflect on his life despite being mandated into treatment.

Can Jake feel safe for more than a moment at a time? At the symptom/situational level, whether at home, on the job, or at recreational activities, there are cues that trigger a rage response in Jake. He is aware of the immediate precipitants of his anger and violence. For example, he can state that "being pushed" at a football game can trigger an aggressive response. He is unaware, however, of how his violent behavior has terrorized Jamie. Although it may seem as if his only response to perceived threat is violence, he can at times stop and think. For example, although terrified of his own father, he was able to plan how to defend himself. In addition, within the present mandated treatment situation, he has been able to think about the impact of his losing control with a CPS worker. He has also been able to perceive that the clinician, though making him angry, is not a threat to his security. The research literature on violence suggests a priming effect of violent TV, alcohol use, and other environmental forces. Thus, it will be important to assess these and other variables to determine what helps versus hinders Jake's ability to control his aggression. Jake will need to become aware of the immediate and long-term impact of his violent discipline on his son's thoughts and behavior if he wants to improve their relationship; this might motivate him to consider change at this level.

Can Jake be safe if he listens to himself? At the maladaptive cognitions level, Jake indicates that he has a mental stream of self-talk that "screams abuse" at him whenever he makes a mistake. Like many violent individuals, he views the world as a hostile place, interpreting neutral events as aggressive. In relating to others, their behavior is interpreted through a negative lens. In his words, people are always trying to get him to "screw up" or "get the drop on him." An exception to this is his wife. He perceives her as being a good person and caring about him. He denies any hostile thoughts toward her and doesn't appear to have thoughts of interfering with or degrading her parenting as is common within battering relationships. Overall, his hostile thoughts toward coworkers and strangers serve as predisposing factors for further violent behavior.

Can Jake be safe if he interacts with people? At the interpersonal level, Jake has no close friendships with his peers. His code requires him to take an aggressive posture with others to prevent their "getting the drop" on him. This has led to physical confrontations at work and has cost him several jobs. He is presently unaware of how his violence scares others off or brings out their own hostile and/or aggressive behavior. However, there are positive signs that Jake can improve his interpersonal functioning. He may have ignored his code in interactions with his wife; he firmly denies ever responding violently to her. Within the home, he can recognize that she takes good care of him and his son and doesn't want his marriage to end. This wish may not be reciprocal. Jennifer is at least a witness to his child-abusive behavior, and he may be verbally abusive to her. Violent men who are controlling their physical aggression often continue to express their aggression verbally. There are indications that this may be occurring in Jake's home. For example, he states that Jennifer always does what he asks her to do, carefully attends to him, and begged him, rather than asked him, to follow through with the CPS recommendations so that Jamie would return home from foster care. Other forms of violence, such as spouse abuse or verbal abuse, are common correlates of child physical abuse and will need to be assessed further as rapport builds within the treatment relationship. Jake has been abusing Jamie, but he perceives himself to be working toward a good father-son relationship. He is in the preparation stage of change for his own parenting behavior. He knows what he won't do—he won't disappear as his father did—but he is currently stymied as to what he needs to do to develop a better relationship with his son; he tried to share with Jamie the bike riding that he finds so relaxing and enjoyable; however, this backfired. Through self-reevaluation, following the incident in the emergency room, Jake has realized that he has a poor relationship with his son, and he is committed to changing this so that his son will not hate him as he hated his own father. At this time he is willing to "talk" about it with the clinician. Other strengths are that he has shown an ability to observe his wife, recognize that her parenting strategies differ from his, and periodically follow her lead without resorting to violence.

Could Jake, the child, be safe at home? At the family/systems level, as Jake was maturing, the power to survive was centered on whoever could most effectively use physical force. For a long time, Jake's father threatened both Jake's and his mother's physical survival. An 8-year-old Jake moved temporarily from precontemplation into preparation and tested whether he could fight back against his father's violence. He had a small success and recognized, if he planned carefully, he could free himself from his dad's violence. His mother, the invisible person, was never involved in the major decision of who was in the family and what the family rules would be. Thus, Jake's experience taught him that to be safe in a family, you needed to be successful at using violence. The survival struggle at home shifted when Jake was 14 and big enough to seize the power firmly from his father. Jake is unaware how the violent code he learned within his family to protect himself is now serving to alienate him from the very person he most desires to connect with—his son. He is aware of his son's fear but unaware that he is reenacting the role of his own father within his new family. Although he literally kicked his father out of his life, his father's violence continues to victimize him through shaping his relationships with other people and preventing him from ever feeling "safe" in the world. Although Jake can talk about his family relationships and evaluate how he felt about them, he is precontemplative about the role of his father's victimizing behavior in his own current behavior.

How can Jake survive? At the intrapersonal level, Jake feels that he must constantly fight to survive. Unable to protect his integrity without violence, he has intimidated most of the people whom he relates to. Presently, he is struggling with the issue of how to be close to people while still being physically safe. Jake is precontemplative about how his fears for his own security have led him to behavior that blocks him from forming positive emotional attachments. This combination has led him to become in many ways just like the figure he most hates and dreads, his own father. He is precontemplative about the similarity between his current lifestyle and personality and that of his father's. His strengths lie in his clear recognition that his father's lifestyle was unacceptable and his desire to not be like him.

Must Jake remain violent? As a child, Jake had to use violence to survive. As an adult, he continues to use violence as a mechanism for feeling safe in the world. Violence has become deeply embedded in every aspect of his life, and he is unaware of how this violence is blocking his ability to relate positively to others, particularly his son. Although he is precontemplative about his need to end his violent behavior at most levels of change, he is in the preparation stage about making changes in "something" so that he can develop a more positive relationship with his son; this greater openness to change may serve as a window of opportunity for modifying Jake's code. A potential barrier to Jake's progression in the change process is that his level of dangerousness to others is not static; it fluctuates due to both situational and interpersonal factors. While Jake is precontemplative about change at the symptom/situational level, if he loses control of his anger he could lose both his marriage and custody of his son. Thus, increasing his immediate ability to control his anger, in addition to working on his father-son relationship, is critical at this time. There are several environmental pressures supporting this type of change at this time. Jake recognizes the power CPS has to keep his child from him. Jake recognizes the look of terror he brought to his son's face and doesn't want to see this look again. Jake respects his wife's mothering skills and doesn't dismiss her input out-of-hand. The clinician may be able to use these pressures and strengths to help Jake contemplate the benefits of a life free from violence.

Transtheoretical Treatment Plan: Theme-Based Style

Treatment Plan Overview. It will be difficult to assess accurately how dangerous Jake is until genuine therapeutic rapport has been developed, so close collaboration with CPS and the court system will be needed, and a *maximum impact strategy* will be used to try and decrease the risk of violence as much as possible. Goals will target the symptom/situational and current interpersonal relationships levels of change. The long-term goals will be initiated in numerical order. The short-term goals are labeled to indicate which stage of change they target and the level of change that is the focus of the intervention; this is done as a teaching tool for the reader. When two levels are worked on for the same stage of change, the short-term goals may be accomplished in an intermixed fashion. The treatment plan will follow the *problem format.*

PROBLEM: Jake's code is interfering in his developing the relationship he wants with his son.

LONG-TERM GOAL 1: Jake will consider whether he can relate safely with others without resorting to his code and if this could help him develop a closer relationship with his son.

Short-Term Goals (Precontemplation to Contemplation at the Symptom/ Situational Level of Change)

1. Jake will increase his awareness of the immediate cues/behaviors on the part of others that make him feel unsafe, and strategies for avoiding the cues that trigger him to feel unsafe will be discussed.

2. Jake will increase his awareness of what he does to inhibit his aggressive behavior, for example, with CPS workers even when the cues/behaviors for eliciting anger are present.

3. Jake will increase his awareness of the specific behaviors CPS needs to see to consider it safe to return Jamie home.

4. Jake will increase his awareness of the negative consequences to further aggressive behavior by discussing foster care with the CPS worker and how foster care would decrease his time with Jamie.

5. Other insight-focused goals will be added if needed to move Jake to the contemplation stage of change at this level.

LONG-TERM GOAL 2: Jake will consider whether another code exists for resolving interpersonal conflicts that would keep him feeling safe and in control yet help improve his relationship with Jamie.

Short-Term Goals (Contemplation to Preparation at the Symptom/Situational Level of Change)

1. Jake will observe role models (the clinician, his wife, coworkers) and increase his awareness of how they display or respond to anger, and he will discuss the pros and cons of using these strategies himself.

2. Jake will read about nonviolent strategies for responding to provocation such as passive, aggressive, assertive, and humorous strategies and consider if any of these strategies might help him stay safe yet not decrease Jamie's or other people's safety.

3 Jake will consider the situations he finds provocative within the treatment relationship and discuss which of the strategies he read about earlier might be effective in responding to these provocative situations without jeopardizing his safety or that of the clinician.

4. Jake will observe the behavior of his wife, his coworkers, and CPS staff and, during the treatment session, discuss his perceptions of their behavior as positive, neutral, and/or negative and consider how accurate his perceptions are in distinguishing truly provocative from not provocative behaviors.

5. Jake will read about relaxation strategies and consider whether any of these might be valuable to him to use when he is beginning to become angry yet recognizes that his safety is not jeopardized.

6. Jake will keep a record of his level of anger before and after he engages in his typical media experiences, including television, video games, and music, and determine when these media calm his anger or intensify it.

7. Jake will consider using the media that decrease his anger to calm himself down at times he recognizes the cues he is getting angry. If he finds some of his media experiences intensify his anger, he will consider avoiding them and finding instead media that help him feel calm and relaxed.

8. Other insight-focused goals will be developed if needed to move Jake into the preparation stage of change.

LONG-TERM GOAL 3: Jake will consider whether he can feel safe and more emotionally connected to his son and other people when interacting with them using a different code of conduct.

Short-Term Goals (Preparation to Action at the Symptom/Situational Level of Change)

1. Jake will have opportunities to practice responding nonaggressively, within sessions, whenever he experiences the clinician's behavior as provocative and discuss whether he felt safe.

2. Jake will ask the clinician to verbalize the motivation behind the "provocative" behavior to explore whether it was truly provocative or whether it was "neutral" or "positive," and Jake will consider how he feels during this discussion.

3. Jake will develop a list of behaviors during the week, involving his current interpersonal relationships, that he finds provocative and then explore with the clinician whether these behaviors might or might not have been intended to be provocative.

4. Jake will select a strategy that he would like to use for relaxing when he recognizes that he is getting angry yet the behavior of the other person is not intended to be provocative.

5. Jake will have opportunities to use these strategies within sessions with the clinician, after being warned that intentional provocation will occur, and consider afterward whether he felt safe and in control.

6. Jake will become aware of what cues/behaviors his wife uses that make him feel good in his interactions with her and consider using them himself.

7. Jake will become aware of the cues/behaviors his wife uses when interacting with Jamie that appear to make Jamie comfortable/happy and consider using them with Jamie himself.

8. Jake will become aware of what cues/behaviors occur within the treatment setting that make him feel good and consider using them himself in his interactions with Jamie and others.

9. Jake will read about effective communication strategies and consider which of these he might be able to use while still maintaining his own safety and that of others.

10. Other insight-focused goals or small action steps will be developed if needed to move Jake into the action stage at the symptom/situational level of change.

Short-Term Goals (Preparation to Action at the Current Interpersonal Level of Change)

1. Jake will practice, within role-plays with the clinician and then with his wife in conjoint sessions, how to use positive cues/behaviors to make others feel good.

2. Jake will discuss how he would like his father-son relationship to change, first in role-plays with the clinician and then in conjoint sessions with his wife where he assertively asks for her advice.

3. Jake will first practice with the clinician and then implement with his wife asking what behaviors of his she perceives as having pushed Jamie away from him, using relaxation strategies if he feels provoked by her opinions.

4. Jake will practice effective communication skills to use with Jamie and his wife first within role-plays with the clinician, then with his wife in conjoint sessions, and finally with his son and Jennifer in family sessions with the clinician pointing out any positive or negative consequences of these new behaviors within the session.

5. Other insight-focused goals and small action steps will be developed if needed to move Jake into the action stage of change at the current interpersonal level.

LONG-TERM GOAL 4: Jake will help his son, and others, feel safe and emotionally secure through responding to them using his new code of nonviolence even when he is angry.

Short-Term Goals (Action to Maintenance at the Symptom/Situational Level)

1. Jake will learn to identify whenever his aggressive urges become strong and ride his motorcycle to calm down if possible.

2. Jake will use other relaxation strategies to calm down whenever the situation does not allow for riding his bike yet he feels his anger rising.

3. Jake will avoid his son when he knows that his anger level is high in order to keep his son from feeling unsafe.

4. Jake will avoid his wife and other people when he knows that his anger level is high in order to keep them from feeling unsafe.

5. Jake will read a book on parenting and decide if anything in the book might be valuable to try within his interactions with his son.

Short-Term Goals (Action to Maintenance at the Current Interpersonal Level of Change)

1. Jake will assertively ask Jamie what he likes to play and explain to his son how riding a motorcycle is play to him.

2. Jake will practice how to play with Jamie within role-plays with the clinician.

3. Jake will generate a list, during the treatment session, of things Jamie might do, during a play session, that could frustrate him or make him angry and consider how he could calm himself down in this situation.

4. Jake will invite his son to play, will notice if his son looks afraid, and if he does, will assertively remove himself from the play session if he becomes angry about this.

5. Jake and his wife will talk about the parenting strategies they want to use with their son, and the clinician will help them compromise when needed. Jake will calm himself down if he finds the need to compromise makes him angry.

6. Jake will practice assertive strategies for disagreeing with his wife over parenting decisions first within role-plays with the clinician and then at home with his wife using his relaxation strategies, or avoidance strategies, whenever necessary to keep his anger under control.

7. Jake will use his new communication and anger management strategies outside of his family life, reminding himself that these strategies can keep Child Protective Services, and the police, from becoming involved in his life again.

8. Other action-focused goals will be added if Jake has not progressed securely to the maintenance stage of change at the current interpersonal level.

Practice Case for Student Conceptualization: Integrating the Domain of Race and Ethnicity

It is time to do a transtheoretical analysis of Kayla. There are many domains of complexity that might provide insights into her behavior. You are asked to integrate the Domain of Race and Ethnicity into your case conceptualization and treatment plan.

Information Received From Brief Intake

Kayla is a 24-year-old single Lakota Sioux. She is a journalist working for Greenpeace. She travels worldwide in helping this organization publicize environmental concerns. She is presently on a leave of absence because of ill health. While on leave, she is living in an apartment in Watertown, Massachusetts (a suburban area of Boston). Kayla has referred herself for treatment, within a private practice setting, because of an overall feeling of malaise and perceived lack of direction to her life. Kayla initiated contact at this time because of situational constraints. Although she has been feeling the need for help for the last year, only in the past week did she return to the United States and find herself in a position to seek help.

During a brief mental status exam, Kayla showed signs of depression and anxiety but not at clinical levels. There were also no signs of suicidal or homicidal ideation or severe psychopathology. Kayla was open to help from whichever clinician at your practice had the first opening. Greenpeace will be sending her abroad in 6 months.

Interview With Kayla (K)
From a Transtheoretical Perspective

C: Kayla, I understand that you are coming in because you are dissatisfied with the general direction your life is taking. Can you tell me more?

K: (forlornly) Well, I have been working for Greenpeace since I graduated from college. It's a great organization, and they are doing work that is full of personal meaning for me. Yet, I feel an emptiness . . . a disconnectedness from everyone. I can't really put my finger on it. I have always felt this way. I thought that this malaise would go away once I had my degree and some important work to do.

C: You've had this feeling your whole life?

K: (forlornly) My family was poor. I never had the same clothes as everyone else. The community was small. Everyone seemed to belong to the Protestant Church but us. I was a Sioux; they were all White. I was always bullied or rejected by the other kids.

C: It sounds like a traumatic experience.

K: (thoughtfully) It was. No one, not even my family, seemed to understand what I was going through until my high school guidance counselor came along. He realized I needed help and sent me to treatment for the first time.

C: First?

K: (calmly) I have been in treatment three times now. Each time it really helped me through a life crisis. However, they never really made me feel like I was part of this world. I always continued to feel that I was disconnected.

C: What parts of the treatment helped you?

K: (reminiscently) In my first round, I learned about relaxation. I had never really known what it was like to relax before. I was always tense, on edge, ready to fight for little or no reason at all. The sessions taught me a lot of relaxation exercises and anger control strategies. This clinician was great, one of the few people I have ever felt connected to. I still use many of those relaxation exercises. If anyone at work or at home gets me going, I just give myself a personal time-out. I haven't had any real fight with anyone since I was about 15 years old.

C: No fights?

K: (satisfied) None that really count. I might get a little irritated with someone, but if it goes beyond that, I immediately withdraw and pull myself back together.

C: Does anyone think he or she fights with you?

K: (confusedly) No, and that's the ironic thing. This lack of fighting is actually what my old boyfriend said blew up our relationship.

C: The relationship is over?

K: (sadly) Yes. We both worked for Greenpeace and had been living together for 2 years. He said that I was too emotionally cold—a ghost, there but not there.

C: Do you know what he meant by that?

K: (pause, hesitantly) He complained that I was only there for the good times. There were a lot of times when he felt that I wasn't around when he needed me.

C: Were you around?

K: (adamantly) I was physically there. But when he was in trouble I felt overwhelmed with anger at whoever or whatever was causing the problem and I needed to cool off before I exploded. He saw my coping as pulling back from him and not allowing myself to care deeply about anything. (long pause) He left Greenpeace.

C: Is there anybody new in your life?

K: (dejectedly) No, I don't think I can handle a relationship right now. I have never been really good at closeness. In college, I only had what my last clinician called superficial friends. We would joke around a lot together, but we made it a point to always keep our emotions under control.

C: What did you feel was beneficial about that treatment experience?

K: (calmly) It really helped me understand interpersonal relationships better. I realized that I had been purposefully distancing myself from others because I was afraid of rejection. I had never experienced any close attachments—I hadn't thought I needed them. But, I came to see how very lonely and isolated I was. I learned how to reach out to people and developed my first real friendships.

C: What changed so that your friendships became real rather than superficial?

K: (reflectively) I had been living a kind of hermit-like existence. I was always holed away in my room writing for hours on end. I loved to write, and I was doing something I thought was meaningful. Yet, I was getting a lot of feedback from my English professors that my work seemed to be lacking a sense of purpose. At first, I thought that my professors were rejecting my work because I was a Sioux. But treatment helped me realize that I was rejecting criticism because I was afraid I didn't have enough talent to write. I forced myself to express these fears to my professors and the students in class and began to feel closer to them. They seemed to show a greater interest in me too; I made real friends.

C: By being vulnerable you established more connections.

K: (calmly) Yes, and I know I still need more connections, but it can be so hard. You guys always seem to know what I'm thinking and what I need to learn next; it's easier to relate to you than anyone else.

C: What about your family?

K: (calmly, sighing) I am a reject to them. (pause) I am not exaggerating. I had to give up completely on them. I did try. In fact, that was a major focus of my second treatment experience. I was really struggling with trying to understand my identity. My high school teachers had helped me get to college on a full scholarship. I wanted so much to be there, but my family was against it. They saw it as my rejecting my Sioux background and completely cut me off for a while.

C: How did that feel?

K: (sadly) I felt traumatized at first that I had lost my family. But in treatment, I realized that nothing had changed that much. I have really always been an outcast in my family. I had always tried to develop a balance between what they wanted for me and what I wanted so that they would accept me. My clinician encouraged me to learn about the Lakota Sioux and draw on my heritage for strength. I read up on everything I could. I began to realize that my confusion over family rituals was because my parents themselves were confused.

C: What do you mean?

K: (seriously) Many Indians in my grandparents' generation were forced away from traditional Indian life, sent to boarding schools, punished for speaking their native language. How could they have taught my parents how to be Sioux? I think my parents are trying to recapture their traditional ways, but they don't know exactly how to do it except to hate outsiders. I approached my mother about this. (pause) I told her I was trying to understand, (pause) but she just walked away from me.

C: You felt rejected. You were trying to understand, and she walked away.

K: (confusedly) I always seem to repel them. (pause) I have become more of an American than an Indian in some ways, but I did learn things maybe they don't even know by reading about the Sioux. After graduation, I picked Greenpeace because it values the land; it was the right amount of connectedness for me.

C: Connectedness is important to you.

K: (emphatically) My family and our people value nature and the environment. My family always talked of how much the land means, although they left our Sioux reservation after my grandmother died and bought our tree farm in Maine. I always worked so hard on the farm, to show I cared too; my dad never seemed to notice.

C: What do you mean?

K: The only attention I got was from the teachers at school. When I applied to go to college, my family accused me of betraying our people and continuing to prefer the company of outsiders. I tried to explain my love for writing to them, but they just said I was turning my back on them. I tried to show them that the land was important to me, using my writing. (pause) I thought they would see my work with Greenpeace as important since its aim is to protect the earth.

C: How do they see it?

K: (dully) It's just following a White path, not a Sioux one. Coming to school was my dream, but I should have put my family's welfare first. I did try to do this during my childhood, but I couldn't fit in. (anxiously) I had to find a place to fit in. After my first semester at the university, my uncle came after me. He said to come home now and listen or to never come home again.

C: Does your uncle speak for everyone?

K: (resignedly) Yes, he always has. My parents, my older sisters, and my uncle and aunt had a meeting to discuss my final insult to the family and decided I was out.

C: Everyone but you was there.

K: (resignedly) Even when I was at home, I was never included.

C: (long pause) Unconnected. (pause) Were you always that way?

K: (resignedly) Spiritually, yes. Physically, we were together every day after school, and every weekend, we would go into the woods together and plant or harvest trees. We also have to cut wood to use in heating our house. If our wood supply gets low, we get cold. Self-sufficiency is very important to my family. We hunt in the woods, although my mother does go to the supermarket for some things. We use as little of the White community services as we can.

C: You and your family have life skills that few people have these days.

K: (sadly) Yes, I was also the best wood chopper in the family, but no one ever said anything. I know it's not the Sioux way to expect thanks for your work, but I just wanted some sign I counted for something; I only got disapproval.

C: Disapproval hurts.

K: (sadly) It did hurt. Whatever I did, starting as far back as I can remember, they accused me of preferring outsiders—particularly Whites. Calling me a White is the biggest insult they can come up with.

C: Why?

K: (intently) My parents hate all of our White neighbors. I think there was some trouble about my parents getting the tree farm, but I don't know what. My parents just always told me that we can't trust Whites and I should stay away from them.

C: Do your mother and father always agree?

K: (intently) Yes. My father makes all the decisions. My mother goes along. Sometimes, I feel she doesn't really agree, and I beg her to take my side. She won't. Later, she will say, "Learn silence, or you will always be in conflict."

C: What does learning silence mean?

K: She meant if I stuck up for myself I would always be in conflict. If I was quiet, there would be no conflict.

C: Does your mother always follow the rule to be silent?

K: She does now, but I think there was a time when she wasn't so silent. I have vague memories of my parents fighting when I was really young. After one big fight, I was sent to live with my aunt and uncle for 3 years. My sisters stayed at home. No one would tell me why I'd been sent away. The first night I was with them, I overheard talk about my mother being in a hospital. I got really scared and ran into the room. They were very angry about this and wouldn't discuss it with me. I wondered if my mom was sent to the hospital for not being silent.

C: How did it feel to be sent away and cut off from your parents and sisters?

K: (anxiously) I was scared and confused, but I knew that if I wanted to get home I had to be silent. I was sent home when it was time for kindergarten. When I got there, they acted as if I had never left. I had so many questions. Why was I sent away and not my sisters; why had my mother gone to the hospital; why had I been sent back; why was it so important to always be silent?

C: Some people are very curious, and some people are not.

K: (emphatically) I'm the curious kind. I loved kindergarten from the very first day because the teachers always encouraged and answered my questions. My parents have always believed I respected my teachers more than them.

C: Did you?

K: (resignedly) I just fit in there better. I wasn't alone like I was at home. I tried to understand what it meant to be a Sioux, but family holidays never made sense. It's weird; my parents say particular days are special to the Sioux, but they don't seem to do anything on these days but smoke and drink. They always get mad if I ask any questions. I'm not sure they know what they're celebrating.

C: They didn't respond to direct questions, but did they ever try to teach you about the holidays through stories or some other teaching ritual?

K: (disgustedly) They seemed to just sit in a circle and get drunk.

C: Who are they?

K: (disgruntledly) My parents, my older sisters, my uncle, and his wife. They just sit in silence. That is what they always said they wanted from me.

C: How much do they drink?

K: (calmly) Until they pass out. But, they aren't alcoholics if that's what you think.

C: There are a lot of families where alcohol is a big problem.

K: (insistently) I don't drink, and I don't think my family drinks too much except maybe on the holidays.

C: I can feel your loyalty to your family. Do you think I assume they are drunks because they are Sioux? Or, do you feel they don't have a drinking problem?

K: (sadly) I don't drink at all. (pause) Maybe, alcohol is part of their problems.

C: Do you think turning to school is what separated you from the family?

K: (emphatically) It made it worse, but my father has always treated me differently from my sisters. He is a quiet man, but he does talk to them. To me, he has always been cold. I can still remember as a small child following him around trying to help him on the farm. He never acknowledged that I was there. I loved school because it's not wrong to talk there.

C: At home you felt different and alone; at school you felt connected, but it took you even further from your parents.

K: (intently) I was always speaking up despite my mother's injunctions to be silent and my father's obvious disapproval. I wanted to fit in like my sisters, but I couldn't be quiet like them. I always had this independent spirit. I fit in with my coworkers at Greenpeace. I am Sioux. I am not trying to make money to collect things; I'm trying to help keep the earth healthy for everyone. I have caused a lot of conflict in my family; a good Sioux should not do that, but it's not against our culture to try and find your own path. (pause) It's not. (long pause, dejectedly) Sometimes I think that if my work at Greenpeace was really of value, my father would talk to me. Why would I feel so empty if my work had meaning?

C: Since you feel empty, you think your work can't be important?

K: (determinedly) I wrote a particularly good article for Greenpeace—I received a literary award for it; I sent it to my parents. Shouldn't they respect how I'm trying to protect the earth? Maybe they thought I sent the article to impress them; that is not our way. (bright red, embarrassedly) I think about this a lot. I have this voice in my head that seems to drone on, "Do something important and your parents will want you back." There are times when I feel like I must be going nuts because I have arguments with this voice; I say, "I am doing something important; they just don't want me." Just talking about it aloud makes me feel tired and worn out.

C: The voice demands a level of perfection and importance that no one can reach.

K: (adamantly) Yes, and it never stops.

C: And your response to the voice is to feel tired?

K: (resignedly) It's so hard to keep trying, but I know that I must.

C: Why?

K: (forcefully) I guess I have always been a fighter—even as a kid. It is one of those things about me that made me so visible to my parents when they wanted me to be invisible; I can't give up. You guys sometimes play this game suggesting I can stop trying, but really you always demand that I be strong.

C: Are we perfectionistic too?

K: (calmly, smiling) Yes, you won't let me be weak and fall apart. That's one thing that keeps me coming back to treatment; you like it when I'm strong.

C: You have told me a lot about yourself, and you seem to have a lot of insight into your own difficulties. Why do you need to be here?

K: (thoughtfully) I'm feeling stuck and lost. I can't seem to move on with my life. This has happened before, and treatment has really helped me regain direction.

C: What do you think is behind this stuckness and lost feeling?

K: (nervously) I can't say right now. (pause) You're the first one I've told everything to. The others didn't ask about as many things. I've kept some secrets from them. I answered any questions they asked, but if they didn't ask . . . (long pause)

C: What secrets?

K: (nervously) I didn't mention to any of them that I had been in treatment before. I thought they would think I was a real loser needing treatment repeatedly.

C: You're a loser if you need treatment more than once?

K: (emphatically) Even coming once was a sign of weakness—I'm supposed to be self-sufficient.

C: So, you feel that coming to treatment is turning your back on your traditions?

K: (emphatically) Absolutely! I'm supposed to be self-sufficient and silent and do what I'm told. Instead, I'm living with outsiders, needing help, asking questions, and ignoring my family's wishes!

C: Is everyone who isn't a Sioux an outsider?

K: (resignedly) The clinicians, the teachers, my friends, and my coworkers.

C: What would other American Indians outside your family think about you?

K: (confusedly) I don't know. There are other Indians involved politically, like those in the American Indian movement. I could contact them, (pause) but I have found a place I fit—it's Greenpeace. It's where I want to be connected. But . . . (long pause)

C: But even from these most connected people you have kept secrets. (K nods) What important secret is left to tell me today?

K: (nervously) I must handle it alone.

C: What will happen if I know this secret?

K: (panicky) I will lose the little connection that I have. You will kick me out.

C: Kicking you out is not an option.

K: (panicky) You would! You would realize what an outcast I am.

C: I know a lot about you now, and I respect you. It's hard for me to imagine that I could learn something now that would lead me to cast you out.

K: (confusedly) What opinion can you have of me? This is our first session!

C: There is a lot I don't know about you. But, what I do know is that you are a tremendously creative and hardworking person, a courageous person, a lonely person. Your family has rejected you, and in a way you have rejected yourself. Could you forgive yourself—for whatever the secret is—and let yourself be connected to me, your colleagues, and other people?

K: (determinedly) I want to, but I don't know if I can.

C: Maybe we could work it out together, or maybe you could work it out for yourself.

K: (panicky) Am I such a loser you won't accept me for treatment?

C: You are such a winner I'm not sure I have anything to offer you that you don't already know you need to do for yourself.

K: (panicky) I can't be alone anymore.

C: You need to be connected to others. But, do you need me to help you?

K: (pleadingly) Yes, I told you I can't handle things anymore on my own.

C: You are not alone. I'm here. Let's each do something important for next week. I will think about what you've shared with me so far and have some ideas to suggest to you. You think about your secret and think about your strengths. Come up with some ideas to suggest to me about your plan of action to end this empty feeling.

K: (calmly) I can do that.

Exercises for Developing a Case Conceptualization of Kayla

Exercise 1 (4-page maximum)

GOAL: To verify that you have a clear understanding of transtheoretical theory.

STYLE: An integrative essay addressing Parts A–C.

NEED HELP?   Review this chapter (pages 327–334).

A. Develop a concise overview of the assumptions of the Transtheoretical Model (the theory's hypotheses about key dimensions in understanding how clients change; think broadly, abstractly).

B. Develop a thorough description of how each of these assumptions is used to understand a client's progression through the change process (for each assumption provide specific examples).

C. Describe the role of the clinician in helping the client change (consultant, doctor, educator, helper; treatment approach; technique examples).

Exercise 2 (5-page maximum)

GOAL: To aid application of the transtheoretical theory to Kayla.

STYLE: A separate sentence outline for each section, A–C.

NEED HELP?   Review this chapter (pages 327–334).

A. Create a list of Kayla's problems (concerns, weaknesses, problems, symptoms, skill deficits, treatment barriers) and for each discuss:

1. At what level of change is Kayla defining the problem?

2. Which stage of change is Kayla in for the problem at this level?

3. Are there any processes of change she has used to try and overcome the problem, and has this produced effective, ineffective, or mixed results? Have the processes of change she used been appropriate considering 1–2 above?

B. Create a list of Kayla's strengths (strong points, positive features, successes, skills, factors facilitating change) and for each discuss:

1. How aware is Kayla of the strength, and in what ways is it benefiting her?

2. Is Kayla using this strength in an attempt to overcome any of her problems (be specific)?

a. A strength could help her *understand* her problem at one or more levels of change.

b. A strength could be used as a *process of change* to move her through a stage of change.

c. A strength could enable her to *make effective use* of a process of change.

C. Based on Part A, what is Kayla most motivated to change at this time? For each of these discuss the following:

1. The treatment strategy you would select for each problem that will be a focus of treatment and why you chose it.

2. The specific change processes that are needed to support change on each problem, within each treatment strategy, and why you chose them.

3. Considering Part B, how might Kayla's strengths be used within your treatment strategy for each problem?

Exercise 3 (3-page maximum)

GOAL: To develop an understanding of the potential role of her Sioux heritage in Kayla's life.

STYLE: A separate sentence outline for each section, A–E.

NEED HELP?   Review Chapter 2 (pages 55–61).

A. Assess the role of Kayla's self-identified Sioux heritage in her life in terms of the strengths, resources, and power it may be bringing to her within the following spheres as appropriate: personal, family, social, educational, vocational, and political.

    B. Consider how current or historical events have influenced the Sioux people and assess if any of Kayla's current problem(s) could be a result of direct or indirect oppression or trauma, her responses to this oppression, assimilation stress, and/or a mismatch in values with the dominant society and its institutions.

    C. Assess how well Kayla is functioning at this time, including a comparison of her functioning through the lens of her Sioux heritage with that of the lens of the dominant cultural group. Consider if there are realistic constraints influencing Kayla at this time and discuss if any of her behavior within the dominant society might represent a healthy adaptation to injustice that would be supported by the Sioux community.

    D. Assess Kayla's personal worldview and the role of her Sioux heritage within it; consider if there are any culturally specific resources, treatment strategies, or helpers that she would value at this time; and consider how these might be used within your treatment plan.

    E. Assess whether any aspects of your identity and cultural conditioning or implicit bias within your treatment approach could lead to communication problems, values conflict, difficulty understanding Kayla's lifestyle or experiences, or invalidation of her strengths and consider how treatment could be made respectful of her heritage to increase the likelihood of a positive outcome (be thoughtful and detailed).

Exercise 4 (7-page maximum)

GOAL: To help you integrate your knowledge of transtheoretical theory and racial and ethnic issues into an in-depth conceptualization of Kayla (who she is and why she does what she does).

STYLE: An integrated essay consisting of a premise, supportive details, and conclusions following a carefully planned organizational style.

NEED HELP? Review Chapter 1 (pages 7–28) and Chapter 2 (pages 55–61).

STEP 1: Consider what style you could use in organizing a transtheoretical understanding of Kayla that would (a) support you in providing a comprehensive and clear understanding of where she is in the change process and what she needs to move forward toward maintenance and (b) support language Kayla might find persuasive as she struggles with her secret.

STEP 2: Develop your concise premise (overview, preliminary or explanatory statements, proposition, thesis statement, theory-driven introduction, hypotheses, summary, concluding causal statements) that explains Kayla's overall level of functioning as an individual struggling to feel connected to others and find meaning in her life. If you need help with Step 2, remember that this should be an integration of the key ideas of Exercises 2 and 3 that (a) might provide a basis for Kayla's long-term goals, (b) is grounded in a transtheoretical perspective and is sensitive to racial and ethnic issues, and (c) highlights the strengths she brings to transtheoretical treatment.

STEP 3: Develop your supporting material (detailed case analysis of strengths and weaknesses, supplying data to support an introductory premise) from a transtheoretical perspective that integrates within each paragraph a deep understanding of Kayla (a woman who has struggled her whole life to fit in). If you need help with Step 3, consider the information you'll need to include in order to (a) support the development of short-term goals, (b) be grounded in transtheoretical theory and sensitive to racial and ethnic issues, and (c) integrate an understanding of Kayla's strengths in the change process whenever possible.

STEP 4: Develop your conclusions and broad treatment recommendations including (a) Kayla's overall level of functioning, (b) anything facilitating or serving as a barrier to her reaching the maintenance stage for each of her problems at this time, and (c) her basic needs in the change process, being careful to consider what you said in Part E of Exercise 3.

Exercise 5 (4-page maximum)

GOAL: To develop an individualized, theory-driven action plan for Kayla that considers her strengths and is sensitive to her Sioux heritage.

STYLE: A sentence outline consisting of long- and short-term goals.

NEED HELP?   Review Chapter 1 (pages 8–28).

STEP 1: Develop your treatment plan overview, being careful to review what you said in Part E of Exercise 3 to try and prevent any negative bias to your treatment plan.

STEP 2: Develop long-term (major, large, ambitious) goals that *ideally* Kayla would reach by the termination of treatment, on each of the problems identified for treatment, so that at the end of treatment she would be interpersonally connected and find meaning in her life. If you are having trouble with Step 2, reread your premise and support topic sentences for ideas to transform into goals that will move Kayla through the change process on each of her identified problems (use the *style* of Exercise 4).

STEP 3: Develop short-term (small, brief, encapsulated, specific, measurable) goals that Kayla and you could expect to see accomplished within a few weeks to chart her progress in the change process for each of her problems, instill hope that she is progressing, and plan time-effective treatment sessions. If you are having trouble with Step 3, reread your support paragraphs looking for ideas to transform into goals that (a) might support her moving through the stages of change on one of her problems using insight- or action-oriented processes of change as appropriate, at the level of change at which each problem is identified, (b) would enhance factors facilitating and decrease factors inhibiting her ability to change and find meaning in her life at this time, (c) utilize strengths she has developed both in and out of treatment whenever possible, and (d) are individualized to her personal journey for meaning rather than generic.

Exercise 6

GOAL: To critique the Transtheoretical Model and the case of Kayla.

STYLE: Answer Questions A–E in essay form or discuss them in a group format.

A. What are the strengths and weaknesses of this model for helping Kayla (a successful professional with acculturation conflicts), and how will you encourage the change process without further encouraging Kayla's *dependence on treatment* to begin the change process?

B. Discuss the strengths and weaknesses of using a relational constructivist approach with Kayla considering her interpersonal problems, her quest for meaning in her life, and her contradictory narratives of being an outcast and being a successful writer.

C. Assume Kayla's secret is that she is a lesbian. Discuss in detail how knowing this might deepen and/or change your understanding of her personal and family dynamics. Discuss how this might influence or change your treatment plan.

D. What ethical dilemmas are raised if Kayla tells you that she feels closer to you than she's ever felt to anyone else and admits to having sexual fantasies involving you? Explore how this makes you feel, particularly as it relates to how attractive you find Kayla as an individual. How will you handle it if she asks you out on a date? (If you are female, assume Kayla is a lesbian; if you are male, assume she is heterosexual.)

E. To use the Transtheoretical Model, you need to be capable of using treatment frameworks and processes of change from many different theoretical orientations, and you must be comfortable with working with Kayla at the stage of change she is in. Discuss the strengths and weaknesses of you using this approach and provide specific examples to back up your points.

Recommended Resources

Allyn & Bacon Professional (Producer). (n.d.). *Part of the brief therapy for addictions hosted by Judy Lewis & Jon Carlson: Stages of Change for Addictions with John Norcross* [Motion picture, ISBN 0–205–31544–5, http://abacon.com/videos]. (Available from Pearson Education Company, 160 Gould Street, Needham Heights, MA)

Pro-change Behavior Systems. http://www.prochange.com/staff/james_prochaska

Prochaska, J. O., & Norcross, J. C. (2009). *Systems of psychotherapy: A transtheoretical analysis.* Pacific Grove, CA: Brooks/Cole.

University of Rhode Island Cancer Prevention Research Center. (2008). *Transtheoretical Model: Detailed overview of the Transtheoretical Model.* Retrieved April 8, 2009, from http://www.uri.edu/research/cprc/TTM/detailedoverview.htm

Eleven

Discussion and Extension of the Model

You have had the opportunity to practice conducting clinical work using eight different theoretical perspectives. What differs between these theories is the lens you give clients for focusing their attention during the change process. Will change happen most effectively if clients are guided to focus on the role of their behaviors (Chapter 3), their thoughts (Chapter 4), society (Chapter 5), their feelings (Chapter 6), their interpersonal style (Chapter 7), their family relationships (Chapter 8), meaning construction (Chapter 9), or motivation for change (Chapter 10)? While each of these theories provides a different lens for understanding clients, to be effective, you will need to integrate certain common factors into your work no matter which theory you use.

Although research continues to discover treatment techniques that might be most effective in working with specific clients or specific client problems, research to date has found that common factors that are independent of theoretical orientation or technique are more important in discriminating effective from ineffective clinicians and in predicting a positive or negative treatment outcome. These common factors include extratherapeutic factors (what the client brings into treatment), which account for 40% of treatment outcome; the therapeutic relationship (whether or not a warm and trusting working relationship is developed), which accounts for 30% of treatment outcome; models and techniques, which account for 15% of treatment outcome; and expectancy and hope, which account for 15% of treatment outcome (Asay & Lambert, 1999; Hubble, Duncan, & Miller, 1999). Since no one theoretical perspective provides you with the truth about the best way to help clients, you can make one of two broad choices. One choice is to use your personal style and beliefs in selecting a theoretical perspective to specialize in and then only work with clients you believe can benefit from this approach. The second choice is to select the theoretical perspective that you feel is most helpful for each client. You should recognize the implications and limitations of your choice and refer to other clinicians as appropriate.

Individualizing Treatment to Ensure Quality Care

An understanding of the complexity of human experience can be used to individualize treatment to the unique characteristics and needs of each client. Deeper and more complex conceptualizations are interesting, but they take more time to develop. Thus, although many domains of human complexity might have value for a particular client, assessing all of them would be an overwhelming, if not impossible, task.

For which clients might it be useful to increase the complexity of your clinical tools? Asay and Lambert (1999) suggest that you make the choice based on the complexity and severity of the client's presenting problems. If the presenting problems are relatively straightforward and symptomatic, then short-term treatment may be called for, and highly complex case conceptualizations and treatment plans may not be needed; research indicates that 50% of clients improve in the first 5 to 10 sessions. In contrast, if the presenting problems are severe and complex, then complex case conceptualizations and treatment plans may be needed to guide long-term treatment; at least 20% to 30% of severe clients need more than 25 sessions and are prone to relapse (Asay & Lambert, 1999).

What if you are unsure of how complex and severe a case is? If the client shows signs of having issues with (a) danger (violence, sexual abuse, suicide, homicide), (b) reality contact, and/or (c) substance abuse, assume the case will be complex. Your client may not trust you enough to allow you to assess these issues accurately in the first interview. When in doubt, assess further after you have had a chance to build more rapport. Early change is an indication that you are on the right path. It doesn't have to be a big change, but it needs to be a step in the right direction. If this isn't happening, then change what you're doing (Asay & Lambert, 1999; Hubble et al., 1999). What if you are unsure if culture or another realm of human complexity is relevant to your case at this time? Consider your clients as partners in the conceptualization endeavor and ask them. If clients say that spirituality is a guiding principle of their lives, then make spirituality a cornerstone of your treatment plan. A strong therapeutic alliance is an important common factor of effective treatment; it is the client's view of the alliance, by the third to fifth session, that is predictive of outcome. Thus, you need to respect the client's point of view, within sessions and within the treatment plan. While it does take more time to write a treatment plan that's individualized to the client, this has been found to enhance the therapeutic alliance (Bachelor & Horvath, 1999).

Case Conceptualization and Treatment Planning Over Time

Effective clinical practice does not require a clinician to develop a flawlessly accurate conceptualization and treatment plan at the beginning of treatment that is carried out unvaryingly until termination. Instead, effective treatment may involve shifting, modifying, or refining the treatment plan over time as new information about clients serves to enhance or reframe their current difficulties. Early in treatment, you must make a judgment about what domain or domains of complexity are most critical to your client at the present time. You then develop a theoretical model for understanding the client that incorporates these domains. If the client can change constructively, this may be the only time that you develop a conceptualization and treatment plan.

If barriers to progress arise in treatment, case conceptualizations and treatment plans may need to be revised. The case of Kayla, introduced in Chapter 10, will be further examined to illustrate how a case conceptualization and treatment plan can evolve over the course of treatment.

The Case of Kayla

Kayla, a 26-year-old Sioux woman, has just referred herself to a clinician with an expertise in family systems treatment. This is the fifth time Kayla has initiated treatment with a clinician. Kayla had been sexually abused by her uncle throughout her childhood and adolescent years. The abuse ended only when she left her home to attend college. Kayla has been in treatment before but never revealed the abuse. She feels she is ready now to face why she has always felt like an outcast.

The Beginning Stage of Treatment

In the first stage of treatment, you and Kayla will work together to form an effective working alliance and develop a clear view of her presenting concerns. A model for understanding Kayla (case conceptualization) will be developed so that a treatment plan can be designed and initiated.

Kayla is intelligent, verbal, and very responsive to your validating comments, and the treatment alliance seems to solidify quickly. Kayla is very articulate in describing her past dysfunctional patterns of relating to others. With support from you, she identifies two areas that she would like to address within treatment. First, she wants to resolve her feelings about her prior sexual abuse so that it no longer influences her relationships with men. Second, in pursuing her own professional goals, she has become alienated from her Sioux parents, and she would like to reconnect with them. At this time, the Domains of Sexual Abuse and Race and Ethnicity seem most relevant to integrate into a family systems perspective on Kayla.

Kayla, similar to other victims of sexual abuse, has trouble trusting other people. Thus, she intentionally keeps some important information from you. This is not unusual. Conceptualizations and treatment plans developed at the beginning of treatment may well lack some relevant information for understanding the client. This may or may not inhibit Kayla's treatment, as not everything needs to be known about her to develop an effective treatment plan.

The Middle Stage of Treatment

In the middle stage of treatment, the major goals of the treatment plan have been broken down into small steps (accomplishments, tasks, etc.), and you are helping Kayla make active progress in goal attainment.

You have developed what you consider to be an effective working relationship with Kayla. She has acquired insight into the role of her prior sexual abuse in her distrust of others, particularly men, and she is reaching out more constructively in interpersonal relationships. No progress has been made, however, on her goal of developing an emotional connection to her parents. In reviewing your case conceptualization, you wonder if, by not being a Sioux, you have been a poor liaison for a family with strong acculturation conflicts. You discuss with Kayla your idea of trying to locate a Sioux healer who might help her in the process of reconnecting with her parents instead of you. She accepts this idea, and you find a healer living in Maine, and he contacts Kayla's parents. They adamantly reject his help and indicate that Kayla is no longer their daughter. The healer then meets with Kayla on several occasions and offers further support to her if she wants it. In his opinion, something besides culture is behind the family's rejection of Kayla. She chooses to continue working on these issues with you rather than the healer. Together, you discuss the need to explore further the structure of her family in terms of its hierarchy, boundaries, and level of emotional attachment. Kayla trusts you more than she did in the beginning stage of treatment. This time, as you obtain a more detailed assessment of her family and her role in it, she reveals that she and her mother had been physically abused by her father.

You develop a deeper conceptualization integrating cultural, sexual abuse, and violence issues. Using this, you redesign your plan with the potential of danger to Kayla and her mother in mind. The first step of the plan is for Kayla to explore what her goals are for this "family reconnection." Kayla comes to recognize that the emotional connection she wants is with her mother. Kayla recontacts her mother when she knows that her father will be absent. Hesitantly, her mother agrees to one meeting.

In the family session, Kayla's mother clarifies the family struggles that ultimately led to Kayla being sexually abused when she was 4 years old. Kayla's parents married young and lived below the poverty line on a reservation. Their family structure revolved around the maternal grandmother, who was a highly respected member of the tribe and at the top of the family hierarchy. When Kayla was 1 year old, this grandmother died suddenly from cancer. The grandmother's presence had kept the family living on the reservation. Her death was instrumental in the family (mother, father, older sisters, Kayla, uncle) resettling in Maine. Their life on the reservation had been difficult. There had been no employment for Kayla's father or uncle on the reservation. Her father and uncle, now the heads of the family, quarreled with the tribal elders over the wisdom of leaving the reservation in search of work. They moved to Maine in response to advertisements for work within the tree industry. When they arrived, however, they faced active discrimination from their White neighbors, but they worked and saved; they felt trapped in Maine by economic necessity. The adults' suspicion of Whites turned into an implacable hatred when they bought a tree farm from a retiring couple amidst community action to stop the sale from being finalized; once their purchase was confirmed, they built strong boundaries between themselves and the community. They had rejected their tribe and thus had no one to turn to for support in their struggles but one another. Kayla's father and uncle turned to alcohol to dampen their feelings of frustration and anger.

As the family grew more and more isolated, the domestic violence and child abuse began. When Kayla was 4, her battered condition was noticed by community members, who reported the family to Child Protective Services (CPS). CPS insisted that Kayla be sent temporarily either to her uncle's home or to an outside foster placement. Although moving in with her uncle seemed at first to be a good solution to the intrusion of the Whites in their lives, Kayla's mother began to suspect the sexual abuse about 2 years later. It still took her another year to get her husband to agree to bringing Kayla back home. CPS did not intervene. Her mother remained silent about both the past physical abuse and the current sexual abuse because she believed that no good would come of discussing them. Kayla's mother had developed a code of silence. When she was silent, she was not beaten; if she was silent, problems could be forgotten. To survive, she felt Kayla must also develop this code.

Kayla and her mother developed a deeper connection with each other during this one session. The emotional neglect Kayla had experienced throughout her childhood was now reframed as her mother's best attempts to teach her to survive in a dangerous world. Kayla wanted further sessions with her mother and expressed fear for her mother's safety. Her mother was not afraid. She said that the domestic violence had ended when Kayla had moved away. Her mother's code of silence had been transformed into a code of loyalty. Her mother believed in the spiritual benefit of enduring hardship and living in balance. She and her husband had survived poverty, discrimination, and loneliness together. She could not come back for further sessions because she believed this would be a betrayal of her husband's trust. She felt strongly that Kayla would never be safe at home and should not return. Discussing the abuse issues had freed Kayla's mother from her torment of silence. She was able to express her love for Kayla directly and to encourage her to find a balance for herself in her new life as a writer.

As a result of this family intervention, Kayla understood her role as "outcast" or "scapegoat" in her family. She symbolized for them their rejection from White society, their poverty, and their pain. Through casting her out, they were distancing themselves from some of the trauma that had engulfed their lives. She recognized her role now and was able to reject its validity for herself as a person. It was true that White society had rejected her parents, but she had had no part in the decision to leave the reservation. CPS had crossed the family's boundaries, but this had been due to her father's physical abuse of her. Her uncle's sexual abuse of her led to a disruption of the family hierarchy because her mother had challenged her father's authority for the first time by bringing Kayla home, but again, the disruption had been a result of her uncle's actions, not Kayla's. She had developed loyalties to White teachers and White clinicians; however, this came as a response to her rejection by her own family.

When Kayla was a child, a feedback loop had developed, with family rejection leading Kayla to identify more strongly with White community members, leading to greater family rejection. In trying to meet her needs for nurturance, Kayla had unintentionally alienated herself from her cultural heritage. As an adult, Kayla's chronic emptiness was relieved when the family code of silence was broken and Kayla could be fully aware of her past traumas. Kayla became able to experience pride in herself as a Sioux professional and experience confidence in her ability to establish emotional connections with others.

The End Stage of Treatment

At the end of treatment, the clinician is helping Kayla consolidate the gains she has made and empowering her with a sense of self-efficacy for addressing any further concerns. Would it be useful at this point to proceed with a deeper case conceptualization? This could be useful in two circumstances. One circumstance would be if Kayla might be returning to treatment. A revised conceptualization could be a resource for guiding her next treatment. Is this likely? Kayla has participated in treatment on many occasions, starting when a school counselor noticed her isolation when she was 14 years old. Each time, she made effective use of treatment and continued in the process of constructive change. Once she developed the necessary skills or insights to move forward, she terminated treatment and continued the process on her own. When her self-change efforts became stymied, she reinitiated treatment. Thus, although Kayla has shown herself to be a bright and resilient individual who can learn effectively both within and outside treatment, her history suggests that she might resume treatment at some point.

A second circumstance that would justify an end-stage conceptualization would be if Kayla's treatment was being reviewed for ethical, insurance, or other professional purposes. An end-stage conceptualization could be used to support your judgments concerning the type and length of treatment that she received. The following is an end-stage premise to support Kayla's long-term treatment.

Premise

Kayla came from a Sioux family consisting of herself, her mother, her father, her two sisters, and her paternal uncle. The family was socially isolated from other tribe members as a result of geographic and economic constraints. The family members intentionally isolated themselves from their White neighbors in reaction to racism and discrimination. The family structure was chaotic. There were few boundaries between adults and children, and family subsystems were emotionally disengaged from one another. The boundaries between the family and the outside world were rigid and inflexible. Within the family, Kayla's developmental needs for nurturance and guidance were either ignored or responded to with physical, sexual, and emotional abuse. She often considered suicide. In reaching out for help to White teachers and clinicians, Kayla received support. These contacts, however, intensified her acculturation conflicts. Despite her traumatic history, Kayla developed many strengths based on her family's cultural emphasis on self-sufficiency and attunement with nature. As an adult, she is an intelligent, self-directed individual with a well-developed social conscience. This is epitomized by her success as a writer for Greenpeace. Kayla attended a total of 44 individual treatment sessions and one family session with her mother. This long-term treatment is justified based on her severe and complex history of victimization, social isolation, and cultural alienation. These factors, coupled with her family history of alcohol abuse, all placed Kayla at risk for suicide or other self-destructive behavior.

Conclusion

Human beings are complex, and our conceptualizations will of necessity consist of only part of the whole picture that is a human being. This book is only an introduction to case conceptualization and treatment planning. There are many other psychological theories, many more domains of complexity, and many more thought-provoking research articles to be mastered as you work toward developing your own personal style as an effective and competent clinician. It is a bias of this book that if you are open to new research developments, you can continue to develop your skills throughout a lifetime of clinical practice.

Red Flag Guidelines for Developing a Case Conceptualization and Treatment Plan

1. Distill the theory down to its major assumptions to ensure you grasp it.

2. Apply these assumptions to the specifics of your client.

3. Review the domain or domains of human complexity that are most relevant and distill them down to guidelines that can be applied to your client.

4. Integrate the information from Steps 2 and 3 into a case conceptualization.

5. Develop a treatment plan that clearly follows from this case conceptualization.

6. Periodically review your work to assess client progress and the appropriateness of your treatment plan.

References

Addis, M. E., & Mahalik, J. R. (2003). Men, masculinity, and the contexts of help seeking. *American Psychologist, 58,* 5–14.

Administration for Children & Families. (2006). *Summary: Child maltreatment 2006.* Retrieved August 22, 2008, from http://www.acf.hhs.gov/programs/cb/pubs/cm06/summary.htm

Albee, G. (1977, February). The Protestant ethic, sex, and psychotherapy. *American Psychologist,* 150–161.

American Civil Liberties Union. (1998, July). *ACLU factsheet: Chronology of Bottoms vs Bottoms, a lesbian mother's fight for her son.* New York: Author. Retrieved June 19, 2008, from http://www.aclu.org/news/n050797c.html

American Institute for Cognitive Therapy. (2003). Retrieved April 8, 2009, from http://www.cognitivetherapynyc.com/

American Psychiatric Association. (1994). *Diagnostic and statistical manual of mental disorders* (4th ed., text rev.). Washington, DC: Author.

American Psychiatric Association. (2000). Commission on Psychotherapy by Psychiatrists (COPP): Position statement on therapies focused on attempts to change sexual orientation (reparative or conversion therapies). *American Journal of Psychiatry, 157,* 1719–1721.

American Psychiatric Association. (2002). *Documentation of psychotherapy via psychiatrists: Resource document* [Ref. #200202]. Washington, DC: Author.

American Psychological Association. (2000a). Guidelines for psychotherapy with lesbian, gay and bisexual clients. *American Psychologist, 55,* 1440–1451.

American Psychological Association. (2000b). Guidelines on multicultural education, training, research, practice, and organizational change for psychologists. *American Psychologist, 58,* 377–402.

American Psychological Association. (2002). Criteria for practice guideline development and evaluation. *American Psychologist, 57*(12), 1048–1051.

American Psychological Association. (2006). *Answers to your questions about transgender individuals and gender identity.* Retrieved May 10, 2008, from http://www.apa.org/topics/transgender.html

American Psychological Association. (2007). Recordkeeping guidelines. *American Psychologist, 62*(9), 993–1004.

American Psychological Association, Commission on Violence and Youth. (1993). *Violence & youth: Psychology's response* (Vol. 1) Washington, DC: American Psychological Association.

American Psychological Association, Committee on Lesbian and Gay Concerns. (1991). *American Psychological Association policy statements on lesbian and gay issues.* Washington, DC: American Psychological Association.

American Psychological Association, Joint Task Force. (2006, July). *Summary of guidelines for psychological practice with girls and women.* Washington, DC: American Psychological Association.

Archer, J. (2002). Sex differences in aggression between heterosexual partners: A meta-analytic review. *Psychological Bulletin, 126,* 651–681.

Asay, T. P., & Lambert, M. J. (1999). The empirical case for the common factors in therapy: Quantitative findings. In M. A. Hubble, B. L. Duncan, & S. D. Miller (Eds.), *The heart & soul of change: What works in therapy* (pp. 23–55). Washington, DC: American Psychological Association.

Association for Lesbian, Gay, Bisexual, and Transgender Issues in Counseling. (n.d.). *Welcome.* Retrieved June 12, 2009, from http://www.algbtic.org/

Atkinson, D. R., Morten, G., & Sue, D. W. (1979). *Counseling American minorities: A cross-cultural perspective.* Boston, MA: McGraw-Hill.

Bachelor, A., & Horvath, A. (1999). The therapeutic relationship. In M. A. Hubble, B. L. Duncan, & S. D. Miller (Eds.), *The heart & soul of change: What works in therapy* (pp. 133–178). Washington, DC: American Psychological Association.

Bacigalupe, G. (2008). *SOAP notes handout.* Retrieved May 23, 2008, from www.umb.edu/forum/1/family_therapy_internship/res/SOAP_Notes_Handout.doc

Bancroft, L., & Silverman, J. (2002). *The batterer as parent: Addressing the impact of domestic violence on family dynamics.* Thousand Oaks, CA: Sage.

Bancroft, L., & Silverman, J. (2004/2005, Fall). The parenting practices of men who batter. *The APSAC Advisor, 11–14.*

Bandura, A. (1986). *Social foundations of thought and action: A social-cognitive theory.* Englewood Cliffs, NJ: Prentice Hall.

Barnett, R. C., & Hyde, J. S. (2001). Women, men, work, and family: An expansionist theory. *American Psychologist, 56,* 781–796.

Bartoli, E., & Gillem, A. R. (2008). Continuing to depolarize the debate on sexual orientation and religion: Identity and the therapeutic process. *Professional Psychology: Research and Practice, 39*(2), 202–209.

Beck, A. T. (1991). Cognitive therapy: A 30-year retrospective. *American Psychologist, 46,* 368–375.

Beck, A. T., & Weishaar, M. (2000). Cognitive therapy. In R. Corsini & D. Wedding (Eds.), *Current psychotherapies* (6th ed., pp. 241–272). Itasca, IL: F. E. Peacock.

Beck Institute for Cognitive Therapy and Research. (2008). Retrieved April 8, 2009, from http://www.beckinstitute.org/Library/InfoManage/Guide.asp?FolderID=200&SessionID={1C10428F-9375-4F78-89AF-E9B106C7DD19}

Beckstead, L., & Israel, T. (2007). Affirmative counseling and psychotherapy focused on issues related to sexual orientation conflicts. In K. J. Bieschke, R. M. Perez, & K. A. DuBord (Eds.), *Handbook of counseling and psychotherapy with lesbian, gay, and transgendered clients* (2nd ed., pp. 221–240). Washington, DC: American Psychological Association.

Berger, K. S. (2009). *The developing person through childhood and adolescence* (8th ed.). New York: Worth Publishers.

Bernal, G., & Enchautegui-de-Jesus, N. (1994). Latinos and Latinas in community psychology: A review of the literature. *American Journal of Community Psychology, 22*(4), 531–557.

Belgrave, F. Z., Chase-Vaughn, G., Gray, F., Addison, J. D., & Cherry, V. R. (2000). The effectiveness of a culture- and gender-specific intervention for increasing resiliency among African American preadolescent females. *Journal of Black Psychology, 26,* 133–147.

Biescheke, K. J., Perez, R. M., & DeBord, K. (2007). *Handbook of counseling and psychotherapy with lesbian, gay, bisexual, and transgender clients* (2nd ed.). Washington, DC: American Psychological Association.

Books, S. (2007). Devastation and disregard: Reflections on Katrina, child poverty, and educational opportunity. In S. Books (Ed.), *Invisible children in the society and its schools* (3rd ed., pp. 1–22). Mahwah, NJ: Lawrence Erlbaum & Associates.

Bowlby, J. (1973). *Attachment and loss: V01.2. Separation, anxiety, and anger.* New York: Basic Books.

Brannon, L. (2002). *Gender: Psychological perspectives.* Boston: Allyn & Bacon.

Brems, C. (2008). *A comprehensive guide to child psychotherapy and counseling* (3rd ed.). Long Grove, IL: Waveland Press, Inc.

Brodkin, K. (2001). How Jews became White. In P. S. Rothenberg (Ed.), *Race, class, and gender in the United States: An integrated study* (5th ed.). New York: Worth Publishers.

Broidy, L. M., Nagin, D. S., Tremblay, R. E., Bates, J. E., Brame, B., Dodge, K. A., et al. (2003). Developmental trajectories of childhood disruptive behaviors and adolescent delinquency: A six-site, cross-national study. *Developmental Psychology, 39*(2), 222–245.

Carpenter, S. (2001, October). Sleep deprivation may be undermining teen health. *Monitor on Psychology,* 42–45.

Caughy, M. O., O'Campo, P. J., & Muntaner, C. (2004). Experiences of racism among African American parents and the mental health of their preschool-aged children. *American Journal of Public Health, 94,* 2118–2124.

Centers for Disease Control and Prevention. (1998). Lifetime annual incidence of intimate partner violence and resulting injuries. *Morbidity and Mortality Weekly Report, 47,* 846–853.

Centers for Disease Control and Prevention. (2006). *Intimate partner violence during pregnancy, a guide for clinicians.* Retrieved October 25, 2008, from http://www.cdc.gov/Reproductivehealth/violence/IntimatePartnerViolence/sld001.htm

Children's Defense Fund. (2008). *The state of America's children 2008.* Washington, DC: Author.

Christian, M. D., & Barbarin, O. A. (2001). Cultural resources and psychological adjustment of African American children: Effects of spirituality and racial attribution. *Journal of Black Psychology, 27*(1), 43–63.

Cochran, S. (2001). Emerging issues in research on lesbian and gay men's mental health: Does sexual orientation really matter? *American Psychologist, 56,* 931–947.

Comas-Diaz, L. (2008). The Black Madonna: The psychospiritual feminism of Guadalupe, Kali, and Monserrat. In L. B. Silverstein & T. J. Goodrich (Eds.), *Feminist family therapy: Empowerment in social context* (pp. 147–160). Washington, DC: American Psychological Association.

Comer, J. P., & Hill, H. (1985). Social policy and the mental health of Black children. *Journal of the Academy of Child Psychiatry, 24*(2), 175–181.

Consortium for Longitudinal Studies of Child Abuse and Neglect. (2006). *LONGSCAN Research Briefs: Volume 2.* Retrieved on August 22, 2008, from http://www.iprc.unc.edu/longscan/pages/researchbriefs/LONGSCAN%20Research%20Briefs%20(Volume%202).pdf

Cooper, L., & Cates, P. (2006). *Too high a price: The case against restricting gay parenting.* New York: American Civil Liberties Union Foundation.

D'Augelli, A. R., & Dark, L. J. (1994). Lesbian, gay, and bisexual youths. In L. Eron, J. Gentry, & P. Schlegel (Eds.), *Reason to hope: A psychosocial perspective on violence and youth* (pp. 177–196). Washington, DC: American Psychological Association.

DeAngelis, T. (2002). A new generation of issues for LGBT clients. *Monitor on Psychology, 33*(2), 42–44.

Delphin, M., & Rowe, M. (2008). Continuing education in cultural competence for community mental health practitioners. *Professional Psychology: Research and Practice, 39*(2), 182–191.

Dixon, L., & Stern, R. K. (2004). *Compensation for losses from the 9/11 attacks* [Monograph MG-264-IC, p. xviii]. Santa Monica, CA: RAND Corporation.

Dixon, S. V., Graber, J. A., & Brooks-Gunn, J. (2008). The roles of respect for parental authority and parenting practices in parent-child conflict among African American, Latino, and European American families. *Journal of Family Psychology, 22*(1), 1–10.

Dodge, K. A., Pettit, G. S., Bates, J. E., & Valente, E. (1995). Social information-processing patterns partially mediate the effect of early physical abuse on later conduct problems. *Journal of Abnormal Psychology, 104,* 632–643.

Du Bois, W. E. B. (1997). *The souls of Black folk.* Boston: Bedford Books. (Original work published 1903)

Dye, M. L., & Davis, K. E. (2003). Stalking and psychological abuse: Common factors and relationship-specific characteristics. *Violence and Victims, 18,* 163–180.

Editors of Consumer Reports. (2004, October). Drugs versus talk therapy. *Consumer Reports,* 22–29.

Egan, G. (2007). *The skilled helper* (8th ed.). Belmont, CA: Brooks/Cole.

Elliott, R., & Greenberg, L. S. (1995). Experiential therapy in practice: The process-experiential approach. In B. Bongar & L. E. Beutler (Eds.), *Comprehensive textbook of psychotherapy: Theory and practice* (pp. 123–139). New York: Oxford University Press.

Emotion-Focused Therapy Organization. (2009). *Welcome to EFT!* Retrieved June 13, 2009, from http://www.emotionfocusedtherapy.org

Erikson, E. H. (1963). *Childhood and society* (2nd ed.). New York: Norton.

Evans, G. W. (2004). The environment of childhood poverty. *American Psychologist, 59*(2), 77–92.

Fantuzzo, J., & Mohr, W. (1999). Prevalence and effects of child exposure to domestic violence. *The Future of Children, 9*(2), 21–32.

Feder, J., Levant, R. F., & Dean, J. (2007). Boys and violence: A gender-informed analysis. *Professional Psychology: Research and Practice, 38,* 385–391.

Ford, D. Y. (1997). Counseling middle-class African Americans. In C. C. Lee (Ed.), *Multicultural issues in counseling* (2nd ed., pp. 81–108). Alexandria, VA: American Counseling Association.

Frankenberg, R. (2008). Whiteness as an "unmarked" cultural category. In K. E. Rosenblum & T. C. Travis (Eds.), *The meaning of difference: American constructions of race, sex and gender, social class, sexual orientation, and disability* (5th ed., pp. 81–87). Boston: McGraw-Hill.

French, L. A. (1997). *Counseling American Indians.* Lanham, MD: University Press of America.

Frieze, I. H. (2005). Female violence against intimate partners: An introduction. *Psychology of Women Quarterly, 29,* 229–237.

Fuligni, A. (1998). Authority, autonomy, and parent-adolescent conflict and cohesion: Study of adolescents from Mexican, Chinese, Filipino, and European backgrounds. *Developmental Psychology, 34,* 782–792.

Garbarino, J. (1999). *Lost boys: Why our sons turn violent and how we can save them.* New York: Free Press.

Gondolf, E. W., & Jones, A. S. (2002). The program effect of batterer programs in three cities. *Violence and Victims, 16,* 693–704.

Goodrich, T. J. (2008). A feminist family therapist's work is never done. In L. B. Silverstein & T. J. Goodrich (Eds.), *Feminist family therapy: Empowerment in social context* (pp. 3–15). Washington, DC: American Psychological Association.

Graham-Kevan, N., & Archer, J. (2005). Investigating three explanations of women's relationship aggression. *Psychology of Women Quarterly, 29*(3), 270–277.

Greenberg, L., & Goldman, R. (2007). Case-formulation in emotion-focused therapy. In T. D. Eells (Ed.), *Handbook of psychotherapy case formulation* (2nd ed., pp. 379–411). New York: Guilford Press.

Greene, B. (1997). Psychotherapy with African American women: Integrating feminist and psychodynamic models. *Journal of Smith College Studies in Social Work—Theoretical, Research, Practice and Educational Perspectives for Understanding and Working With African American Clients, 67*, 299–322.

Haas, E., Hill, R., Lambert, M. M., & Morrell, B. (2002). Do early responders to psychotherapy maintain treatment gains? *Journal of Clinical Psychology, 58*, 1157–1172.

Halberstadt, A. G., & Eaton, K. L. (2003). A meta-analysis of family expressiveness and children's emotion expressiveness and understanding. *Marriage & Family Review, 34*, 35–62.

Haldeman, D. (2000). Therapeutic responses to sexual orientation: Psychology's evolution. In B. Greene & G. L. Croom (Eds.), *Education, research, and practice in lesbian, gay, bisexual, and transgendered psychology: A resource manual* (pp. 244–262). Newbury Park, CA: Sage.

Hall, C. C. I. (2003). Not just Black and White: Interracial relationships and multicultural individuals. In J. S. Mio & G. Y. Iwamasa (Eds.), *Culturally diverse mental health* (pp. 231–248). New York: Brunner-Routledge.

Hall, R. L., & Greene, B. (2008). Contemporary African American families. In L. B. Silverstein & T. J. Goodrich (Eds.), *Feminist family therapy: Empowerment in social context* (pp. 107–120). Washington, DC: American Psychological Association.

Hanson, R. F., Self-Brown, S., Fricker-Elhai, A. E., Kilpatrick, D. G., Saunders, B. E., & Resnick, H. S. (2006). The relations between family environment and violence exposure among youth: Findings from the National Survey of Adolescents. *Child Maltreatment, 11*, 3–15.

Hays, P. (2008). *Addressing cultural complexities in practice: Assessment, diagnosis, and therapy* (2nd ed.). Washington, DC: American Psychological Association.

Hershberger, S. L., & D'Augelli, A. R. (2000). Issues in counseling lesbian, gay, and bisexual adolescents. In R. Perez, K. DeBord, & K. Bieschke (Eds.), *Handbook of counseling and psychotherapy with lesbian, gay, and bisexual clients* (pp. 225–247). Washington, DC: American Psychological Association.

History Learning Site. (2008). *Family life.* Retrieved August 13, 2008, from www.historylearningsite.co.uk/familylife.htm

Holmes, S. A., & Morin, R. (2006, June). *Being a Black man: The poll.* Washington, DC: *The Washington Post.* Retrieved June 5, 2009, from http://www.washingtonpost.com/wp-dyn/content/discussion/2006/06/02/DI2006060201012.html

Hubble, M. A., Duncan, B. L., & Miller, S. D. (1999). Directing attention to what works. In M. A. Hubble, B. L. Duncan, & S. D. Miller (Eds.), *The heart and soul of change: What works in therapy* (pp. 407–447). Washington, DC: American Psychological Association.

Human Rights Campaign. (2000). *Finally free* [Research report]. Washington, DC: Author.

Ignatieff, M. (2005, September 25). The broken contract. *The New York Times.* Retrieved June 13, 2009, from http://www.nytimes.com/2005/09/25/magazine/25wwln.html?_r=1&scp=1&sq=Ignatieff%20broken%20contract&st=cse

Ignatiev, N. (1995). *How the Irish became White.* New York: Routledge.

Ingram, B. L. (2006). *Clinical case formulations* (pp. 157–190). Hoboken, NJ: John Wiley & Sons, Inc.

Jackson, J. (2000). What ought psychology to do? *American Psychologist, 55*(3), 328–330.

Jaffe, P., & Geffner, R. (1998). Child custody disputes and domestic violence: Critical issues for mental health, social service, and legal professionals. In G. Holden, R. Geffner, & E. Jouriles (Eds.), *Children exposed to marital violence: Theory, research, and applied issues* (pp. 371–408). Washington, DC: American Psychological Association.

Johnson, M. P. (1995). Patriarchal terrorism and common couple violence: Two forms of violence against women. *Journal of Marriage and the Family, 75,* 283–294.

Johnson, M. P., & Leone, J. M. (2005). The differential effects of intimate terrorism and situational couple violence: Findings from the National Violence Against Women Survey. *Journal of Family Issues, 26,* 322–349.

Johnson, S. (2007). *International Centre for Excellence in Emotion Focused Therapy [ICEEF].* Retrieved June 12, 2009, from http://www.eft.ca/home.htm

Kantor, G. K., & Little, L. (2003). Refining the boundaries of child neglect: When does domestic violence equate with parental failure to protect? *Journal of Interpersonal Violence, 18*(4), 338–355.

Keenan, J. M. (2008). *Review of SOAP note charting.* Retrieved May 23, 2008, from http://www.meded.umn.edu/students/residency/documents/06_Keenan_Review_SOAP_Note_Charting.pdf

Kelly, G. A. (1955). *The psychology of personal constructs.* New York: Norton.

Kimmel, M. S. (2008). The gendered society. In K. E. Rosenblum & T. C. Travis (Eds.), *The meaning of difference: American constructions of race, sex and gender, social class, sexual orientation, and disability* (5th ed., pp. 81–87). Boston: McGraw-Hill.

Koss, M. P., Bailey, J. A., Yuan, N. P., Herrera, V. M., & Lichter, E. L. (2003). Depression and PTSD in survivors of male violence: Research and training initiatives to facilitate recovery. *Psychology of Women Quarterly, 27,* 130–142.

Krugman, P. (2005, September 19). Tragedy in black and white. *The New York Times,* p. A25.

Lambert, M. J., Garfield, S. L., & Bergin, A. E. (2004). Overview, trends, and future issues. In M. J. Lambert (Ed.), *Bergin and Garfield's handbook of psychotherapy and behavior change* (5th ed., pp. 805–821). New York: John Wiley & Sons, Inc.

Lansford, J. E., Miller-Johnson, S., Berlin, L. J., Dodge, K. A., Bates, J. E., & Pettit, G. S. (2007). Early physical abuse and later violent delinquency: A prospective longitudinal study. *Child Maltreatment, 12,* 233–245.

LaRue, A., & Majidi-Ahi, S. (1998). African-American children. In J. T. Gibbs & L. N. Huang (Eds.), *Children of color: Psychological interventions with culturally diverse youth* (pp. 143–170). San Francisco Jossey-Bass.

Ledley, D. R., Marx, B. P., & Heimberg, R. G. (2005). *Making cognitive-behavioral therapy work: Clinical process for new practitioners.* New York: Guilford Press.

Levenson, H., & Strupp, H. H. (2007). Cyclic maladaptive patterns: Case formulation in time-limited dynamic psychotherapy. In T. D. Eells (Ed.), *Handbook of psychotherapy case formulation* (2nd ed., pp. 164–197). New York: Guilford Press.

Lipton, E., & Nixon, R. (2005, September 26). Many contracts for storm work raise questions. *The New York Times,* p. A1.

Lott, B. (2002). Cognitive and behavioral distancing from the poor. *American Psychologist, 57*(2), 100–110.

Mann, C. C. (2005). *1491 new revelations of the Americas before Columbus.* New York: A. A. Knopf.

Masten, A. S. (2001). Ordinary magic: Resilience processes in development. *American Psychologist, 56,* 227–238.

Mazure, C. M., Keita, G. P., & Blehar, M. C. (2002). *Summit on women and depression: Proceedings and recommendations.* Washington, DC: American Psychological Association.

McIntosh, P. (2008). White privilege: Unpacking the invisible knapsack. In K. E. Rosenblum & T. C. Travis (Eds.), *The meaning of difference: American constructions of race, sex and gender, social class, sexual orientation, and disability* (5th ed., pp. 368–372). Boston: McGraw–Hill.

Michael, J. L. (2004). *Concepts and principles of behavior analysis* (Rev. ed.). Kalamazoo, MI: Society for the Advancement of Behavior Analysis.

Minuchin, S. (1974). *Families and family therapy.* Cambridge, MA: Harvard University Press.

Minuchin, S., & Fishman, H. (1981). *Family therapy techniques.* Cambridge, MA: Harvard University Press.

Minuchin, S., Nichols, M. P., & Lee, W.-Y. (2007). *Assessing couples and families: From symptom to system.* Boston: Allyn & Bacon.

Monroe, C. R. (2005). Why are "bad boys" always Black? Causes of disproportionality in school discipline and recommendations for change. *The Clearing House, 79,* 45–50.

Myers, J. E. B., Berliner, L., Briere, J., Hendrix, C. T., Jenny, C., & Reid, T. A. (2002). *The APSAC handbook on child maltreatment* (2nd ed.). Thousand Oaks, CA: Sage.

National Center for Health Statistics. (2002, April 24). Deaths: Injuries, 2002. *National Vital Statistics Reports, 54*(10). Retrieved February 3, 2009, from http://www.cdc.gov/nchs/data/nvsr/nvsr54/nvsr54_10.pdf

Neal-Barnett, A. M., & Crowther, J. H. (2000). To be female, middle class, anxious, and Black. *Psychology of Women Quarterly, 24,* 129–136.

Neimeyer, R. A. (1995). An invitation to constructivist psychotherapies. In R. A. Neimeyer & M. J. Mahoney (Eds.), *Constructivism in psychotherapy* (pp. 1–8). Washington, DC: American Psychological Association.

Neimeyer, R. A. (2000). Narrative disruptions in the construction of the self. In R. A. Neimeyer & J. D. Raskin (Eds.), *Constructions of disorder: Meaning-making frameworks for psychotherapy* (pp. 207–242). Washington, DC: American Psychological Association.

Nelson, S. (2008). *Welcome message to iask.inc.* Retrieved July 24, 2008, from www.iaskinc.org

New York Life. (2008). *African American wealth: Powerful trends and new opportunities.* Retrieved June 14, 2008, from http://www.newyorklife.com/cda/0,3254,13767,00.html

Newsweek. (2000). *Post super Tuesday/gays & lesbians (United States).* Storrs, CT: Roper Center for Public Opinion Research.

Ng, F. F., Pomerantz, E. M., & Lam, S. (2007). European American and Chinese parents' response to children's success and failure: Implications for children's responses. *Developmental Psychology, 43*(5), 1239–1255.

Nichols, M. P. (2008). *Family therapy: Concepts and methods* (8th ed.). Boston: Pearson Education, Inc.

Nolen-Hoeksema, S. (2000). The role of rumination in depressive disorders and mixed anxiety/depressive symptoms. *Journal of Abnormal Psychology, 109,* 504–511.

Ogbu, J. (2003). *Black American students in an affluent suburb: A study of academic disengagement.* Mahwah, NJ: Lawrence Erlbaum & Associates.

Papp, P. (2008). *Gender, marriage, and depression.* In L. B. Silverstein & T. J. Goodrich (Eds.), *Feminist family therapy: Empowerment in social context* (pp. 211–223). Washington, DC: American Psychological Association.

Pavlov, I. (1927). *Conditioned reflexes.* London: Oxford University Press.

Pedrotti, J. T., Edwards, L. M., & Lopez, S. J. (2008). Working with multiracial clients in therapy: Bridging theory, research, and practice. *Professional Psychology: Research and Practice, 39,* 192–201.

Perls, F., Hefferline, R., & Goodman, P. (1951). *Gestalt therapy.* New York: Dell.

Piaget, J. (1952). *The origins of intelligence in children* (M. Cook, Trans.). Oxford, England: International Universities Press. (Original work published 1936)

Pincus, F. L. (2001/2002, Winter). The social construction of reverse discrimination: The impact of affirmative action on Whites. *Journal of Intergroup Relations, 38*(4), 33–44.

Pinderhughes, E. E., Dodge, K. A., Bates, J. E., Pettit, G. S., & Zelli, A. (2000). Discipline responses: Influences of parents' socioeconomic status, ethnicity, beliefs about parenting, stress, and cognitive-emotional processes. *Journal of Family Psychology, 14,* 380–400.

Pro-change Behavior Systems. (2008, March). *About us.* Retrieved April 8, 2009, from http://www.prochange.com/staff/james_prochaska

Prochaska, J. (1999). How do people change, and how can we change to help many more people? In M. A. Hubble, B. L. Duncan, & S. D. Miller (Eds.), *The heart and soul of change: What works in therapy* (pp. 227–255). Washington, DC: American Psychological Association.

Prochaska, J. (2005). Reply to Callaghan: Stages of change and termination from psychotherapy. *Psychotherapy: Theory, Research, Practice, Training, 42*(2), 247–248.

Prochaska, J., & DiClemente, C. (1984). *The transtheoretical approach: Crossing traditional boundaries of change.* Homewood, IL: Dorsey.

Prochaska, J., & DiClemente, C. (1986). The transtheoretical approach. In J. Norcross (Ed.), *Handbook of eclectic psychotherapy* (pp. 163–200). New York: Brunner/Mazel.

Prochaska, J. O., & Norcross, J. C. (1999). Comparative conclusions: Toward a transtheoretical therapy. In J. O. Prochaska & J. C. Norcross (Eds.), *Systems of psychotherapy: A transtheoretical analysis* (4th ed., pp. 487–532). Pacific Grove, CA: Brooks/Cole.

Prochaska, J. O., & Norcross, J. C. (2009). *Systems of psychotherapy: A transtheoretical analysis.* Pacific Grove, CA: Brooks/Cole.

Quinn, D. M., & Crocker, J. (1999). When ideology hurts: Effects of belief in the Protestant affect and feeling overweight on the psychological well-being of women. *Journal of Personality and Social Psychology, 77*(2), 402–414.

Ramirez, O. (1998). Mexican American children and adolescents. In J. T. Gibbs, L. N. Huang, & Associates (Eds.), *Children of color: Psychological interventions with culturally diverse youth* (2nd ed., pp. 215–239). San Francisco, CA: Jossey-Bass.

Riggle, E. D. B., Whitman, J. S., Olson, A., Rostosky, S. S., & Strong, S. (2008). The positive aspects of being a lesbian or gay man. *Professional Psychology: Research and Practice, 39*(2), 210–217.

Rodriguez, C. E. (2008). Latinos and the U.S. race structure. In K. E. Rosenblum & T. C. Travis (Eds.), *The meaning of difference: American constructions of race, sex and gender, social class, sexual orientation, and disability* (5th ed., pp. 81–87). Boston: McGraw-Hill.

Rogers, C. (1951). *Client-centered therapy.* Boston: Houghton Mifflin.

Samuelson, S. L., & Campbell, C. D. (2005). Screening for domestic violence: Recommendations based on a practice survey. *Professional Psychology: Research and Practice, 36*(3), 276–282.

Santana, S., & Santana, F. (2001). An introduction to Mexican culture: For rehabilitation service providers. Retrieved August 5, 2008, from http://cirrie.buffalo.edu/monographs/mexico.pdf

Savin-Williams, R. C. (2001). *Mom, Dad, I'm gay. How families negotiate coming out.* Washington, DC: American Psychological Association.

Schneider, M. S., Brown, L. S., & Glassgold, J. (2002). Implementing the resolution on appropriate therapeutic responses to sexual orientation: A guide for the perplexed. *Professional Psychology: Research and Practice, 33*(3), 265–276.

Shapiro, I., Greenstein, R., & Primus, W. (2001, May 31). *Pathbreaking CBO study shows dramatic increases in income disparities in 1980s and 1990s: An analysis of CBO data.* Retrieved June 12, 2008, from the Center on Budget and Policy Priorities Web site at http://www.cbpp.org/5-31-01tax.htm

Shidlo, A., & Schroeder, M. (2002). Changing sexual orientation: A consumers' report. *Professional Psychology: Research and Practice, 33*(3), 249–259.

Skinner, B. F. (1938). *The behavior of organisms: An experimental analysis.* New York: Appleton.

Smith, L., Constantine, M. G., Graham, S. V., & Diz, B. (2008). The territory ahead for multicultural competence: The "spinning" of racism. *Professional Psychology: Research and Practice, 39*(3), 337–345.

Snow Owl. (2004, September). *Native American people/tribes: The great Sioux nation.* Retrieved August 13, 2008, from http://www.snowwowl.com/peoplesioux.html

Society for Constructivism in the Human Sciences. (2008). Retrieved April 13, 2008, from http://constructingworlds.googlepages.com/?popup=1

Solorzano, D., Ceja, M., & Yosso, T. (2000, Winter). Critical race theory, racial microaggressions, and campus racial climate: The experiences of African American college students. *Journal of Negro Education, 69*, 60–73.

Strupp, H., & Binder, J. (1984). *Psychotherapy in a new key: A guide to time-limited dynamic treatment.* New York: Basic Books.

Stuart, R. B. (2005). Treatment for partner abuse: Time for a paradigm shift. *Professional Psychology: Research and Practice, 36*(3), 254–263.

Sudak, D. M. (2006). *Psychotherapy in clinical practice: Cognitive behavioral therapy for clinicians.* Philadelphia: Lippincott Williams & Wilkins.

Sue, D. W. (2005). Racism and the conspiracy of silence. *Counseling Psychologist, 33*, 100–114.

Sue, D. W., Arredondo, P., & McDavis, R. J. (1992). Multicultural counseling competencies and standards: A call to the profession. *Journal of Counseling and Development, 70*, 477–486.

Sue, D. W., Capodilupo, C. M., Torino, G. C., Bucceri, J. M., Holder, A. M. B., Nadal, K. L., et al. (2007). Racial microaggressions in everyday life. *American Psychologist, 62*, 271–286.

Sue, D. W., & Sue, D. (2008). *Counseling the culturally diverse: Theory and practice* (5th ed., pp. 95–121, 259–283, 345–357). Hoboken, NJ: John Wiley & Sons.

Surgeon General. (2001). *Youth violence: Report from the Surgeon General.* Retrieved August 1, 2007, from http://www.surgeongeneral.gov/library/youth/report.html

Tutwiler, S. W. (2007). How schools fail African-American boys. In S. Books (Ed.), *Invisible children in the society and its schools* (3rd ed., pp. 1–22). Mahwah, NJ: Lawrence Erlbaum & Associates.

University of Rhode Island Cancer Research Center. (2008). *Transtheoretical Model.* Retrieved April 8, 2009, from http://www.uri.edu/research/cprc/TTM/detailedoverview.htm

U.S. Bureau of Labor Statistics. *Monthly Labor Review*. (2009, February). *The changing impact of marriage and children on women's labor force participation*. Retrieved June 5, 2009, from http://www.bls.gov/opub/mlr/2009/02/art1full.pdf

U.S. Census Bureau. (2000a). *American factfinder: Demographic profile highlights: White alone* [Summary file 2 (SF2) and summary file 4 (SF4)]. Retrieved May 21, 2008, from http://factfinder.census.gov

U.S. Census Bureau. (2000b). *Marital status: 2000*. Retrieved June 3, 2008, from http://www.census.gov/prod/2003pubs/c2kbr-30.pdf

U.S. Census Bureau 2000. (2001). *Gender: 2000*. Retrieved June 3, 2008, from http://www.census.gov/prod/200/pubs/c2Kbr01–9.pdf

U.S. Census Bureau 2000. (2003). *Married-couple and unmarried-partner households*. Retrieved June 3, 2008, from http://www.census.gov/prod/2004pubs/censr-5.pdf

U.S. Census Bureau 2000. (2004a). *Ancestry: 2000*. Retrieved June 3, 2008, from http://www.census.gov/prod/2004pubs/c2kbr-35.pdf

U.S. Census Bureau 2000. (2004b). *Children and the households they live in*. Retrieved June 3, 2008, from http://www.census.gov/prod/2004pubs/censr-14.pdf

U.S. Census Bureau 2000. (2004c). *U.S. interim projections by age, sex, race, and Hispanic origin*. Retrieved May 30, 2008, from http://www.census.gov/ipc/www/usinterimproj/

U.S. Census Bureau 2000. (2004d). *We the people: Hispanics in the United States*. Retrieved June 3, 2008, from http://www.census.gov/prod/2004pubs/censr-18.pdf

U.S. Census Bureau 2000. (2005). *We the people: Blacks in the United States*. Retrieved June 3, 2008, from http://www.census.gov/prod/2005pubs/censr-25.pdf

U.S. Census Bureau 2000. (2006a). *State and county quick facts*. Retrieved May 21, 2008, from http://www.census.gov

U.S. Census Bureau 2000. (2006b). *We the people: American Indians and Alaska Natives in the United States*. Retrieved June 3, 2008, from http://www.census.gov/prod/2006pubs/censr-28.pdf

U.S. Census Bureau. (2007). *The American community—Blacks: 2004*. Retrieved May 21, 2008, from http://factfinder.census.gov/home/en/datanotes/exp_acs2004.html

U.S. Department of Health and Human Services. (1999). *Report of the Surgeon General's Conference on Children's Mental Health: A National Action Agenda*. Retrieved February, 6, 2001, from http://www.surgeongeneral.gov/cmh/default.htm

U.S. Department of Health and Human Services. (2001). *National strategy for suicide prevention: Goals and objectives for action* [Inventory # SMA01-3517]. Retrieved June 19, 2009, from http://www.mentalhealth.samhsa.gov/suicideprevention/strategy.asp

U.S. Department of Health and Human Services, Administration on Children, Youth and Families. (2006). *Child maltreatment 2004*. Washington, DC: Government Printing Office.

U.S. Department of Health and Human Services, Federal Interagency Forum on Child and Family Statistics 2000. (2008). *American's children in brief: Key national indicators of well-being.* Retrieved June 19, 2009, from http://www .childstats.gov/americaschildren

U.S. Department of Health and Human Services, The Office of Minority Health. (2006a). *American Indian/Alaska Native profile.* Retrieved June 2, 2008, from http://www.omhrc.gov/templates/browse.aspx?lvl=3&Ivlid=26

U.S. Department of Health and Human Services, The Office of Minority Health. (2006b). *Hispanic/Latino profile.* Retrieved May 21, 2008, from http://www .omhrc.gov/templates/browse.aspx?lvl=3&Ivlid=31

U.S. Department of Health and Human Services, The Office of Minority Health. (2008). *Hispanic/Latino profile.* Retrieved May 21, 2008, from http://www .omhrc.gov/templates/browse.aspx?lvl=3&Ivlid=31

U.S. Department of Justice. (2002). *American Indians and crime: A BJS statistical profile, 1992–2002.* Retrieved June 3, 2008, from http://www.ojp.usdoj.gov/bjs/ abstract/aic02.htm

U.S. Department of Justice. (2006a). *Lifetime likelihood of going to state or federal prison.* Retrieved June 3, 2008, from http://www.ojp.usdoj.gov/bjs/ abstract/llgsfp.htm

U.S. Department of Justice. (2006b). *Prison statistics.* Retrieved June 3, 2008, from http://www.ojp.usdoj.gov/bjs/prisons.htm

Vygotsky, L. S. (1978). *Mind in society: The development of higher psychological processes* (M. Cole, V. John-Steiner, S. Scribner, & E. Souberman, Eds.). Cambridge, MA: Harvard University Press. (Original work published 1935)

Washington, A. T. (2005). Katrina riles, rallies Black America. *Bellingham Herald,* p. A3.

Watson, D. L., Andreas, J., Fischer, K., & Smith, K. (2005). Patterns of risk factors leading to victimization and aggression in children and adolescents. In K. Kendall-Tackett & S. Giacomoni (Eds.), *Child victimization* (pp. 1–23). Kingston, NJ: Civic Research Institute.

Weber, M. (1958). *The Protestant ethic and the spirit of capitalism* (T. Parsons, Trans.). New York: Scribner's. (Original work published 1904–1905)

Wolak, J., & Finkelhor, D. (1998). Children exposed to partner violence. In J. Jasinski & L. Williams (Eds.), *Partner violence: A comprehensive review of 20 years of research* (pp. 73–111). Thousand Oaks, CA: Sage.

Worell, J., & Remer, P. (2003). *Feminist perspectives in therapy: Empowering diverse women.* New York: John Wiley & Sons, Inc.

World Health Organization. (2000, June 21). *World Health Organization assesses the world's health systems* [World Health Organization Press Release WHO/44]. Retrieved June 12, 2008, from http://www.who.int/inf-pr-2000/en/ pr2000-44.html

World Health Organization. (2001). *Violence against women* [WHO Fact Sheet No. 239]. Geneva, Switzerland: Author.

World Health Organization. (2002). *World report on violence and health: Summary* [NLM classification: HV6625]. Geneva, Switzerland: Author.

Zorza, J. (2006). *Violence against women Volume III: Victims and abusers.* Kingston, NJ: Civic Research Institute.

Zweig, M. (2008). What's class got to do with it? In K. E. Rosenblum & T. C. Travis (Eds.), *The meaning of difference: American constructions of race, sex and gender, social class, sexual orientation, and disability* (5th ed., pp. 81–87). Boston: McGraw-Hill.

About the Author

Pearl S. Berman, PhD, is a licensed psychologist who is a professor of psychology and a clinical supervisor within the doctoral program in psychology at Indiana University of Pennsylvania. She received her BA in psychology from Brandeis University in 1977 and her PhD in clinical psychology from Bowling Green State University in 1983. Her areas of clinical and research expertise include child physical and sexual abuse, neglect, spousal violence, violence prevention, and professional training. She is the author of three doctoral-level books. Her first book is titled *Therapeutic Exercises for Victimized and Neglected Girls: Applications for Individual, Family, and Group Psychotherapy* (Professional Resource Press, 1994). Her second book was the first edition of *Case Conceptualization and Treatment Planning: Exercises in Integrating Theory With Clinical Practice* (SAGE Publications, 1997); this book was translated into Korean by Hak Ji Sa in 2007. Her third book is *Interviewing and Diagnostic Exercises for Clinical and Counseling Skills Building* with her colleague Susan Shopland, PsyD (Lawrence Erlbaum & Associates, 2005). She has also published six book chapters and nine professional articles. She has presented 40 professional papers and 12 professional workshops in her areas of expertise. In addition, she has taught 3 undergraduate and 10 doctoral-level courses in psychology. Finally, she is a member of many professional groups working toward the cessation of victimization, including the American Psychological Association, the American Association of Applied and Preventive Psychology, the American Professional Society on the Abuse of Children, the Southern Poverty Law Center, and the National Organization for Women.

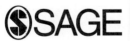
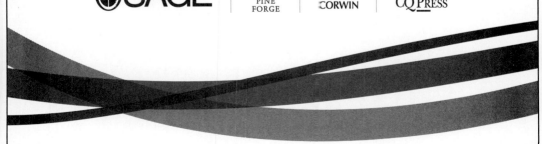